THERAPEUTIC EXERCISE for

Physical
Therapist
Assistants

SECOND EDITION

THERAPEUTIC EXERCISE for Physical Therapist Assistants

SECOND EDITION

WILLIAM D. BANDY, PT, PhD, SCS, ATC
Professor
Department of Physical Therapy
University of Central Arkansas
Conway, Arkansas

BARBARA SANDERS, PT, PhD, SCS
Professor and Chair
Department of Physical Therapy
Texas State University–San Marcos
Associate Dean
College of Health Professions
San Marcos, Texas

Photography by **MICHAEL A. MORRIS**, FBCA
University of Arkansas for Medical Sciences

Wolters Kluwer | Lippincott Williams & Wilkins
Health
Philadelphia • Baltimore • New York • London
Buenos Aires • Hong Kong • Sydney • Tokyo

Acquisitions Editor: Peter Sabatini
Managing Editor: Andrea M. Klingler
Marketing Manager: Allison M. Noplock
Associate Production Manager: Kevin P. Johnson
Creative Director: Doug Smock
Compositor: Maryland Composition
Printer: Quebecor Dubuque

Printed in the United States of America
First Edition, 2001, Lippincott Williams & Wilkins
Library of Congress Cataloging-in-Publication Data

Therapeutic exercise for physical therapist assistants / [edited by]
    William Bandy, Barbara Sanders ; photography by Michael A. Morris.
    – 2nd ed.
       p. ; cm.
    Rev. ed. of: Therapeutic exercise. c2001.
    Includes bibliographical references and index.
    ISBN-13: 978-0-7817-9080-2
    ISBN-10: 0-7817-9080-8
    1. Musculoskeletal system–Diseases–Exercise therapy.   I. Bandy,
William D. II. Sanders, Barbara. III. Therapeutic exercise.
    [DNLM: 1. Exercise Therapy–methods.   WB 541 T39804 2007]
RC925.5.T48 2007
616.7'062--dc22

                                            2006023960

To Beth, Melissa, and Jamie for providing constant love, patience, and inspiration.
WDB

To Mike and Whitney, whose love and support allow me to do the things I enjoy.
BS

The first two physical therapist assistant (PTA) education programs, at Miami Dade Community College in Florida and St Mary's Campus of the College of St. Catherine in Minnesota, opened their doors in 1967. In 1969 the first 15 PTAS graduated from these two schools. Since that time the number of these very important technical assistants to the physical therapist (PT) has grown to include an estimated 50,000 PTAs currently licensed in the United States. To date a plethora of textbooks exist defining therapeutic exercises and describing the role of therapeutic exercise in the treatment of patients and clients. But no textbook exists on the topic of therapeutic exercise written specifically for the PTA. The purpose of *Therapeutic Exercise for the Physical Therapist Assistant* is to provide descriptions and rationale for the use of a variety of therapeutic exercise techniques that are frequently delegated to the PTA by the PT for the rehabilitation of an individual with impairment or for the prevention of potential problems.

We are excited to write the first textbook devoted totally to the use of therapeutic exercise for the PTA. Instead of using a therapeutic exercise book written for the PT and making changes to make the content appropriate to the PTA, it is our goal that *Therapeutic Exercise for the Physical Therapist Assistant* will meet the needs of educators who are training the future PTAs.

The primary audience for this textbook is individuals in a PTA curriculum. Although written primarily for PTA students, this textbook can also provide experienced clinicians with background and illustrations of specific exercise techniques, allowing even the experienced clinician to add to their repertoire of therapeutic exercises used.

As indicated in the *Guide to Physical Therapist Practice* (published by the American Physical Therapy Association), therapeutic exercise is the most important procedural intervention provided in the field of physical therapy. We believe that this textbook is an excellent choice for teaching this important topic to the PTA in a therapeutic exercise course in the curriculum or as unit in a musculoskeletal course. The basic assumption of this textbook is that the patient has been examined by the PT, the impairment has been identified, and the plan of care has been established by the PT. This textbook focuses on the implementation of the treatment plan using therapeutic exercise techniques that the PTA will provide under the direction and supervision of the PT.

ORGANIZATION

A look at the Table of Contents shows that the book is divided into seven sections. Section I lays the foundation for the next six sections of the book. A history of therapeutic exercise is provided and an understanding of where therapeutic exercise fits into the realm of all interventions is explained. Using current policies held by the American Physical Therapy Association, important terms related to the management of the patient are defined and the role of the PTA within the healthcare team is clarified. Additional information presented in to these first two chapters includes the reaction of the various tissues to exercise, the use of complementary modalities, and effective use of communication with patients.

Section II presents information for increasing mobility by performing range of motion techniques (passive, active-assistive, and active) and stretching activities. Information on increasing strength and power, ranging from frequently used therapeutic exercise techniques (open-chain and closed-chain exercises) to more sophisticated and aggressive exercises (PNF and plyometrics), is presented in Section III.

Important information needed for understanding the concept of balance and providing therapeutic exercise techniques for treatment of balance dysfunction is presented in Section IV. A unique concept, reactive neuromuscular training, is presented in Section IV as well. Section V addresses the practice area of cardiopulmonary, with information presented on aerobic conditioning for the unfit but healthy individual, cardiac rehabilitation for the patient after a cardiac accident, and enhancement of breathing for the person with respiratory dysfunction.

Section V integrates information from the previous five sections in order to treat patients with dysfunction of the upper and lower extremities and the spine. Finally, the unique applications of aquatic therapy and a new concept, contextual fitness for the elderly, are presented in Section VI.

CHAPTER STRUCTURE

Each Chapter in Sections II through VII is set up using a consistent format (excluding Chapter 5). We believe that this consistent format allows a nice flow to the book from one Chapter to the next and adds to the ease of reading and clarity. The standard headings are presented in the following order:

Objectives have been added to the beginning of each chapter to clarify the content that will be presented.

Scientific Basis includes background information and a brief discussion of the benefits of the intervention being presented—supported by evidence, when available.

Clinical Guidelines provide information such as how, why, and when to use the techniques.

Techniques provide illustrations of frequently used therapeutic exercise techniques.

Case Studies not only provide examples as to how to use the therapeutic exercise techniques on patients, but demonstrate how the treatment is advanced as the patient progresses.

Summary contains a bulleted list of key concepts.

References contain the most current evidence available.

Geriatric and Pediatric Perspectives offer information specific to the pediatric and geriatric patient (using "boxes") that is important for understanding the appropriate use of therapeutic exercise across the lifespan.

CHANGES FROM THE FIRST EDITION

The major change in the Second Edition is the change in focus to the PTA. All chapters from the first edition were updated and the focus changed from treatment provided by a PT and an athletic trainer to the use of therapeutic exercise by the PTA. In addition, new chapters on enhancement of breathing (Chapter 13) and a new concept, contextual fitness (Chapter 17), have been added to include more information on respiratory care and unique intervention for the elderly. Chapters have been expanded and include added units on reaction of the various tissues to exercise and complementary modalities (Chapter 1), communication with patients (Chapter 2), and cardiac rehabilitation (Chapter 12). In addition, a glossary with the definitions of more than 120 words was added to allow a quick reference to frequently used terms contained within the text.

Feedback from reviewers of the first edition was very complimentary of the use of case studies in each chapter. An important part of practicing efficiently, ethically, and legally is that the PTA provides therapeutic exercise within the plan of care developed by the PT. To illustrate the appropriate relationship between the PT and PTA, each case study has been rewritten to describe appropriate (and sometimes inappropriate) interventions performed by the PTA and the interaction between the PT and the PTA. In addition, at the end of each case study, a "Summary—An Effective PT-PTA Team" section has been added which provides feedback as to whether the interaction between the PTA and PT was appropriate.

SPECIAL FEATURES

In addition to updating all chapters for the student, new ancillary materials have been added to assist the PTA educator. The educator who adopts this textbook will be provided with a PowerPoint presentation and sample test questions for every chapter. These PowerPoint presentations and tests can be edited to meet the specific needs of the instructor; it is hoped that these supplementary materials provide a base with which the instructor can present the information in the chapter. In addition, PowerPoint presentations provide a sample of the use of the figures contained in the text. Additional ancillary information for the instructor includes an image bank containing all the figures from the text. This image bank allows the instructor to further individualize instruction presented to the PTA students. All ancillary material is available on CD (0-7817-6982-5) and online (http://thepoint.lww.com/bandy2e).

SUMMARY

Therapeutic exercise can be considered a craft. As such, therapeutic exercise must be learned by doing, not by reading. This textbook provides ideas and techniques; however, to fully learn therapeutic exercise, the PTA student must practice the techniques under the supervision of an experienced educator. To gain this practical experience, the student should begin by practicing on an individual who is free from dysfunction before trying the techniques on patients with impairments; the student should always practice in a supervised environment. It is our hope that you find *Therapeutic Exercise for the Physical Therapist Assistant* a valuable asset to the initial and ongoing education of the PTA.

ACKNOWLEDGMENTS

We expected the writing of a revision to a textbook to be a large undertaking. But writing a revision and changing the target audience turned out to be a bigger task than expected. The support that our family, friends, and colleagues provided for writing the first edition of this textbook was outstanding. Allowing us to pursue a second edition, knowing how much work the task would involve, is even more appreciated.

In writing a book and a revision over the last 5 years, our publisher, Lippincott Williams & Wilkins, has gone through some tremendous reorganization and growth. Karen Ruppert and Andrea Klingler were the glue that held it all together, and we really appreciate all the work they put into this project.

Despite a change in his employment, we were thankful to retain Michael Morris, FBCA, as our photographer. Michael took all the pictures in the text, and working together again was as easy as putting on an old favorite pair of jeans—a very comfortable fit. Related to the photographs, we would also like to thank all the models for this book: Michael Adkins, Melissa Bandy, Laura Cabrera, Rachel Cloud, Emily Devan, Dot East, Neil Hattlestad, Renatto Hess, Jean Irion, Verdarhea Langrell, Nancy Reese, and Trigg Ross. A very special thank you goes to Ben Downs from the Respiratory Therapy Department at Arkansas Children's Hospital for his assistance for the pictures in Chapter 13.

We are grateful to all the authors of chapters in the first edition for agreeing to allow us to make changes for the second edition. We appreciate them for their trust in us as we edited their work and made the transition from a textbook for the PT and athletic trainer to a book for the PTA. In addition, we are very appreciative to authors of new chapters, Chris Russian and Reta Zabel, as well as the contribution of new units by Beth McKitrick-Bandy, Dennis O'Connell, Erin O'Kelley, and David Taylor.

A special thank you needs to go out to Russell Stowers and Michele Voight, two very hard-working PTAs who recreated the case studies from the first edition. Their work at giving the case studies a PTA focus is appreciated—and we think these case studies are a strength of the book.

The writing of this revision was made easier due to the support of graduate assistants from the University of Central Arkansas and their work with Medline searches, editing, writing objectives, organizing the glossary, and constant word processing. Our thanks go to Kelly Free, Leah Lowe, Emily Devan, Marie Charton, Mieke Corbitt, and Carnie Blankenship.

We would be remiss if we did not acknowledge two outstanding physical therapy faculties: Departments of Physical Therapy at the Texas State University–San Marcos and the University of Central Arkansas. We really appreciate such a supportive group of colleagues, a group that makes it fun to come in to work every day. We want to give a special thanks to Dr. Nancy Reese for her continued guidance, experience, and support of us as we worked on this project.

Finally, writing a textbook takes time from our families. We again wish to thank our families—our spouses (Beth and Mike) and our girls (Jamie, Melissa, and Whitney)—for their love, patience, and support.

William D. Bandy, PT, PhD, SCS, ATC
Professor
Department of Physical Therapy
University of Central Arkansas
Conway, Arkansas

Janet Bezner, PT, PhD
Senior Vice President for Education
American Physical Therapy Association
Alexandria, Virginia

James P. Fletcher, PT, MS, ATC
Assistant Professor
Department of Physical Therapy
University of Central Arkansas
Conway, Arkansas

Barbara Hoogenboom, PT, EdD, SCS, ATC
Associate Professor
School of Health Professions
Grand Valley State University
Allendale, Michigan

Jean M. Irion, PT, EdD, SCS, ATC
Assistant Professor
Department of Physical Therapy
University of South Alabama
Mobile, Alabama

Ginny Keely, PT, MS, OCS, FAAOMPT
Ronning Physical Therapy
Santa Cruz, CA

Beth McKitrick-Bandy, PT, PCS, MBA
Director of Rehabilitation Services
Arkansas Children's Hospital
Little Rock, Arkansas

Dennis O'Connell, PT, PhD, FACSM
Professor
Department of Physical Therapy
Hardin-Simmons University
Abilene, Texas

Erin O'Kelley, MSPT, ATC
Lecturer
Department of Physical Therapy
Texas State University–San Marcos
San Marcos, Texas

Michael M. Reinold, PT, DPT, ATC
Facility Director & Coordinator of Rehabilitative
Research
Champion Sports Medicine
American Sports Medicine Institute
Birmingham, Alabama

Chris Russian, RRT, MEd
Assistant Professor
Department of Respiratory Care
Texas State University–San Marcos
San Marcos, Texas

Barbara Sanders, PT, PhD, SCS
Professor and Chair
Department of Physical Therapy
Texas State University–San Marcos
San Marcos, Texas

Michael Sanders, EdD
Director, Life Skills
Department of Intercollegiate Athletics
University of Texas
Austin, Texas

Marcia H. Stalvey, PT, MS, NCS
Director of Physical Therapy
Edwin Shaw Hospital for Rehabilitation
Akron, Ohio

Russell Stowers, PTA, MS
Director and Assistant Professor
Physical Therapist Assistant Program
Del Mar College
Corpus Christi, Texas

J. David Taylor, PT, PhD
Assistant Professor
Department of Physical Therapy
University of Central Arkansas
Conway, Arkansas

Steven R. Tippett, PT, PhD, SCS, ATC
Associate Professor
Department of Physical Therapy and Health Science
Bradley University
Peoria, Illinois

Michael L. Voight, PT, DHSc, OCS, SCS, ATC
Professor
Department of Physical Therapy
Belmont University
Nashville, Tennessee

Michele Voight, PTA, BS
Coordinator of Professional Development
CHRISTUS Spohn Rehabilitation Services
Corpus Christi, Texas

Bridgett Wallace, PT
Balance Therapy of Texas
Austin, Texas

Kevin E. Wilk, PT, DPT
Clinical Director
Champion Sports Medicine
American Sports Medicine Institute
Birmingham, Alabama

Reta J. Zabel, PT, PhD, GCS
Associate Professor
Department of Physical Therapy
University of Central Arkansas
Conway, Arkansas

TABLE OF CONTENTS

THERAPEUTIC EXERCISE for

Physical
Therapist
Assistants

SECOND EDITION

Foundations of Therapeutic Exercise

Introduction to Therapeutic Exercise

William D. Bandy, PT, PhD, SCS, ATC, Barbara Sanders, PT, PhD, SCS, Erin O'Kelley, MSPT, ATC, and J. David Taylor, PT, PhD

OBJECTIVES

Upon completion of this chapter, the reader will be able to:

- Define therapeutic exercise.

- Discuss the role of therapeutic exercise as an intervention in patient care.

- Identify the effect of therapeutic exercise on specific soft tissues.

- Identify physical agents and electrotherapeutic interventions that would be appropriate in support of therapeutic exercise.

DEFINITION OF THERAPEUTIC EXERCISE

In a 1967 survey of more than 100 clinicians and faculty who were using or teaching therapeutic exercise, Bouman[1] collected 53 definitions of therapeutic exercise. Bouman[1] concluded, "I think we all know what therapeutic exercise is. It is just difficult to define." Before providing an operational definition of therapeutic exercise, a brief discussion of the historical development of the field is presented.

Historical Perspective

The following review of the significant highlights in the history of therapeutic exercise provides the reader with a perspective of the progression of the use of therapeutic exercise by clinicians. For an extensive history of the field, see Licht,[2] who defined therapeutic exercise as "motions of the body or its parts to relieve symptoms or to improve function."

The use of therapeutic exercise (then referred to as medical gymnastics) was recorded as early as 800 BC in the *Atharva-Veda,* a medical manuscript from India. According to the manuscript, exercise and massage were recommended for chronic rheumatism. However, most historians in the field believe that therapeutic exercise first gained popularity and widespread use in ancient Greece. Herodicus is believed to be the first physician to write on the subject (ca. 480 BC) and is considered the Father of Therapeutic Exercise. Herodicus claimed to have used exercise to cure himself of an "incurable" disease, and he developed an elaborate system of exercises for athletes. Hippocrates, the most famous of Herodicus' students, wrote of the beneficial effects of exercise and its value in strengthening muscle, improving mental attitude, and decreasing obesity.

Galen, considered by some as the greatest physician in ancient Rome, wrote of exercise in the 2nd century AD. He was appointed the physician for the gladiators and classified exercise according to intensity, duration, and frequency. In the 5th century AD another Roman physician, Aurelianus, recommended exercise during convalescence from surgery and advocated the use of weights and pulleys. In 1553 in Spain Mendez wrote *Libro Del Exercicio,* the first book on exercise. The book emphasized exercises to improve hygiene.

Therapeutic exercise in modern times appears to have originated in Sweden in the 19th century with a fencing instructor named Pehr Henri Ling. Ling believed that a good fencer should also be a good athlete, and he developed and taught a system of specific movements. His system of therapeutic exercise included dosage, counting, and detailed instruction for each exercise. He demonstrated that precise movements, if scientifically applied, could serve to remedy disease and dysfunction of the body.[3] In 1932 McMillan[4] wrote, "it is Peter Henry Ling and the Swedish systematical order that we owe much today in the field of medical gymnastics and therapeutic exercise."

About the same time that Ling developed his system, Swiss physician Frenkel[5] wrote a controversial paper in 1902. Frenkel proposed an exercise program for ataxia that incorporated repetitive activities to improve damaged nerve cells. No weights or strengthening activities were used, and the program became very popular. Although Frenkel's program is not as popular as it once was, his greatest contribution to the development of therapeutic exercise was the insistence on repetition.

Several individuals made major contributions to the development of therapeutic exercise in the 20th century. In 1934 Codman[6] developed a series of exercises to alleviate pain in the shoulder; these exercises are now referred to as Codman's, or pendulum, exercises. One of the most important advances was the adaptation of progressive resistance exercises (PRE) by Delorme[7] in 1945. This exercise program was developed in a military hospital in an effort to rehabilitate patients after knee surgeries. According to Licht,[2] PRE was adapted more widely and rapidly than any other concept of therapeutic exercise in the century, except for early ambulation.

Kabat[8] took therapeutic exercise out of the cardinal plane by introducing diagonal movement and the use of a variety of reflexes to facilitate muscle contraction. His work was further developed by Knott and Voss,[9] who published the textbook *Proprioceptive Neuromuscular Facilitation* in 1956.

Using the principles of vector analysis on the flexor and extensor muscles that control the spine, Williams[10] developed a series of postural exercises and strengthening activities to alleviate back pain and emphasize flexion. In 1971 McKenzie[11] introduced a program to treat patients with back pain that focused on extension to facilitate anterior movement of the discs.

Hislop and Perrine[12] introduced the concept of isokinetic exercise in 1967, which was quite popular in the 1970s and 1980s. Finally, the work of Maitland,[13] Mennell,[14] and Kaltenborn[15]—who introduced the basic concepts of arthrokinematics and the use of mobilization and manipulation to decrease pain and capsular stiffness—cannot be overlooked as important contributions in the 20th century.

It is impossible to name all the accomplishments related to therapeutic exercise, but some of the more important events and concepts were highlighted. This textbook was written by current experts in the field of therapeutic exercise. Each chapter focuses on a specialized field of therapeutic exercise and includes background information and references to the major researchers and scholars in that area. In addition, all the authors are clinicians and therefore have firsthand knowledge and understanding of the exercise techniques presented. When Licht's[2] history of therapeutic exercise is revised, it may well refer to the authors of the chapters of this textbook.

Physical Therapy Perspective: Guide to Physical Therapist Practice

In November 1997 the American Physical Therapy Association first published the *Guide to Physical Therapist Practice*.[16] The *Guide* provides an outline of the body of knowledge for physical therapists (PT) and delineates preferred practice patterns. In addition, the *Guide* describes boundaries within which the PT may select appropriate care. It represents the best efforts of the physical therapy profession to define itself. The document was developed over 3 years and involved the expert consensus of more than 1,000 members of the physical therapy community.

The *Guide* defines intervention as "the purposeful and skilled interaction of the PT with the patient/client." According to the *Guide*, physical therapy intervention has the following three components, listed in order of importance:

Coordination, communication, and documentation

Patient/client-related instruction

Procedural interventions

    Therapeutic exercise

    Functional training in self-care and home management (activities of daily living, instrumental activities of daily living)

    Functional training in work (job, school, play) community and leisure integration or reintegration

    Manual therapy

    Prescription, application, and fabrication of devices and equipment

    Airway clearance techniques

    Integumentary repair and protective techniques

    Electrotherapeutic modalities

    Physical agents and mechanical modalities

Note that therapeutic exercise is considered the most important procedural intervention. Table 1-1 presents a definition of therapeutic exercise and a detailed account of the types of therapeutic exercises used in the practice of physical therapy. The operational definition of therapeutic exercise used in this textbook is the one given in Table 1-1.

EFFECT OF THERAPEUTIC EXERCISE ON SPECIFIC SOFT TISSUES

Before information is provided on the role of the physical therapist assistant (PTA) and the description of the wide variety of therapeutic exercises that the PTA can use in the treatment of their patients and clients, an understanding of injuries, the healing process, and how therapeutic exercise relates to specific soft tissues of the body is needed. This section will provide information which is important to understanding how therapeutic exercise is integrated into the total treatment plan and management of the patient.

Injury Classification

Tissue is injured either with a single injurious force referred to as macrotrauma or by a series of small forces referred to as microtrauma. With a macrotrauma injury the pain and tissue destruction occurs simultaneously. However, with microtrauma the tissue incurs several small injuries prior to the patient experiencing pain. In both instances pain is not an accurate indicator of the health of the tissue. The chemical mediators relaying the message of pain are often dissipated long before the tissue is healthy enough to respond to the forces such as those that led to the initial injury.

Phases of Healing

Although three phases of the healing process exist, healing is actually an ongoing process until resolution with no clear delineation of one phase from the other. *Phase I* is the inflammatory response phase. An injury occurs and the body tries to respond by stabilizing the injured site; the inflammation begins and usually lasts 24 to 48 hours but can last up to 7 to 10 days. The acute inflammatory reaction begins with vasoconstriction of small vessels. As the acute phase resolves, vasodilatation of the vessels occurs which increases the blood and plasma flow to the area of injury. This vasodilatation is followed by increased permeability, which leads to edema. These changes allow the increase in the number of white blood cells to combat foreign bodies and instigate the process of debris removal. The inflammatory process is a time of many complex events which manifest themselves with the signs of inflammation including redness, swelling, pain, increased temperature, and loss of normal function.

Phase II is considered the repair sequence, or the proliferation phase, and begins after Phase I, anytime from 48 hours to 6 weeks after injury. Tissue regeneration occurs with vascularization and cell growth to fill any tissue voids. The fibroblastic activity provides proliferation of the reparative cells for wound closure and regeneration of any small vessels. These events are complex and interactive among cells and chemicals in the area. The collagen produced during this phase is type III collagen, which is weak and thin but lays down the foundation for further collagen replacement with type I collagen.

Phase III is the stage of connective tissue formation and remodeling, and it begins from 3 weeks to 12 months after injury. During this phase there is a balance between

TABLE 1-1 Procedural Interventions

Therapeutic Exercise

Therapeutic exercise is the systematic performance or execution of planned physical movements, postures, or activities intended to enable the patient/client to (1) remediate or prevent impairments, (2) enhance function, (3) reduce risk, (4) optimize overall health, and (5) enhance fitness and well-being. Therapeutic exercise may include aerobic and endurance conditioning and reconditioning; agility training; balance training, both static and dynamic; body mechanics training; breathing exercises; coordination exercises; developmental activities training; gait and locomotion training; motor training; muscle lengthening; movement pattern training; neuromotor development activities training; neuromuscular education or reeducation; perceptual training; postural stabilization and training; range-of-motion exercises and soft tissue stretching; relaxation exercises; and strength, power, and endurance exercises.

Physical therapists select, prescribe, and implement exercise activities when the examination findings, diagnosis, and prognosis indicate the use of therapeutic exercise to enhance bone density; enhance breathing; enhance or maintain physical performance; enhance performance in activities of daily living (ADL) and instrumental activities of daily living (IADL); improve safety; increase aerobic capacity/endurance; increase muscle strength, power, and endurance; enhance postural control and relaxation; increase sensory awareness; increase tolerance to activity; prevent or remediate impairments, functional limitations, or disabilities to improve physical function; enhance health, wellness, and fitness; reduce complications, pain, restriction, and swelling; or reduce risk and increase safety during activity performance.

Clinical Considerations

Examination findings that may direct the type and specificity of the procedural intervention may include:

- *Pathology/pathophysiology (disease, disorder, or condition), history (including risk factors) of medical/surgical conditions, or signs and symptoms (e.g., pain, shortness of breath, stress) in the following systems:*
  — cardiovascular
  — endocrine/metabolic
  — genitourinary
  — integumentary
  — multiple systems
  — musculoskeletal
  — neuromuscular
  — pulmonary

- *Impairments in the following catergories:*
  — aerobic capacity/endurance (e.g., decreased walk distance)
  — anthropometric characteristics (e.g., increased body mass index)
  — arousal, attention, and cognition (e.g., decreased motivation to participate in fitness activities)
  — circulation (e.g., abnormal elevation in heart rate with activity)
  — cranial and peripheral nerve integrity (e.g., difficulty with swallowing, risk of aspiration, positive neural provocation response)
  — ergonomics and body mechanics (e.g., inability to squat because of weakness in gluteus maximus and quadriceps femoris muscles)
  — gait, locomotion, and balance (e.g., inability to perform ankle dorisflexion)
  — integumentary integrity (e.g., limited finger flexion as a result of dorsal burn scar)
  — joint integrity and mobility (e.g., limited range of motion in the shoulder)
  — motor function (e.g., uncoordinated limb movements)
  — muscle performance (e.g., weakness of lumbar stabilizers)
  — neuromotor development and sensory integration (e.g., delayed development)
  — posture (e.g., forward head, kyphosis)
  — range of motion (e.g., increased laxity in patellofemoral joint)
  — reflex integrity (e.g., poor balance in standing)
  — sensory integrity (e.g., lack of position sense)
  — ventilation and respiration/gas exchange (e.g., abnormal breathing patterns)

- *Functional limitations in the ability to perform actions, tasks, and activities in the following categories:*
  — self-care (e.g., difficult with dressing, bathing)
  — home management (e.g., difficulty with raking, shoveling, making bed)
  — work (job/school/play) (e.g., difficulty with keyboarding, pushing, or pulling, difficulty with play activities)
  — community/leisure (e.g., inability to negotiate steps and curbs)

- *Disability—that is, the inability or restricted ability to perform actions, tasks, or activities of required roles within the individual's sociocultural context—in the following categories:*
  — work (e.g., inability to assume parenting role, inability to care for elderly relatives, inability to return to work as a police officer)
  — community/leisure (e.g., difficulty with jogging or playing golf, inability to attend religious services)

- *Risk reduction/prevention in the following areas:*
  — risk factors (e.g., need to decrease body fat composition)
  — recurrence of condition (e.g., need to increase mobility and postural control for work [job/school/play] actions, tasks and activities)
  — secondary impairments (e.g., need to improve strength and balance for fall risk reduction)

- *Health, wellness, and fitness needs:*
  — fitness, including physical performance (e.g., need to improve golf-swing timing, need to maximize gymnastic performance, need to maximize pelvic-floor muscle function)
  — health and wellness (e.g., need to improve balance for recreation, need to increase muscle strength to help maintain bone density)

(continued)

TABLE 1-1 (continued)

Interventions

Therapeutic exercise may include:

- Aerobic capacity/endurance conditioning or reconditioning
  — aquatic programs
  — gait and locomotion training
  — increased workload over time
  — movement efficiency and energy conservation training
  — walking and wheelchair propulsion programs

- Balance, coordination, and agility training
  — developmental activities training
  — motor function (motor control and motor learning) training or retraining
  — neuromuscular education or reeducation
  — perceptual training
  — posture awareness training
  — sensory training or retraining
  — standardized, programmatic, complementary exercise approaches
  — task-specific performance training
  — vestibular training

- Body mechanics and postural stabilization
  — body mechanics training
  — postural control training
  — postural stabilization activities
  — posture awareness training

- Flexibility exercises
  — muscle lengthening
  — range of motion
  — stretching

- Gait and locomotion training
  — developmental activities training
  — gait training
  — implement and device training
  — perceptual training
  — standardized, programmatic, complementary exercise approaches
  — wheelchair training

- Neuromotor development training
  — developmental activities training
  — motor training
  — movement pattern training
  — neuromuscular education or reeducation

- Relaxation
  — breathing strategies
  — movement strategies
  — relaxation techniques
  — standardized, programmatic, complementary exercise approaches

- Strength, power, and endurance training for head, neck, limb, pelvic-floor, trunk, and ventilatory muscles
  — active assistive, active, and resistive exercises (including concentric, dynamic/isotonic, eccentric, isokinetic, isometric, and plyometric
  — aquatic programs
  — standardized, programmatic, complementary exercise approaches
  — task-specific performance training

Anticipated Goals and Expected Outcomes

Anticipated goals and expected outcomes related to therapeutic exercises may include:

- Impact on pathology/pathophysiology (disease, disorder, or condition)
  — Atelectasis is decreased.
  — Joint swelling, inflammation, or restriction is reduced.
  — Nutrient delivery to tissue is increased.
  — Osteogenic effects of exercise are maximized.
  — Pain is decreased.
  — Physiological response to increased oxygen demand is improved.
  — Soft tissue swelling, inflammation, or restriction is reduced.
  — Symptoms associated with increased oxygen demand are decreased.
  — Tissue perfusion and oxygenation are enhanced.

- Impact on impairment
  — Aerovic capacity is increased.
  — Airway clearance is improved.
  — Balance is improved.
  — Endurance is increased.
  — Energy expenditure per unit of work is decreased.
  — Gait, locomotion, and balance are improved.
  — Integumentary integrity is improved.
  — Joint integrity and mobility are improved.
  — Motor function (motor control and motor learning) is improved.
  — Muscle performance (strength, power, and endurance) is increased.
  — Postural control is improved.
  — Quality and quantity of movement between and across body segments are improved.
  — Range of motion is improved.
  — Relaxation is increased.
  — Sensory awareness is increased.
  — Ventilation and respiratory/gas exchange are improved.
  — Weight-bearing status is improved.
  — Work of breathing is decreased.

- Impact on functional limitations
  — Ability to perform physical actions, tasks, or activities related to self-care, home management, work (job/school/play), community, and leisure is improved.
  — Level of supervision required for task performance is decreased.
  — Performance of and independence in ADL and IADL with or without devices and equipment are increased.
  — Tolerance of positions and activities is increased.

- Impact on disabilities
  — Ability to assume or resume required self-care, home management, work (job/school/play), community, and leisure roles is improved.

- Risk reduction/prevention
  — Preoperative and postoperative complications are reduced.
  — Risk factors are reduced.
  — Risk or recurrence of condition is reduced.
  — Risk of secondary impairment is reduced.

(continued)

TABLE 1-1 (continued)

Anticipated Goals and Expected Outcomes (continued)

- — Safety is improved.
- — Self-management of symptoms is improved.
- Impact on health, wellness, and fitness
  - — Fitness is improved.
  - — Health status is improved.
  - — Physical capacity is increased.
  - — Physical function is improved.
- Impact on societal resources
  - — Utilization of physical therapy services is optimized.
  - — Utilization of physical therapy services results in efficient use of health care dollars.
- Patient/client satisfaction
  - — Access, availability, and services provided are acceptable to patient/client.

- — Administrative management of practice is acceptable to patient/client.
- — Clinical proficiency of physical therapist is acceptable to patient/client.
- — Coordination of care is acceptable to patient/client.
- — Cost of health care services is decreased.
- — Intensity of care is decreased.
- — Interpersonal skills of physical therapist are acceptable to patient/client, family, and significant others.
- — Sense of well-being is improved.
- — Stressors are decreased.

Source: Reprinted with permission from the American Physical Therapy Association.

proteolytic degradation of excess collagen and deposition, organization, and modification of the collagen in preparation for the maturation process. Type III collagen is converted to type I collagen, which strengthens and provides much more cross-lineage to develop tensile strength. Remodeling is the process by which the architecture of tissue changes in response to stress.

Tissue repair is an adaptive intrinsic and extrinsic process. Physical therapy cannot accelerate the process but can support and not delay or disrupt it. There needs to be a balance between protection and application of controlled functional stresses.

As more specific make-up of the various tissues in the body is described, it is important to gauge the stage of healing and also understand that tissues have different rates of healing. Tissues must receive nutrients to heal. The most efficient and therefore strongest determinant of tissue healing rate is blood supply. However, when blood supply is either absent or low, it is important to understand the available avenues to supply the tissue with nutrients and how to incorporate this information into safe rehabilitation techniques. The various soft tissues of the body that can be affected by therapeutic exercises will now be described: joint capsule, ligament, tendon, and muscle.

Joint Capsule

The joint capsule exists in all synovial joints. Dysfunction of the joint capsule may be due to a tensile force leading to connective tissue failure and secondly joint instability. The joint capsule may also contribute to dysfunction by restricting normal arthrokinematic motions by decreased extensibility from previous injury or tissue disease.

The joint capsule consists of two distinct layers. The external layer, stratum fibrosum, is often referred to as the fibrous capsule. Functionally the stratum fibrosum contributes to joint stability. The functional role is achieved by the dense irregular connective tissue which has a large percentage of type I collagen fiber bundles oriented in several directions to combat the multidirectional tensile loads. Although the stratum fibrosum connects to the periosteum of the bone, the tissue is poorly vascularized. Conversely, the stratum fibrosum is highly innervated with both pain and mechanoreceptors. These mechanoreceptors are very important from a rehabilitation perspective. The use of exercises such as simple active or passive range of motion (ROM; presented in Chapter 3) will help maintain and reeducate the sensory organs after injury. Higher levels of exercises such as progressive rhythmic stabilization to functional open-chain and closed-chain exercises (presented in Chapters 5 through 9) with increases in speed and difficulty are essential to a comprehensive rehabilitation program.

The internal layer of the capsule, stratum synovium, is highly vascularized yet poorly innervated. The stratum synovium is crucial to joint health for delivery of lubrication and nutrition to joint surfaces and accessory bodies such as menisci. The specialized cells of the stratum synovium are responsible for manufacturing synovial fluid. Synovial fluid contains hyaluronic acid, which acts like a lubricator filling the joint space, lubricating the synovium, and is responsible for the synovial fluid's viscosity.[17]

Each of us has experienced a change in shape of the stratum fibrosum and the effects of decreased lubrication. If you sit in a chair and have your knee fully extended by placing your foot on another chair for an extended period of time, you will experience pain and a resistance to the initiation of knee flexion. The time in the extended position places the stratum fibrosum on stretch and initiates pain. Additionally, during the elongated position the synovial fluid becomes stagnant, making your knee feel stiff. To overcome this uncomfortable sensation, we naturally gently move out of the extended position and then repeatedly flex the knee. The repetitive motion promotes synovial bathing and motion becomes easier and less painful. With this simple daily example, you should be able to clearly imagine the results of prolonged immobilization.

Ligaments

Ligaments vary widely in the amount of blood supply and fiber make-up based on location and function. Most commonly, ligaments function as passive connectors and stabilizers between two bones. Similarly to the capsule, ligaments also house neurosensory organs. Location of a ligament is a key factor in its nutritional supply. Ligaments are often interwoven in the stratum fibrosum and considered capsular ligaments. In capsular ligaments, the amount of blood supply is limited. Other ligaments are extracapsular or intracapsular but are extrasynovial and receive blood supply from small vessels which allows a better blood supply.

When the stability of a joint has been compromised by joint capsule or ligamentous injury, the healing time is between 6 and 8 weeks. Full healing of ligamentous tissue may extend beyond this initial time to 12 to 14 weeks. A fibrous scar will replace the defect. Stress during the healing process will strengthen the repair of the ligamentous tissue when applied in a controlled manner. The goal of rehabilitation is to control the inflammation in the acute stage, provide a healthy environment with pain-free motion, utilize muscles crossing the injured joint to help stabilize the area, and finally provide controlled stresses to help align newly laid collagen fibers in an organized and efficient direction.

Tendons

Mechanically, tendons are similar in biologic make-up to ligaments. However, because tendons do not have to resist forces from multiple angles, the collagen fiber alignment is a tightly packed parallel configuration. The tendon attaches to the bone via mineralized fibrocartilage known as Sharpy's fibers. The musculotendinous junction is a critical zone as the collagen fibers of the tendon merge with the contractile units of the muscle. It is the musculotendinous zone that has the greatest vascular contribution. However, the remaining portions of the tendon have relatively poor blood supply available for healing.

Injuries to the tendon may be either from macrotrauma or microtrauma. Most macrotrauma injuries, which occur at the bony insertion or below the musculotendinous junction, will require surgical intervention. Microtrauma

injuries are often due to repetitive overload, commonly of an eccentric nature. For example, tennis elbow is caused by eccentric overloading of the tendon with the recurrent nature of the swing and ball hit. This type of injury may also occur with an industrial worker who is constantly performing the same repetitive lifting motion. It is important to realize that the tissue injury is present long before the patient identifies the start of pain. Perhaps more importantly, the patient's pain will subside prior to the conclusion of healing, leaving the patient at risk for repeat episodes of injury, inflammation, and pain if the patient returns to full activity too soon after injury. A therapeutic exercise program should begin within the first 24 hours of pain onset. Active ROM exercises (presented in Chapter 3) should be initiated only in the pain-free range. Early on, exercise should avoid eccentric loading and be limited to no more than two exercises to the injured tissue. However, as the patient is able to achieve full pain-free ROM and concentric strength, a gradual eccentric loading and rate must be initiated.[18] (The concepts of eccentric and concentric loading will be presented in Chapters 5 and 6.) The tendon responds to loads with increases in tensile strength and efficiency.[19]

Cartilage

There are three distinct types of cartilage in the human body: hyaline cartilage, fibrocartilage, and elastic cartilage. Elastic cartilage is found in the ears and epiglottis and, as the name implies, has a significantly higher ratio of elastin than the other types of cartilage to allow greater amounts of deformation without permanent alteration in resting shape. Fibrocartilage is found between bones that require little motion, such as the intervertebral disk, menisci, and labrums. Hyaline cartilage is a specialized substance found at the ends of bones in synovial joints and functions to provide a smooth, low-friction surface.

Hyaline cartilage serves to evenly disperse compressive and shearing forces. In combination with the synovial fluid, hyaline cartilage provides a low coefficient of friction with a surface that is five to twenty times more slippery than ice.[20]

The hyaline cartilage is both aneural and avascular. Nourishment to this tissue comes only from the synovial fluid and through diffusion of nutrients from the subchondral bone. This nourishment occurs in a milking action through intermittent compression of the joint surface.

Because the articular cartilage is aneural and avascular, early indications of injury in the form of pain and swelling do not occur until the articular lesion reaches the subchondral bone. However, with advancements in imaging and often identification of cartilage lesions during surgical procedures initiated to address other injuries, early identification of cartilage injury is now common.

Fibrocartilage functions as a shock absorber, as noted above, and can be found in both weight-bearing and non-weight-bearing joints. Fibrocartilage has similar properties to hyaline cartilage but is less distensible due to the dense collagen fibers. Fibrocartilage is avascular, alymphatic, and aneural. It is designed to sustain a large and repeated stress load.

Although the classification of articular damage and methods to repair the damage are beyond the scope of this chapter, the defects generally are filled with fibrocartilage, which is mechanically less advantageous than hyaline cartilage. However, based on the understanding of how articular cartilage receives nutrition, some rehabilitation guidelines can be provided. The goal is to provide the injured area with a large amount of synovial flushing and to use the milking action to receive nutrients from the subchondral bone without further compromising the area. It is important to recognize that with the advances in surgical procedures consisting of articular transplant and laboratory cell growth, alterations in the rehabilitation process are vast and should follow the physician's guidelines.

Skeletal Muscle

Skeletal muscle is the basis for human movement. Muscle strains are graded in accordance to the amount of fiber destruction. A grade 1 strain is characterized as an adverse stretching of the fibers leading to a minimal tear, no palpable defect, and minor loss of function. A grade 2 strain indicates that up to half of the muscle fibers are torn and leads to painful dysfunction that limits full ROM and activity. A grade 3 muscle strain is considered a rupture of all of the muscle fibers. Commensurate with this type of injury is major disability and often a palpable defect.

Muscle also has viscoelastic properties. It is easy to focus on the contractile units of myosin and actin and forget that muscle is surrounded by fascia (information on actin and myosin is presented in Chapter 5). In addition, within the actual muscle unit (sarcomere) resides connective tissue that contributes to the viscoelastic properties. The muscle cell membrane and protein titin provide the parallel elastic properties of muscle. When the muscle is lengthened, these units lengthen with the muscle and then, through their elastic properties, help return the muscle to its resting length. The tendon works in series to provide elastic characteristics. When a muscle is contracted, the parallel properties are on slack; however, the tendon becomes tense. When a muscle is elongated fully over the joint it crosses, both the series and parallel components are under tension. Collectively, the elastic components found in the muscle and in the tendon provide the spring-like action, or stiffness, of a muscle.[17,21]

Mechanically, increasing the tension of the muscle and adjoining tendon is similar to stretching a rubber band. After taking up the resting slack in the muscle, both the parallel and serial properties endure an increase in tension that builds exponentially until tissue failure. An abnormal amount of passive tension secondary to a decrease in the elastic properties of the muscle can contribute to a functional decrease in ROM. For example, a woman who only wears high-healed shoes will demonstrate a decrease in ankle dorsiflexion secondary to a tight gastrocnemius/Achilles complex. The inability of a joint to move through a full ROM due to loss of elastic extensibility of the connective tissue components is known as passive insufficiency. Passive insufficiency can cause dysfunction similar to that of the high-heeled patient just described.

Therapeutic Exercise and Soft Tissues—Summary

Rarely is only one soft tissue affected in a patient. A patient with articular cartilage damage is also likely to present with decreased capsular mobility or a hamstring injury perhaps accompanied by nerve irritation. It is the PT's responsibility in following the rehabilitation plan to address each soft tissue and not allow a certain intervention on one soft tissue to exacerbate the symptoms and condition of the other tissues involved. Following the stages of healing will assist in a successful intervention. Careful recognition of signs such as decreased ROM, strength, and pain, despite the likely stage of healing, must be addressed by decreasing the load and/or increasing the amount of rest.

COMPLEMENTARY INTERVENTIONS TO THERAPEUTIC EXERCISE

In the physical therapy management of individuals with diagnoses, various impairments, and functional limitations, the PTA administers a variety of interventions. Physical therapy interventions administered by the PTA are defined as the "purposeful interaction of the PTA with the patient/client using various physical therapy procedures including therapeutic exercise, physical agents, and electrotherapeutic modalities."[16] Physical agents and electrotherapeutic modalities are often used to promote healing and complement therapeutic exercise to improve physical performance in people with impairments and functional deficits.

Physical Agents

Physical agents are a group of procedures using various forms of energy (acoustic, aqueous, or thermal) that are applied to tissues in a systematic manner. PTAs implement

TABLE 1-2 Physical Agents	
Thermotherapy	***Hydrotherapy***
Dry heat	Contrast bath
Hot packs	Whirlpool
Paraffin bath	
	Sound agents
Cryotherapy	Phonophoresis
Cold packs	Ultrasound
Ice massage	
Vapocoolant spray	

physical agents to increase connective tissue extensibility, increase the healing rate of soft tissue, modulate pain, reduce swelling and inflammation, and enhance physical performance in individuals with impairments and loss of function. The therapeutic goal of physical agents is to complement the role of therapeutic exercise in improving strength, power, endurance, aerobic capacity, ROM, and physical performance that is impaired due to injury or disease.[16]

Physical agents may include thermotherapy, cryotherapy, hydrotherapy, and sound agents (Table 1-2). Thermotherapy (e.g., dry heat, hot packs, paraffin baths) is the treatment of damaged tissue by therapeutic application of heat. Cryotherapy (e.g., cold packs, ice massage [Fig. 1-1], vapocoolant spray) is the use of cold in the treatment of tissue injury. Hydrotherapy (e.g., contrast bath, whirlpool tanks) is the external application of water as a liquid, solid, or vapor for therapeutic purposes. A sound agent (e.g., phonophoresis, ultrasound; Fig. 1-2) is used as an intervention to treat tissue injury by transmitting vibrations

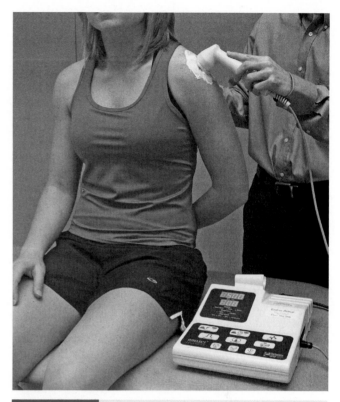

Figure 1-2   Ultrasound to the shoulder.

produced by a sounding body through a conductive medium.[16]

Use of Physical Agents to Complement Therapeutic Exercise

The *Guide to Physical Therapist Practice*[16] indicates that the use of physical agents in the absence of other interventions should not be considered physical therapy unless documentation exists that justifies the necessity of exclusive use of physical agents. Therefore, this textbook describes the use of physical agents as a group of complementary interventions to therapeutic exercise.

Cryotherapy is an adjunctive intervention to therapeutic exercise. Bleakley et al[22] performed a systematic review of randomized, controlled trials (RCTs) assessing the efficacy of cryotherapy in the treatment of acute soft-tissue injuries. After a review of 22 RCTs, the authors concluded that ice in addition to exercise was effective in the treatment of ankle sprains and surgical-related impairments.

Yanagisawa et al[23] conducted a clinical trial that investigated the effects of ice and exercise on shoulder ROM after subjects threw a baseball. The control group and experiment group showed a significant decrease in shoulder ROM immediately after throwing a baseball; however, shoulder ROM in the experimental group significantly

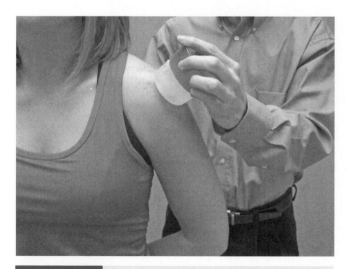

Figure 1-1   Ice massage to the shoulder.

improved after the intervention with ice in conjunction with exercise when compared with the control group.

Ultrasound is a physical agent that may be used to support therapeutic exercise in improving ROM. Knight et al[24] conducted a clinical trial to evaluate the effect of hot packs, ultrasound, and active exercise warm-up prior to stretching compared with stretching alone on the extensibility of the plantar-flexor muscles. The results of the study indicated that the use of ultrasound prior to stretching was the most effective for increasing ankle dorsiflexion ROM.

Esenyel et al[25] investigated the effectiveness of ultrasound treatment and trigger point injections in combination with neck-stretching exercises on myofascial trigger points of the upper trapezius muscle. Subjects were randomly assigned to receive either ultrasound therapy to trigger points in conjunction with neck-stretching exercises (group 1), trigger point injections and neck-stretching exercises (group 2), or neck-stretching exercises only (control group). When compared with the control group, subjects in groups 1 and 2 had a statistically significant reduction in pain and increase in ROM. No statistically significant differences between groups 1 and 2 were found. The study concluded that in patients with myofascial pain syndrome, ultrasound in combination with stretching was as effective as combined trigger point injections and stretching, and the addition of ultrasound or trigger point injections was more effective than stretching alone.

The Philadelphia Panel[26-29] conducted a series of meta-analysis studies on the effects of various interventions on shoulder, neck, knee, and low back pain. The meta-analysis studies indicated that evidence does exist to support the use of thermotherapy and therapeutic exercise for musculoskeletal pain. Yet the meta-analysis studies also indicated that the research supporting the use of thermotherapy in conjunction with therapeutic exercise is limited. The Philadelphia Panel[26-29] concluded that good evidence exists to support the use of therapeutic exercise alone as an intervention for musculoskeletal pain but evidence is insufficient for the combined interventions of thermotherapy and therapeutic exercise.

Electrotherapeutic Modalities

Electrotherapeutic modalities are a group of agents that use electricity and are intended to assist functional training, assist muscle force generation and contraction, decrease unwanted muscular activity, maintain strength after injury or surgery, increase circulation, reduce edema, decrease pain, reduce swelling, reduce inflammation, and assist in wound healing. The PTA uses electrotherapeutic modalities to increase joint mobility, improve muscle and neuromuscular impairments, enhance physical performance, and improve upon loss of physical function.[16] As in the case of physical agents, the therapeutic goal of electrotherapeutic modalities is to complement therapeutic exercise in improving strength, power, endurance, aerobic capacity, ROM, and physical performance that is impaired due to injury or disease.[16]

Electrotherapeutic modalities include biofeedback and electrical stimulation (e.g., electrical muscle stimulation [Fig. 1-3], functional electrical stimulation, neuromuscular electrical stimulation, transcutaneous electrical nerve stimulation).[16] Biofeedback is a training technique that promotes

Figure 1-3 Electrical muscle stimulation to the knee.

gain in voluntary control based on the principle that a desired response is learned when received information (feedback) indicates that a specific action has produced the desired response.[16] Electrical stimulation, as referred to in this textbook, is defined as an intervention that is used to stimulate muscle contraction.

Use of Electrotherapeutic Modalities to Complement Therapeutic Exercise

As with physical agents, the *Guide to Physical Therapist Practice*[16] indicates that the use of electrotherapeutic modalities in the absence of other interventions should not be considered physical therapy unless documentation exists that justifies the necessity of its exclusive use. Therefore, this textbook describes the use of electrotherapeutic modalities as a group of complementary interventions to therapeutic exercise.

Biofeedback in combination with therapeutic exercise has been shown to be effective in the clinical management of orthopaedic impairments. A recent systematic review of RCTs by Bizzini et al[30] assessed nonoperative treatments for patellofemoral pain syndrome. Based on the results of RCTs exhibiting a sufficient level of quality, the combination of exercise with patellar taping and biofeedback was found to be effective in decreasing pain and improving function in patients with patellofemoral pain syndrome.

Ingersoll and Knight[31] studied the changes in the patellofemoral biomechanics as a result of biofeedback training that emphasized vastus medialis oblique (VMO) strengthening, strength training only, and no exercise. The results of this study suggested that the use of biofeedback training to selectively strengthen the VMO was beneficial in correcting faulty patellar tracking and biomechanics.

Researchers have investigated the use of electrical stimulation in the context of exercise programs to develop strength and physical performance. Improvements in muscle strength are explained on the basis of electrical stimulation of motor units. Electrical stimulation of motor units during exercise promotes synchronous recruitment of muscle fibers. Significant increases in muscle fiber cross-sectional areas, isokinetic peak torque, maximal isometric and dynamic strength, and motor performance skills have been found using combined electrical stimulation and exercise.[32]

Complementary Interventions—Summary

Physical agents and electrotherapeutic modalities are a collection of interventions that the PTA can use to complement therapeutic exercise. Yet physical agents and electrotherapeutic modalities should not be used exclusively without appropriate documentation that justifies their sole use. Using the best evidence available, the PT should determine the optimum combination of physical agents or electrotherapeutic

modalities with therapeutic exercise. The PT can then provide instruction and direction to the PTA for implementation of physical agents and electrotherapeutic modalities in the therapeutic exercise treatment program. In conjunction with therapeutic exercise, physical agents and electrotherapeutic modalities can be an effective group of interventions in the physical therapy plan of care.

SUMMARY

The *Guide to Physical Therapist Practice*[16] notes that therapeutic exercise is a vital component of patient intervention and is a core element in the care of patients with dysfunctions and of clients who require preventative measures. This textbook emphasizes the specific techniques used in programs of care for individuals with dysfunction, as well as prevention of dysfunction.

References

1. Bouman HD. Delineating the dilemma. *Am J Phys Med.* 1967;46:26–41.
2. Licht S, ed. *Therapeutic exercise.* New Haven, CT: Licht; 1965.
3. Taylor GH. *An exposition of the Swedish movement-cure.* New York: Fowler & Wells; 1860.
4. McMillan M. *Massage and therapeutic exercise.* Philadelphia: WB Saunders; 1932.
5. Frenkel HS. *The treatment of tabetic ataxia.* Philadelphia: Blakeston; 1902.
6. Codman EA. *The shoulder.* Philadelphia: Harper & Row; 1934.
7. Delorme TL. Restoration of muscle power by heavy resistance exercises. *J Bone Joint Surg Am.* 1945;27:645–650.
8. Kabat H. Studies in neuromuscular dysfunction XIII: new concepts and techniques of neuromuscular reeducation for paralysis. *Perm Found Med Bull.* 1950;8:112–120.
9. Knott M, Voss DE. *Proprioceptive neuromuscular facilitation.* Philadelphia: Harper & Row; 1956.
10. Williams PC. Examination and conservative treatment for disc lesion of the lower spine. *Clin Orthop.* 1955;5:28–39.
11. McKenzie RA. *The lumbar spine: mechanical diagnosis and therapy.* Upper Hutt, New Zealand: Spinal; 1971.
12. Hislop HJ, Perrine JA. The isokinetic concept of exercise. *Phys Ther.* 1967;47:114–118.
13. Maitland GD. *Vertebral manipulation.* 4th ed. London: Butterworth; 1977.
14. Mennell JM. *The musculoskeletal system: differential diagnosis from symptoms and physical signs.* Gaithersburg, MD: Aspen; 1992.
15. Kaltenborn FM. *The spine.* 2nd ed. Oslo: Olaf Norris; 1993.
16. American Physical Therapy Association. *Guide to physical therapist practice.* 2nd ed. Alexandria, VA; 2003.
17. Levangie PK, Norkin C. *Joint structure and function: a comprehensive analysis.* 3rd ed. Philadelphia: FA Davis Co; 2001.

18. Sandrey MA. Acute and chronic tendon injuries: factors affecting the healing response and treatment. *J Sport Rehabil.* 2003;12:70–91.

19. Young MA, Cook JL, Purdam CR, et al. Eccentric decline squat protocol offers superior results at 12 months compared with traditional eccentric protocol for patellar tendinopathy in volleyball players. *Br J Sports Med.* 2005;39:102–105.

20. Mow FC, Flatow EL, Foster RJ, et al. Biomechanics. In Simon SR, ed. *Orthopaedic basic science.* Rosemont, IL: American Academy of Orthopaedic Surgeons;1994.

21. Neumann DA. *Kinesiology of the musculoskeletal system: foundations for physical rehabilitation.* Philadelphia, PA: Mosby;2002.

22. Bleakley C, McDonough S, MacAuley D. The use of ice in the treatment of acute soft-tissue injury: a systematic review of randomized controlled trials. *Am J Sports Med.* 2004;32:251–261.

23. Yanagisawa O, Miyanaga Y, Shiraki H, et al. The effects of various therapeutic measures on shoulder range of motion and cross-sectional areas of rotator cuff muscles after baseball pitching. *J Sports Med Phys Fitness.* 2003;43:356–366.

24. Knight CA, Rutledge CR, Cox ME, et al. Effect of superficial heat, deep heat, and active exercise warm-up on the extensibility of the plantar flexors. *Phys Ther.* 2001;81:1206–1214.

25. Esenyel M, Caglar N, Aldemir T. Treatment of myofascial pain. *Am J Phys Med Rehabil.* 2000;79:48–52.

26. Philadelphia Panel. Philadelphia Panel evidence-based clinical practice guidelines on selected rehabilitation interventions for shoulder pain. *Phys Ther.* 2001;81:1719–1730.

27. Philadelphia Panel. Philadelphia Panel evidence-based clinical practice guidelines on selected rehabilitation interventions for neck pain. *Phys Ther.* 2001;81:1701–1717.

28. Philadelphia Panel. Philadelphia Panel evidence-based clinical practice guidelines on selected rehabilitation interventions for knee pain. *Phys Ther.* 2001;81:1675–1700.

29. Philadelphia Panel. Philadelphia Panel evidence-based clinical practice guidelines on selected rehabilitation interventions for low back pain. *Phys Ther.* 2001;81:1641–1674.

30. Bizzini M, Childs JD, Piva SR, et al. Systematic review of the quality of randomized controlled trials for patellofemoral pain syndrome. *J Orthop Sports Phys Ther.* 2003;33:4–20.

31. Ingersoll CD, Knight KL. Patellar location changes following EMG biofeedback or progressive resistive exercises. *Med Sci Sports Exerc.* 1991;23:1122–1127.

32. Requena Sanchez B, Padial Puche P, Gonzalez-Badillo JJ. Percutaneous electrical stimulation in strength training: an update. *J Strength Cond Res.* 2005;19:438–448.

The Role of the Physical Therapist Assistant

William D. Bandy, PT, PhD, SCS, ATC, and Beth McKitrick-Bandy, PT, PCS, MBA

OBJECTIVES

Upon completion of this chapter, the reader will be able to:

- Describe the roles of the physical therapist (PT) and the physical therapist assistant (PTA) in the provision of physical therapy, including appropriate PT-PTA supervision.

- Define the five elements of patient/client management: examination, evaluation, diagnosis, prognosis, and intervention.

- Describe the interventions that are appropriate for the PTA to perform—and not to perform.

- Define the terms impairment, functional limitation, and disability.

- Explain the importance of appropriate communication with, and respect for, all patients across all ages, languages, and cultures.

According to the policies and positions of the House of Delegates of the American Physical Therapy Association (APTA), "physical therapy is a health profession whose primary purpose is the promotion of optimal health and function. This purpose is accomplished through application of scientific principles to the processes of examination, evaluation, diagnosis, prognosis, and intervention to prevent or remediate impairments, functional limitations, and disabilities as related to movement and health."[1] PTs are the only professionals who examine, diagnose, and provide prognoses for patients receiving physical therapy.[2]

The purpose of this chapter is to define the important role that the PTA plays in assisting the PT in the delivery of physical therapy. To that end, the role of the PTA will be defined, including suggestions for appropriate supervision; the five elements of patient care will be described, with an emphasis on the interventions that are appropriate for the PTA to provide; the disablement model will be introduced; and the importance of effective communication across all ages and cultures will be discussed.

PHYSICAL THERAPIST ASSISTANT DEFINED

The APTA defines the PTA as "a technically educated health care provider who assists the physical therapist in the provision of physical therapy. The PTA is a graduate of a physical therapist assistant associate degree program accredited by the Commission on Accreditation in Physical Therapy Education (CAPTE)."[3] The PTAs provide selected physical therapy interventions under the direction and supervision of the PT.[2] The PT remains responsible for the physical therapy services provided by the PTA. The PTA can only modify or change an intervention outside the plan of care developed by the PT if the patient is in an unsafe situation or is in pain.[3] Any changes made in the plan of care by the PTA for reasons of patient safety or comfort must be communicated to the PT immediately.

Supervision

Selected physical therapy interventions performed by the PTA are under the direction and general supervision of the PT. "In general supervision, the physical therapist is not required to be on site for the direction and supervision, but must be available at least by telecommunications. The ability of the physical therapist assistant to perform the selected intervention as directed shall be assessed on an ongoing basis by the supervising physical therapist."[3]

Although it may be appropriate for the PTA to work in a different location than the PT (after the plan of care is established by the PT), the PT and PTA should have established a good working relationship and discussed proper

---

TABLE 2-1 Requirements for Supervision of the Physical Therapist Assistant When Off Site[3]

"When supervising the physical therapist assistant in any off-site setting, the following requirements must be observed:

- A physical therapist must be accessible by telecommunications to the physical therapist assistant at all times while the physical therapist assistant is treating patients/clients.

  There must be regularly scheduled and documented conferences with the physical therapist assistant regarding patients/clients, the frequency of which is determined by the needs of the patient/client and the needs of the physical therapist assistant.

  In those situations in which a physical therapist assistant is involved in the care of a patient/client, a supervisory visit by the physical therapist will be made:

- Upon the physical therapist assistant's request for a reexamination, when a change in the plan of care is needed, prior to any planned discharge, and in response to a change in the patient's/client's medical status.

  At least once a month, or at a higher frequency when established by the physical therapist, in accordance with the needs of the patient/client.

A supervisory visit should include:

- An on-site reexamination of the patient/client.
- On-site review of the plan of care with appropriate revision or termination.
- Evaluation of need and recommendation for utilization of outside resources."

---

options for communication (such as oral, written, or electronic) prior to the PTA working off site. When determining the appropriate extent of independence for the PTA, the PT and PTA should consider the education, training, experience, and skill level of the PTA. In addition, the independence of the PTA may vary depending on the criticality, acuity, stability, and complexity of the patients. The condition of a patient with an acute injury may change significantly and quickly, requiring more frequent re-examination by the PT than a patient with a chronic condition that may be more stable over time. The APTA policy on the requirements for supervision when the PTA is not in the same setting as the PT is provided in Table 2-1.

FIVE ELEMENTS OF PATIENT/CLIENT MANAGEMENT

Before a detailed account and in-depth discussion on therapeutic exercise can be undertaken, terms that are commonly used in the practice arena must be defined so that

PTs and PTAs from diverse backgrounds can understand not only this text but each other. Think about the last new patient who was seen in your clinic. What did the *interpretation* of the test results indicate? Did the *evaluation* performed by the PT indicate an individual with an anterior cruciate ligament-deficient knee or was the *assessment* that the patient had a meniscus injury? Or did the PT think that, based on the *examination*, the patient had damage to the medial collateral ligament? Regardless of what the clinical decision-making skills of the PT tell you about the patient's knee, do you realize that, based on the italicized words, we may not even be talking the same language. How do we understand each other when we do not use a language that is consistent among PTs and PTAs in the same treatment venue, much less among clinicians in different states or across different professions?

The APTA defined key terms used in the field of patient rehabilitation and presented them as the "five elements of patient/client management."[4] The APTA's definitions serve as the operational definitions used throughout this text. Examination, evaluation, and establishment of a diagnosis and a prognosis performed by the PT are all part of the process that guides the PT in determining the most appropriate intervention that should be performed by the PT or delegated by the PT to the PTA.

Examination. Required before any intervention (treatment); must be performed by the PT on all patients and clients; consists of three components.

History. Account of past and current health status; specific mechanism of injury, if available.

Systems review. Brief or limited examination that provides additional information about the general health of the patient/client; includes a review of the four systems: cardiopulmonary, integumentary, musculoskeletal, and neuromuscular.

Tests and measures. Special tests or tools that determine the cause of the problem (e.g., for a patient with knee dysfunction, may include a Lachman test, valgus and varus tests, and anterior and posterior drawer tests to the knee).

Evaluation. Thought process of the PT that accompanies each and every examination procedure; information gained from the outcome of a particular test (e.g., the actual performance of a valgus test to the knee is an examination procedure; because the patient's knee does not have a tight end feel and the knee gives, the PT determines that the patient has a positive test—the evaluation).

Diagnosis. Encompasses a cluster of signs, symptoms, syndromes, and categories; the decision reached by the PT as a result of the evaluation of information obtained during the examination (e.g., after the examination and evaluation of the knee, the PT determines that the cluster of

signs—positive valgus test, negative Lachman test, negative anterior drawer and posterior drawer test, negative varus test—indicates a diagnosis of medial collateral ligament damage to the knee).

Prognosis. The predicted optimal level of improvement in function and amount of time needed to reach that level; at this point the physical therapist establishes a plan of care, including goals (e.g., a patient with second-degree medial collateral ligament damage to the knee is expected to return to full, unrestricted activity within 3 to 6 weeks).

Intervention. The treatment or rehabilitation program, which may be performed by the PT or PTA at the clinic or independently; includes strength work, increasing range of motion, manual therapy, aerobic conditioning, appropriate sequence of exercise.

Interventions Delegated to the Physical Therapist Assistant

The interventions performed by the PTA are those delegated to the PTA by the PT. The role of the PTA is not to develop a treatment program independently of the PT. The *Evaluative Criteria for Accreditation of Education Programs for the Preparation of Physical Therapist Assistants* provides the minimal standard that all education programs must meet to be accredited by the CAPTE, which is the only accrediting body for PTAs.[5] Table 2-2 presents all the interventions that PTA educational programs must teach to become accredited. As indicated in Table 2-2, therapeutic exercise is a required intervention for a PTA program to achieve accreditation through CAPTE.

In 2000 the House of Delegates of the APTA further defined the interventions that are appropriate for a PTA to perform. This group determined that spinal and peripheral joint mobilization/manipulation (components of manual therapy) and sharp selective debridement (a component of wound management) require immediate and continuous examination and evaluation throughout the intervention. Due to this need for continuous examination during the performance of interventions, the House of Delegates determined that it was inappropriate for a PTA to perform these interventions.[6] CAPTE concurred, and these topics are not included in the *Evaluation Criteria* for the PTA.[5] Therefore, these topics of mobilization/manipulation and sharp debridement are not presented in this textbook.

In addition to performing the delegated interventions as determined by the PT, the PTA must recognize when a change in the patient's status (physical or psychologic) occurs and should report this change to the supervising PT. (Refer to next section on data collection skills.) This change may be a significant improvement in a patient, requiring a more aggressive plan of care to be developed by the PT, or it could be that an intervention should not be provided by

TABLE 2-2 Interventions listed in the *Evaluative Criteria for Accreditation of Education Programs for the Preparation of Physical Therapy Assistant*[5]

Plan of Care

3.3.2.6 Communicates an understanding of the plan of care developed by the physical therapist to achieve short and long term goals and intended outcomes.

3.3.2.7 Demonstrates competence in implementing selected components of interventions identified in the plan of care established by the physical therapist.

Functional Training
Activities of daily living
Assistive/adaptive devices
Body mechanics
Developmental activities
Gait and locomotion training
Prosthetics and orthotics
Wheelchair management skills

Infection Control Procedures
Isolation techniques
Sterile technique

Manual Therapy Techniques
Passive range of motion
Therapeutic massage

Physical Agents and Mechanical Agents
Thermal agents
Biofeedback
Compression therapies
Cryotherapy
Electrotherapeutic agents
Hydrotherapy
Superficial and deep thermal agents
Traction

Therapeutic Exercise
Aerobic conditioning
Balance and coordination training
Breathing exercises and coughing techniques
Conditioning and reconditioning
Posture awareness training
Range of motion exercises
Stretching exercises
Strengthening exercises

Wound Management
Application and removal of dressing or agents
Identification of precautions for dressing removal

the PTA due to a regression in the status of the patient. In both scenarios, the PTA should notify the PT of the change in status. In addition, the PTA must recognize when the directions from the PT as to a delegated intervention are beyond what is appropriate for a PTA to perform and the PTA should initiate clarification from the PT. As indicated earlier in this chapter, the PT is ultimately responsible for the plan of care for the patient and remains responsible for the physical therapy services provided by the PTA. The PTA cannot independently modify the plan of care developed by the PT.

Data Collection Skills

As indicated previously, when the PTA recognizes a significant change in the status of the patient, this change must be reported to the PT. The PT may then make a change to the patient's plan of care. To recognize these potential changes, the PTA must monitor the responses of the patient to the interventions being performed. This patient monitoring by the PTA is referred to as data collection skills, and these are essential skills for the PTA to possess to carry out the plan of care delegated by the PT. The PTA uses information from this data collection to progress the intervention within the plan of care established by the PT and to report changes to the supervising PT as needed.

A list of suggested data collection skills that the PTA should be able to perform upon graduation from an accredited program are listed in Table 2-3.[7] Using these data collection skills allows the PTA to:

- Assist the supervising PT in components of the patient examination process by performing selected data-collection tests and measures, as delegated by the supervising PT, within legal guidelines and educational preparation.

- Differentiate normal and abnormal responses to interventions.

- Inform the PT of the patient's response to intervention, results of data collected, progress toward patient's goals, and/or need to modify interventions.

- Document change in patient status in progress notes.

- Provide a consistent, organized application of specific delegated tests and measures through ongoing data collection.

THE DISABLEMENT MODEL

Before specifically addressing the role of the PTA in providing therapeutic exercise, a few more terms need to be introduced. Understanding these terms will enable the PTA to better communicate with the PT.

TABLE 2-3 Data Collection Skills Listed in *Evaluative Criteria for Accreditation of Education Programs for the Preparation of Physical Therapy Assistant*[5]

3.3.2.8. Demonstrates competency in performing components of data collection skills essential for carrying out the plan of care.

These data collection skills are performed within the context of the interventions implemented by the physical therapist assistant under the direction and supervision of the physical therapist. These data collection skills are performed for the purpose of monitoring the response of a patient or client to the interventions delegated to the physical therapist assistant by the physical therapist.

Aerobic Capacity and Endurance
Measures standard vital signs.
Recognizes and monitors responses to positional changes and activities.
Observes and monitors thoracoabdominal movements and breathing patterns with activity.

Anthropometric Characteristics
Measures height, weight, length, and girth.

Arousal, Mentation, and Cognition
Recognizes changes in direction and magnitude of patient's state of arousal, mentation, and cognition.

Assistive, Adaptive, Orthotic, Protective, Supportive, and Prosthetic Devices
Identifies the individual's and caregiver's abilities to care for the device.
Recognizes changes in skin condition while using devices and equipment.
Recognizes safety factors while using the device.

Gait, Locomotion, and Balance
Describes the safety, status, and progression of patients while engaged in gait, locomotion, balance, wheelchair management, and mobility.

Integumentary Integrity
Recognizes absent or altered sensation.
Recognizes normal and abnormal integumentary changes.
Recognizes activities, positioning, and postures that can aggravate or relieve pain or altered sensations, or that can produce associated skin traumas.
Recognizes viable versus nonviable tissue.

Joint Integrity and Mobility
Recognizes normal and abnormal joint mobility.

Muscle Performance
Measures muscle strength by manual muscle testing.
Observes the presence or absence of muscle mass.
Recognizes normal and abnormal muscle length.
Recognizes changes in muscle tone.

Neuromotor Development
Recognizes gross motor milestones.
Recognizes fine motor milestones.
Recognizes righting and equilibrium reactions.

Pain
Administers standardized questionnaires, graphs, behavioral scales, or visual analog scales for pain.
Recognizes activities, positioning, and postures that aggravate or relieve pain or altered sensations.

Posture
Describes resting posture in any position.
Recognizes alignment of trunk and extremities at rest and during activities.

Range of Motion
Measures functional range of motion.
Measures range of motion using a goniometer.

Self-care and Home Management and Community or Work Reintegration
Inspects the physical environment and measures physical space.
Recognizes safety and barriers in home, community, and work environments.
Recognizes level of functional status.
Administers standardized questionnaires to patients and others.

Ventilation, Respiration, and Circulation Examination
Recognizes cyanosis.
Recognizes activities that aggravate or relieve edema, pain, dyspnea, or other symptoms.
Describes chest wall expansion and excursion.
Describes cough and sputum characteristics.

Disablement refers to "the various impact(s) of chronic and acute conditions on the functioning of specific body systems, on basic human performance, and on people's functioning in necessary, usual, expected, and personally desired roles in society."[8] Several conceptual schemes or models for disablement exist, including those developed by Nagi,[9] the World Health Organization,[10] and the National Center for Medical Rehabilitation Research.[11] For a detailed comparison of these models, see Jette.[8] This textbook uses the Nagi model and definition.

In the Nagi classification model of the disablement process, clinicians provide services to patients and clients with impairment, functional limitation, and disability. *Impairment* is an abnormality or loss of an anatomic, physiologic, or psychologic origin.[12] Examples of impairments are decreased range of motion, strength, and endurance; hypomobility of the joint; and pain.

Functional limitation is defined as a limitation in the ability of the individual to perform an activity in an efficient or competent manner.[4] Inability to take an object from an overhead shelf, to walk without a limp, and to sit without pain are examples of functional limitations.

Disabilities are restrictions to function within normal limits[12] and represent any inability to perform socially defined roles expected of an individual in a sociocultural and physical environment.[9] Examples of disabilities include inability to perform the normal duties associated with work, school, recreation, and personal care.

Two examples illustrate these definitions. First, consider a lawyer who has back pain (impairment). Because of the back pain, the lawyer is unable to sit in a chair for more than 10 minutes and cannot walk for more than 5 minutes (functional limitation). As a result of the pain and inability to sit or walk, the lawyer is not able to go to work (disability). One goal for intervention is to use therapeutic exercise—such as instruction in posture, body mechanics, and spinal stabilization (Chapter 14)—to treat the impairment of pain, alleviating the functional limitation and disability.

Second, consider a college athlete who has undergone anterior cruciate ligament surgery. After surgery, the athlete has decreased range of motion and decreased strength in the quadriceps and hamstring muscles (impairments). Because of these impairments, the athlete cannot run, cut, or jump (functional limitations). Therefore, the individual will not be able to participate in the sport (disability). One goal for intervention is to use therapeutic exercise—such as passive range of motion (Chapter 3), open- and closed-chain exercises (Chapters 6 and 8), aquatic therapy (Chapter 16), and functional progression (Chapter 15)—to treat the impairments of motion and strength, alleviating the functional limitations and disability.

The presence of an impairment does not mean that a functional limitation must occur. Similarly, a disability does not automatically follow from a functional limitation. For example, an individual might present with an anterior cruciate-deficient knee, with hypermobility as the impairment. But the goals of this patient are to play racquetball, hike, and bike. The patient decides to avoid surgery and participate in a therapeutic exercise program. After the intervention, the patient finds that playing racquetball is possible if a brace is worn and that he/she is able to hike and bike without the brace. Therefore, this individual has an impairment (hypermobility); however, through intervention, the patient is able to avoid any functional limitation (running and cutting) or disability (participation in recreational sports).

After considering the examination, evaluation, and diagnosis, the PT works with the PTA to provide interventions for a patient with any level of disablement: to provide services to an individual with a disability, to provide treatment for a client with a functional limitation, or to alleviate an impairment in a patient. Based on a consideration of the interrelationships among impairment, functional limitation, and disability, this textbook focuses on the alleviation of impairments through the creative and effective use of therapeutic exercise.

COMMUNICATION BETWEEN PTA AND PATIENT

Of great importance to the PTA in the effective delivery of therapeutic exercise to the patient is appropriate communication. Effective communication must incorporate respect for all patients irrespective of differences in age, language, or cultures and is vital for a successful outcome. When the clinician and patient understand each other, adherence to the program is enhanced and outcomes are positive. When communication is poor, the patient may be doing an exercise incorrectly, performing the wrong number of repetitions, or not following the appropriate precautions related to his/her condition; in essence, the outcome will be negatively affected. The PTA needs to be aware that communication with the patient can be influenced by difference in personality, values, teaching and learning styles, and culture.

Initially, a more passive listening role by the PTA allows the patient to provide information about their condition, expectations, and goals. Good listening skills include paying attention to what the patient is saying and asking follow up questions for clarification to ensure that the clinician has a full understanding of the patient and his/her needs. Eye contact, along with affirmation and reflection of what the patient has said, can serve to clarify what the clinician hears.[13]

The plan of care and the goals of treatment set by the PT should be shared with the patient. This sharing provides an opportunity for the PTA to discuss the recovery prognosis and the expectations that the PTA has for the patient. In addition, discussing the plan of care and goals will demonstrate to the patient that the PT and PTA have been in communication and will provide the patient with evidence that good quality of care is being provided.

On subsequent visits the PTA should frequently review short- and long-term goals, provide positive feedback to the patient when short-term goals are achieved and motivate and encourage the patient when the patient is not adhering to the physical therapy program. Continued clarification of how progress is defined and reasonable expectations regarding progress can improve patient compliance and satisfaction.

Cultural Considerations

A major criterion for good communication between the PTA and the patient is to respect patients who speak a different language or come from a culture unlike that of the PTA. No longer must one live in a major metropolitan area to be exposed to a wide variety of cultures. If the patient does not speak the same language, even the simplest of activities can become difficult. Use of an interpreter that understands medical terminology should be requested, if possible. Questions about the patient's attitudes and beliefs should be worked naturally and carefully into the initial interaction with the patient. Realize that cultures may differ on things like appropriate eye contact, physical contact, and appropriate types of greeting.[13] Religious observance or customs may prevent a patient from wearing clothing that allows the appropriate body part to be visualized or palpated during the treatment session. In these instances, explain what needs to be done (and why) and ask for permission to perform the techniques in advance. It is important that these cultural differences be addressed early in the treatment plan to the best of the ability of both the PT and PTA so that problems and a lack of trust do not occur later.[13]

Communication with the Elderly

Good communication skills are also important when treating the elderly. Older patients who feel heard and understood are more likely to follow the orders provided, adhere to the treatment, and have positive outcomes. Specifically related to the elderly, the PTA should avoid stereotypes about aging and that problems are an inevitable part of aging. Getting old does not cause illness, and being old does not mean the individual must live with pain and discomfort.[14]

The PTA should establish respect for the patient right away by using formal language. The patient's correct title (Dr., Reverend, Mr., Mrs., Ms., Miss, etc.) and surname should be used unless the patient requests a more casual form of address. The PTA's introduction should be clear, and hurrying the older patient should be avoided. Feeling rushed leads older people to believe they are not being respected and understood.[14]

Keep the treatment plan as simple and straightforward as possible. Avoid providing too much information too quickly. Speaking more slowly will give time for the older patients to process what is being said. Tell the patient what to expect from the treatment and explain how it will improve the patient's overall health. If a home exercise program is in order, provide oral and written instruction and make sure the patient has a full understanding of what is expected of him/her.[13]

Cultural Considerations Specific to the Treatment of the Elderly

It is very important for the PTA caring for older adults to develop an understanding of different ethnic groups to effectively communicate and treat patients. The PTA should keep in mind that older patients are diverse and unique, just like younger patients.[15] Older immigrants or nonnative English speakers may need an interpreter. It is in the best interest of the PTA to have a developed plan as to how to treat the non-English-speaking population. The PTA may need to check with the PT for assistance.

The terms referring to specific cultural groups can change over time, and older individuals may use different terms than younger individuals in the same culture. It is important for the PTA to learn what a patient's preferred terms are related to culture.[15] As indicated earlier, each culture has its own rules about body language and hand gestures. Pointing with one finger and making eye contact may be considered rude. If the PTA is not sure about a patient's preference, the PTA should ask.[13]

Communication with Children

When working with children, the PTA has to be aware that the patient, frequently one or both parents, and any siblings that the patient may have will be present during the therapy session. The PTA should talk at a level both the child and parent can understand. The PTA should tell the pediatric patient about the treatment plan so that the patient feels a part of the plan and not just that something is being done to him/her. To be successful, the PTA should read the child's chart thoroughly to know the age, cognitive level, and functional level of the child prior to talking to the child and caregiver. While all children develop at their own pace, general behaviors can be expected at certain ages, or they at least follow a general sequence. Contributing to the child's unique development are family, environmental, and cultural influences which impact how the child develops in social, cognitive, and motor domains. Any additional medical factors also play a part in how the child develops in the various domains. Just as there is a projected sequence of motor development, there is a projected sequence of cognitive and social development of the individual from child through toddlerhood, preschool, school age and into adolescence. Being aware of those sequences helps with interaction as the PTA treats the patient.

Be sure to check with the evaluating PT to see if there are any specific concerns that may not be reflected in the chart. The PT should have documented any home program and instructions that were sent home with the child. For the younger child or the more involved child who is dependent on the parent to do the home program, let the parent demonstrate the home program. Provide feedback to the parent. If the parent has done the exercise/activity incorrectly, suggest that the parent try it a different way, demonstrate the correct way, and then ask the parent to try again. If the patient is older and is capable of doing the home program independently but may need the supervision of the parent, ask the child to demonstrate how the exercise is being performed with the parent observing. If corrections are needed, be sure and give the patient reinforcement for having done the program, but tell the patient to try something a little differently, then demonstrate, and ask the patient to demonstrate his/her understanding.

Following are general sequences and approximate ages that children develop in the cognitive/social domains. Being aware of the development and being able to adjust conversation and interaction with the pediatric patient accordingly will augment the clinical skills of the PTA and lead to a more successful clinical outcome. Although various ways of looking at age exist, for the sake of this chapter, the groups are infant (birth to 1 year), toddler (13 months to 35 months), preschool (3–5 years) school aged (6–12 years), and adolescents (13–18 years).[16]

Infant (Birth to 1 Year)

Initially PTAs should introduce themselves to the parents and inform them that the program set up at the initial physical therapy evaluation is going to be followed. Ask if there are any questions and if the parents had any difficulty with the home program provided at the initial evaluation. During the course of the conversation with the parents, intermittently engage the child. During the first 8 weeks the infant fixates on faces and will respond to a smiling face. Once the PTA has addressed the parents' concerns, the PTA may focus on the child. Although words may be directed to the parents of the child as an explanation for what is being done, the PTA's voice and expressions are directed to the child. The PTA does not need to use "baby talk" but should talk in an expressive manner to engage the child. Once the child is engaged, the PTA can talk to the parents in a more appropriate manner while maintaining eye contact with the child. Toys used during therapy sessions should be appropriate for the level of the child. The family may have favorite toys that can be used during the therapy session if other available toys do not interest the child. Ideally the toys at home should be different than those used during therapy to allow some novelty. The PTA should ask the parent to entertain the child with toys as the PTA facilitates the movement. At 20 weeks an infant enjoys seeing his/her reflection in a mirror. Working in front of a mirror allows the infant to see him/herself and the PTA as the child is being treated. Using a mirror also models what a parent can do when another person is not available to entertain the infant when the parent is working with the infant.

When the infant is facing the PTA, as might occur on a ball or roll working on righting reactions, vocal play is a way to engage the infant. Sounds like "ba, da, ga" emerge around 28 weeks. In addition, infants during the 28- to 40-week stage enjoy imitation; therefore, imitating sounds and actions like hitting the mat or ball are reinforcing. At around 40 weeks the child enjoys nursery rhymes and finger play games like pat-a-cake. As the child approaches 1 year, he/she begins to understand single words like "mommy" and "daddy" and may understand the names of people or pets to which he/she is exposed regularly.

Stranger anxiety generally emerges around 24 weeks or 6 months. If the PTA has worked with the patient throughout this time, no problems may be experienced. However, as the tasks become more challenging, the infant may turn more and more to the parents to be "rescued" from therapy. Asking the parents to leave the treatment area and watch out of the infant's line of sight or through an observation window may be necessary to maximize the outcome of the treatment session. Generally, once the parents are not in view, the infant will cooperate with the therapy session or allow the PTA to comfort and redirect the infant's anxiety. After a few sessions with the parents outside of the treatment area, ask the parents to come in toward the end of the session to see if the infant will allow the session to continue or if the child becomes too distracted by the parents' presence. If the latter is the case, it may be necessary to continue with the parents outside of the treatment area for a while. Periodically re-introduce having the parents present. Parents should feel like they are a part of the child's therapy.

Toddler (1–3 Years)

The early toddler will point to objects that are wanted and may utter a single syllable that is perceived as the name of what is desired. The child begins to imitate the actions of parents, such as sweeping the floor or wiping the table. If the child of toddler age is not able to do so physically, the child will attempt activities that are easier to perform. By the age of 2 years, the child is "talking" incessantly and will use vocal variety. Incorporating "pretend" into the therapy session will enhance the likelihood of the toddler to cooperate. The toddler can identify body parts so incorporating an action song like "head, shoulders, knees, and toes" can be fun in therapy—even if the toddler is not standing or walking at this point. Just recognizing the toddler's ability to identify head and toes helps bring the child into the therapy session. The toddler also begins to identify colors; therefore, the color of a toy that is being used in the therapy session should be included. It is helpful to use solid-color toys so as not to confuse the toddler with multiple colors on a single object.[17,18]

Preschool (3–5 Years)

During the preschool years, the child's imagination continues to develop. The preschooler tends to tell elaborate stories and may have an imaginary friend. "Pretend" play is very successful in enticing a child of this age. Plan therapy sessions in advance and decide what skills/activities need to be worked on during the therapy session. Arrange the treatment area in a way that the preschooler's favorite story, television, or movie character of the time can be incorporated into the treatment session. For instance, climbing stairs may be climbing up into a spaceship or treehouse to help Spiderman.

School Aged (6–12 Years)

Continue to talk to the patient and learn what the interests of the child are and adjust activities to the level of the child. Make believe may not be as motivational as it was for the preschool child. Games designed for this age may be played while working on balance. Standing on a rocker board while playing Connect Four can challenge balance and also work on eye hand and cognitive skills. For more dynamic balance, a patient can stand on the rocker board and shoot a basketball or stand on one leg while playing floor hockey; these activities can be quite challenging for patient and therapist alike!

Adolescent (13–18 Years)

Skills and activities described for school-aged children can also be used with the adolescent patient. It is important to incorporate the interests of the patient into the treatment session as much as possible. As the adolescent ages, it is more important for the child to be an active participant in establishing goals and recognizing his/her role in performing the home exercise program. Although the parents of the adolescent need to be kept in the loop about what is needed to be done, the adolescent needs to take ownership as much as possible. For the adolescent who is physically dependent on the parent to do the home exercise program, the PTA (and PT) need to make sure that the child is fully aware of the importance of the program and not give his/her parents a hard time when it is time to do the program.

As stated earlier, every child develops at a different speed. Some will develop faster than chronologic age and some slower. It is important to recognize where the child is and structure therapy sessions accordingly. It is also important to understand cultural and family differences that may impact that child's development. Also be aware that children who are nonverbal or have dysarthria are cognitively close to their appropriate chronologic age and should be spoken to as any child that age level. Just because the child cannot speak or is difficult to understand does not mean that the child cannot understand what is said. An individual speaking slower or louder will not make it any easier to understand what the *child* is saying—it will only make the child feel like he/she is being spoken down to.

Cultural Considerations Specific to the Treatment of Children

If the family speaks a language in which the PTA is not proficient, an interpreter who understands medical terminology should be requested. Using a family member should be avoided if possible, especially if that family member is a sibling and an explanation during therapy needs to be given to the parents. In some cultures, the father is considered the primary caregiver and should be addressed only by an adult. Children can take advantage of knowing the language or may not understand terminology and not give a good representation of what is being said. Even if the mother is the primary caregiver, the father should also be told what is needed if he is present.

Family-focused Care

It is very easy to expect families to do everything requested to maximize the time away from therapy and hopefully improve the child's outcome. But one must be very sensitive to what is going on with the family and try to focus on the priorities for the child.

As with any patient, finding time to do a home program is difficult. Ask the patient and family if there is any difficulty with getting the home program completed as recommended by the PT. If difficulty occurs, ask the patient and family what the typical day is like and help them find a way to incorporate the program. Talk with the PT to see if there are exercises that require more emphasis and perhaps decrease the number of exercises or activities, the repetitions, or time spent. Another alternative is to do some exercises on one day and the remainder on another day. Sometimes a chart that can be checked off or using a sticker that can be placed to indicate completion is reinforcing to a child, especially when the child brings it back to show completion.[19]

SUMMARY

- The PTA functions as an important member of the health care team assisting the PT in the provision of physical therapy.

- The PTA is actively involved in providing interventions to the patient after a thorough evaluation of the patient's status by the PT and under the direction and supervision of the PT. These selected interventions performed by the PTA include the provision of therapeutic exercise.

- The goal of the PTA using therapeutic exercise is to treat the patient's impairment and thereby alleviate functional limitation and disability.

- Appropriate communication between the PTA and the patient is vital for a successful outcome. When the PTA and patient understand each other, adherence to the exercise program is enhanced and the outcomes for the patient are positive.

- In today's multicultural society, the PTA must keep in mind that patients, old and young, are diverse and unique. For proper communication, the PTA must remain alert to the differences among individual patients from given cultures and be on guard against stereotyping a person based on ethnic or cultural affiliation.

References

1. American Physical Therapy Association. Physical therapy as a health profession. [HOD 06-99-19-23] House of Delegates Positions, Standards, Guidelines, Policies, and Procedures. October 2005.

2. American Physical Therapy Association. Provision of physical therapy interventions and related tasks. [HOD 06-00-17-28] House of Delegates Positions, Standards, Guidelines, Policies, and Procedures. October 2005.

3. American Physical Therapy Association. Direction and supervision of the physical therapist assistant. [HOD 06-05-18-26] House of Delegates Positions, Standards, Guidelines, Policies, and Procedures. October 2005.

4. American Physical Therapy Association. *Guide to physical therapist practice.* 2nd ed. Alexandria, VA; 2003.

5. American Physical Therapy Association. Commission on Accreditation in Physical Therapy Education. Evaluative criteria for accreditation of education programs for the preparation of physical therapist assistants. Adopted April 26, 2006.

6. American Physical Therapy Association. Procedural interventions exclusively performed by physical therapists. [HOD 06-00-30-36] House of Delegates Positions, Standards, Guidelines, Policies, and Procedures. October 2005.

7. American Physical Therapy Association. *A normative model of physical therapist assistant education.* Version 99. Alexandria, VA; 1999.

8. Jette AM. Physical disablement: concepts for physical therapy research and practice. *Phys Ther.* 1994;74:380–387.

9. Nagi SA. Disability concepts revisited. In: Pope A, Tarlov A, eds. *Disability in America: toward a national agenda for prevention.* Washington, DC: National Academy Press; 1991.

10. World Health Organization. International classification of impairments, disabilities, and handicaps. Geneva: WHO; 1980.

11. National Advisory Board on Medical Rehabilitation Research. Draft V: report and plan for medical rehabilitation research. Bethesda, MD: National Institutes of Health; 1992.

12. Schenkman M, Donavan J, Tsubota J, et al. Management of individuals with Parkinson's disease: rationale and case studies. *Phys Ther.* 1989;69:944–955.

13. Thein Brody L. Principles of self-management and exercise instruction. In: Hall CM, Brody LT. *Therapeutic exercise: moving toward function.* 2nd ed. Philadelphia: Lippincott Williams & Wilkins; 2005:33–41.

14. National Institute on Aging. Working with your older patient: a clinician's handbook. Bethesda, MD: National Institute on Aging; 2004.

15. American Geriatrics Society. *Doorway thoughts: cross-cultural health care for older adults.* Sudbury, MA: Jones and Bartlett Publishers; 2004:3–7.

16. Illingworth R. *The development of the infant and young child: normal and abnormal.* 9th ed. Edinburgh: Churchill Livingstone; 1987.

17. Long T, Toscano K. *Pediatric physical therapy.* 2nd ed. Baltimore: Lippincott Williams & Wilkins; 2002.

18. Mullen EM. *Mullen scales of early learning.* Circle Pines, MN: American Guidance Service, Inc; 1995.

19. Sparling JW, Kolobe TH, Ezzelle L. Family centered intervention. In: Campbell S. *Physical therapy for children.* Philadelphia: WB Saunders; 1995.

Mobility

Range of Motion

James P. Fletcher, MS, PT, ATC

OBJECTIVES

Upon completion of this chapter, the reader will be able to:

■ Identify the functional purpose and benefits of range of motion (ROM) in the positioning and mobility of the body.

■ Identify extrinsic and intrinsic factors affecting the available ROM at a synovial joint.

■ Identify specific categorizations of ROM exercise as found in the *Guide to Physical Therapist Practice.*

■ Identify key factors affecting the application and performance of passive, active-assistive, and active ROM techniques.

■ Apply appropriate techniques for passive, active-assistive, and active osteokinematic movements of the extremities and spine performed in anatomic body planes within the established plan of care.

The concept of ROM specific to the human body brings many thoughts and ideas to the mind of the healthcare professional. Along with strength, endurance, power, balance, and coordination, ROM plays a major role in physical ability and therefore contributes significantly to the overall quality of a person's physical functions.[1] This is obvious when one considers the negative effect a ROM impairment can have on the quality and efficiency of human movement.

One broadly accepted notion is that ROM occurs through the interdependent functions of the musculoskeletal and synovial joint systems, enabling the human body to perform free and easy movements. The basic functional purpose and use of ROM is the effective movement of the extremities, head, and trunk in performing body positioning and mobility.[2] This chapter discusses ROM primarily in the context of osteokinematic movement resulting from synovial joint movement. Issues of muscle length are presented in Chapter 4.

SCIENTIFIC BASIS

Definitions

Much like human anatomy, ROM and its associated terminology are descriptive in nature. A brief introduction of several anatomic and kinesiologic terms is essential. The reader must have a working knowledge of the terminology associated with body planes (e.g., sagittal, frontal, horizontal), anatomic position (e.g., medial, lateral, proximal), and osteokinematic and arthrokinematic movement.[2-5]

The basic definition of ROM differs among published sources.[6-10] One of the clearest descriptions is that ROM is the extent of osteokinematic motion available for movement activities, functional or otherwise, with or without assistance.[6] Osteokinematic motion is the movement of a whole bone resulting from rolling, sliding, or spinning movements (arthrokinematics) among the articulating bony surfaces making up a synovial joint.[3] The assistance in moving a body segment provided by the clinician, as well as effort generated by the patient, requires the division of ROM into three levels of performance: active range of motion (AROM), active-assistive range of motion (AAROM), and passive range of motion (PROM).[6-9]

AROM. Joint movements performed and controlled solely by the voluntary muscular efforts of the individual without the aid or resistance of an external force; the individual is independent in this activity.

AAROM. Joint movement performed and controlled, in large or small part, by the voluntary muscular efforts of the individual combined with the assistance of an external force (e.g., assistance from another body part, another person, or a mechanical device).

PROM. Joint movement performed and controlled solely by the efforts of an external force without the use of voluntary muscular contraction by the person.

Although gravity does act on the mass of the body segment, offering some assistance or resistance to the movement being performed, it is a variable that is controlled by the position of the body segment during the movement. External forces used in the assistance of a movement (AAROM or PROM) are considered nongravitational.

Physical and Physiologic Considerations

The amount of ROM available at a synovial joint depends on many factors, both intrinsic and extrinsic. Intrinsic factors are related to the anatomic composition of the joint, such as shape and congruency of the articulating bony surfaces and pliability of the joint capsule, ligaments, and other collagenous tissues. In addition, the strength and flexibility of musculature acting on or crossing the joint are considered intrinsic factors.[2,3] One or more of these factors create anatomic limits to joint ROM. For example, most osteokinematic motions at the glenohumeral and hip joints are limited by soft-tissue extensibility rather than a bony restriction, except in cases of pathology (e.g., osteoarthritis). Conversely, the limitations to osteokinematic motion at the humeroulnar joint owe more to bony contact. This is not to say that joints with anatomic movement limitations related to bone shape, congruency, and approximation have less ROM than other synovial joints. Zachazewski[10] points out that although the amount of joint ROM is determined primarily by the shape and congruency of the articulating surfaces, the periarticular connective tissues are the limiting factors at the end of the ROM. More detailed discussions of the intrinsic factors affecting joint ROM are available in the literature.[2,3,11]

Other factors affecting joint ROM are extrinsic, which may have a direct effect on the intrinsic factors. One significant factor is age. Decreased pliability in contractile and noncontractile tissues caused by changes in tissue composition and tissue degeneration that occur with aging can decrease joint ROM.[1,3] Body segment size related to muscle or adipose tissue bulk is another extrinsic factor that may affect joint ROM; it often limits osteokinematic motions such as knee flexion and elbow flexion.[12]

Finally, the known effects of disease, injury, overuse, and immobilization on joint tissues and joint ROM must be considered. The well-being of joint tissues depends on a certain amount of use of the joint and stress to the joint structures. For example, hyaline cartilage nutrition depends on the compression and decompression that occurs with joint movement. In addition, maintenance of ligament and capsule strength and pliability depends on a certain amount of tissue stress and strain associated with joint movement.

Common diseases affecting the joints include rheumatoid arthritis and osteoarthritis, which adversely affect the synovial membrane and hyaline cartilage, respectively. These diseases (along with traumatic injuries to ligament, capsule, or hyaline cartilage) result in pain, swelling, and loss of joint motion. Often disease and traumatic injuries alter the biomechanics of the joint, leading to malalignment, abnormal motion, and joint tissue degeneration.

Microtrauma to joint tissues from overuse related to prolonged or repetitive work or athletic activities can lead to problems such as ligament and capsule lengthening and cartilage degeneration. The overall effects of microtrauma are similar to changes resulting from disease and joint tissue injury: pain, swelling, and loss of joint motion. The adverse effects of immobilization and joint disuse are commonly recognized and include regional osteoporosis, cartilage dehydration and degeneration, collagenous tissue fibrosis and adhesion, and muscle tissue contracture and atrophy.[3,13–15]

Immobilization

The immobilization of a joint or body segment is still commonplace and necessary to allow the initial stages of healing when dealing with fractures or acutely traumatized tissues, including tissue trauma caused by surgery. Also, a wide variety of conditions such as paralysis, muscle spasticity, various forms of arthritis, and even pain can result in extended periods of immobilization. However, the effects that immobilization and disuse can have on the musculoskeletal and synovial joint tissues, and thus on mobility and joint motion, are profoundly negative. These effects include regional loss of bone density, cartilage degeneration, collagenous tissue fibrosis and adhesion, and muscle tissue atrophy and contracture; each of these effects will be discussed briefly.[3,13–15]

While not always obvious in clinical presentation, diminished bone density and reduced bone strength secondary to immobilization can begin to occur just a few weeks into the immobilization period because of a lack of mechanical loading on the bone, primarily because of a lack of muscle contraction and weightbearing forces.[16,17] If the immobilization continues for several months, regional osteoporosis will occur and full recovery of bone mass, volume, and strength may be delayed or incomplete.[18,19]

Articular cartilage, being largely avascular and dependent on joint loading for nutrition, can undergo irreversible degeneration when subjected to even short periods (i.e., days) of immobilization.[20,21] The gradual softening and breakup of the surface of the cartilage will reduce the thickness and stiffness of the tissue and result in a reduced ability to absorb and dissipate joint forces without injury to the cartilage.[22]

Connective tissues high in collagen, namely ligaments, joint capsule, fascia, and tendons, demonstrate a tightening and stiffening fibrosis during immobilization, which is primarily caused by the formation of excessive collagen fiber crosslinks. These changes result in reduced joint motion as well as reduced mechanical strength of the connective tissue.[3,9]

A reduction in muscle tissue size and contractile force (both strength and endurance) is the most obvious change in muscle secondary to immobilization. Such changes can begin to develop after just a few days of immobilization and disuse.[23] Additionally, the extent of the atrophy depends on the type of muscle fiber affected, with muscles consisting of more slow-twitch fibers exhibiting greater atrophy than those composed of more fast-twitch fibers.[24] The amount of muscle tissue contracture (adaptive shortening) is dependent on the positioning during immobilization. Different effects on both sarcomere length and number can occur depending on whether the muscle is immobilized in a shortened or lengthened position.[25]

Benefits of Range of Motion Exercise

When AROM, AAROM, or PROM is performed repetitively for the general purpose of maintaining current joint movement and preventing decreased pliability of tissue, the action is called a ROM exercise. ROM exercise also offers a potential benefit to the mechanical properties of noncontractile tissue.[11] For example, performing a movement repetitively, actively, or passively through a full ROM moves a joint into and out of the closed packed position (which is the position that a joint is in when the articulating surfaces are maximally approximated and the ligaments and capsule are tight).[4] Movement into and out of this position results in an intermittent compression and decompression of the articular cartilage, which is the natural mechanism used for nutrition and continuous remodeling of the tissue.[15]

The benefits of ROM exercise, beyond maintaining joint mobility and nutrition and preventing tissue adhesion and contracture, depend on the type of movement. To aid blood circulation, inhibit pain via stimulation of joint mechanoreceptors (gate control), and promote ligament and capsule remodeling, PROM exercises may be used.[26,27] In addition, AROM and AAROM exercises may increase blood circulation, prevent clot formation from venous stasis, increase proprioceptive input, maintain contractility, slow the rate of atrophy of contracting muscles, and improve coordination and motor control specific to the motion performed.[27] Furthermore, as low-level exercises that use gravity for resistance, AROM and AAROM may help reduce an individual's emotional or psychologic stress and depression and improve psychologic outlook while serving as a method of exercise in the early phases of rehabilitation for the patient who is deconditioned secondary to illness, injury, or surgery.

Continuous passive motion (CPM) is essentially PROM exercise that is performed continuously to a joint by a mechanical device for hours at a time. After a surgical procedure, CPM is primarily used to decrease the effects of joint immobilization, help with pain management, and promote early recovery of ROM.[26,28–30] Typically, the range, rate, and duration of the motion can be programmed, and specific recommendations are based on the surgeon's preference, the patient's response, and the surgical procedure. A variety of CPM devices are available on the market, and devices for almost all extremity joints exist.

CLINICAL GUIDELINES

A brief discussion of how the *Guide to Physical Therapist Practice*[31] portrays the role of ROM exercise for direct intervention will allow the reader to appreciate the broad range of applications that these exercises can offer the healthcare professional. The *Guide* notes that the direct interventions of therapeutic exercise and manual therapy can improve ROM. Specifically, the *Guide* categorizes AROM and AAROM as therapeutic exercise and PROM as manual therapy, which is broadly defined as a passive intervention in which the clinician uses his or her hands to administer a skilled movement.[31] A review of the direct interventions listed in the *Guide* for practice patterns in the musculoskeletal, neuromuscular, cardiopulmonary, and integumentary domains reveals that some form of ROM exercise is a potential method of treatment in the majority of practice patterns.

The physical therapist (PT) must carefully examine joint pathologies and ROM impairments to determine the source of the problem(s). Direct interventions such as muscular stretching (Chapter 4) may be more effective than ROM exercise for improving the impairment of a joint's ROM caused by capsule, ligament, or musculotendinous tissue restriction. However, ROM exercise is an appropriate adjunct or complement to these interventions. ROM exercise is a recommended component of the treatment program for postsurgical musculoskeletal conditions; pathologic conditions such as musculotendinous spasm, strain, inflammation, and contu-

sion; and joint sprain, inflammation, degeneration, and contracture.[27,32]

Clinical decision making regarding the use of ROM exercises as a method of intervention is based on a knowledge of the needs of the patient and the potential benefits, precautions, and limitations of the intervention. The primary precaution for performing ROM exercises has traditionally been the presence of acute injury. With the discovery of the benefits of early motion for preventing tissue shortening and degeneration and maintaining joint nutrition after trauma or surgery, ROM exercise in the acute phase of rehabilitation is recommended if it is performed with rigid adherence to specific precautions dictated by the nature of the tissue injury or surgical repair. The primary therapeutic limitations of AROM exercise are that it typically will not increase muscular strength or prevent atrophy. PROM exercise has the additional limitation of little to no potential for even slowing muscle atrophy or maintaining strength. Furthermore, PROM exercise is less effective than AROM exercise at increasing circulation because of the lack of voluntary muscle contraction.[26]

Once the PT determines that ROM exercise is an appropriate intervention for a given patient, a decision must be made on the use of AROM, AAROM, or PROM. PROM exercises are typically used when the patient is not able to perform an active joint movement because of pain, weakness, paralysis, or unresponsiveness. In the event that the patient is not supposed to actively move a joint because of injury, inflammation, or surgical repair, PROM exercises might be carefully performed with strict adherence to all motion precautions and avoidance of pain. In most other situations, AAROM or AROM exercise is preferred because of the added benefits and potential for more independent performance by the patient. Tomberlin and Saunders[27] provide a general recommendation for progressing from PROM to AAROM and AROM exercises as part of an intervention program after traumatic injury and add specific precautions for avoiding muscle guarding and pain.

A session of ROM exercises should emphasize full range of movement within the client's tolerance. Each movement sequence has two phases: (a) beginning position to ending position and (b) reversal. The physical therapist assistant (PTA) should perform these movements slowly and rhythmically. The specific number of sessions per day, repetitions within each session, and inclusion or exclusion of a hold time at the end range depend on the goals of the exercise, underlying pathology, and patient's response to treatment. Keep in mind that a patient's independent performance will be best if sessions and repetitions take only a few minutes to perform and use of equipment is kept to a minimum. Finally, establishing a regimen that ensures consistency and quality of independent performance by a patient requires a committed effort to effective communication between the patient and PTA.

TECHNIQUES

ROM exercise techniques are performed in anatomic body planes with classic osteokinematic movements, in diagonal or combined joint patterns, or in functional patterns that simulate those used in a patient's daily activities. The techniques presented in this chapter primarily emphasize passive, active-assistive, and active osteokinematic motions performed in anatomic body planes, both with and without equipment. The purpose of all these techniques is to maintain or increase joint mobility, joint nutrition, and tissue pliability. (Given that the purposes of all the exercises are the same, they will not be repeated for each technique.)

The PTA who provides assistance with PROM and AAROM exercise techniques should remember the key factors affecting the application and performance of the techniques. These factors include supportive handling of body segments, proper positioning of the patient, and use of appropriate levels of force to avoid causing intense pain when performing the exercise.

Extremities and Spine

Figures 3-1 to 3-31 illustrate common techniques for ROM exercises. Figures 3-1 to 3-23 show the techniques commonly used for the extremities. Figures 3-24 to 3-31 show frequently used techniques for the spine.

Equipment

Figures 3-32 and 3-33 illustrate a sampling of ROM exercise techniques that use equipment, including wands, pulleys, and CPM devices.

Figure 3-1   Hip and knee flexion active-assistive or passive range of motion.

POSITIONING: Patient lying supine with one knee flexed and foot flat on stable surface. Physical therapist assistant (PTA) standing next to leg that is flexed.

PROCEDURE: PTA performs unilateral flexion of hip and knee by grasping patient's limb at knee and under heel and pushing knee toward patient's shoulder on same side.

NOTE: Same positioning can be used for active range of motion hip flexion. Patient actively flexes knee and hip on one side and brings knee toward shoulder. Motion can be performed with self-assistance by having patient grasp top of knee and pull hip and knee into flexion by pulling knee toward shoulder on same side.

Figure 3-2   Hip abduction and adduction active-assistive or passive range of motion.

POSITIONING: Patient lying supine on stable surface with both limbs extended and one limb positioned in slight hip abduction. Physical therapist assistant (PTA) standing adjacent to patient's leg.

PROCEDURE: PTA performs unilateral abduction and adduction by grasping patient's leg under knee and ankle and moving extended, neutrally rotated limb into abduction and adduction.

NOTE: Same position can be used for active range of motion hip abduction and adduction. Patient moves hip by sliding extended, neutrally rotated limb back and forth across surface.

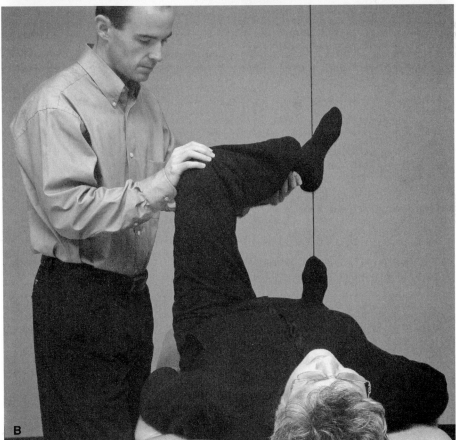

Figure 3-3 Hip rotation active-assistive or passive range of motion.

POSITIONING: Patient lying supine with one knee flexed and foot flat on stable surface. Physical therapist assistant (PTA) standing at side of flexed limb and adjacent to patient's bent leg.

PROCEDURE: PTA performs unilateral medial **(A)** and lateral **(B)** rotation of hip by first grasping patient's limb at knee and heel and positioning patient's limb in 90 degrees of flexion at hip and knee. In this position, PTA stabilizes patient's distal thigh, knee, and leg while rotating hip by performing a swinging motion of leg in a horizontal plane.

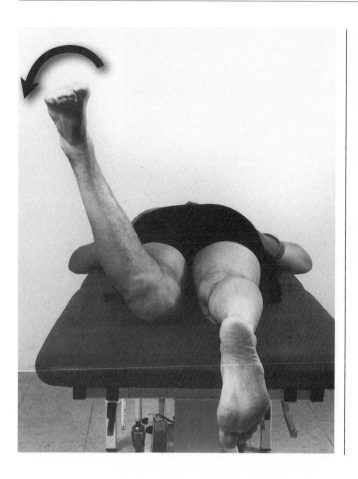

Figure 3-4	Hip rotation active range of motion.

POSITIONING: Patient lying prone on stable surface with one knee flexed to 90 degrees.

PROCEDURE: Patient performs unilateral active medial and lateral rotation of hip by moving leg toward floor, keeping thigh and pelvis flat and knee neutral regarding flexion and extension.

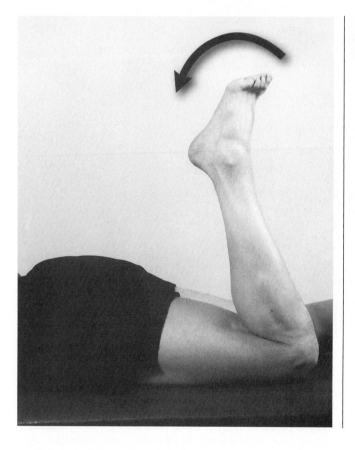

Figure 3-5	Knee flexion and extension active range of motion.

POSITIONING: Patient lying prone on stable surface with both legs extended.

PROCEDURE: Patient performs unilateral active flexion and extension of knee by moving leg toward and away from hip in sagittal plane, keeping thigh and pelvis flat.

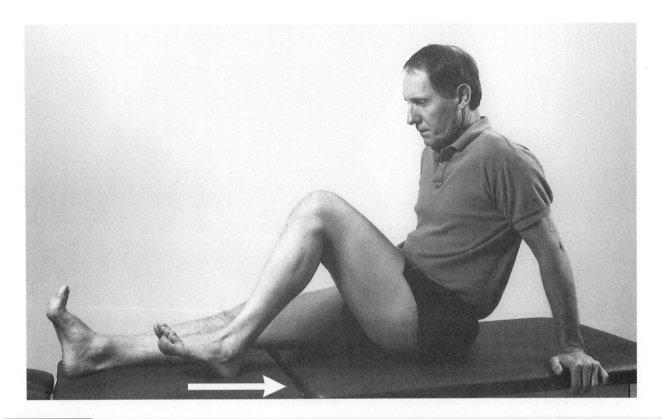

Figure 3-6 Knee and hip flexion and extension active range of motion (heel slides).

POSITIONING: Patient in long-sitting position on stable surface with back supported or with patient leaning back on extended arms (tripod sitting).

PROCEDURE: Patient performs active unilateral flexion and extension of knee by moving heel of leg toward and away from hip in sagittal plane, keeping pelvis in neutral position.

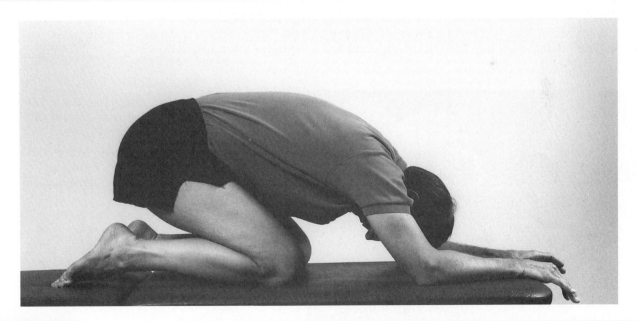

Figure 3-7 Combined thoracic, lumbar, hip, and knee flexion.

POSITIONING: Patient kneeling on hands and knees (quadruped).

PROCEDURE: Patient performs combined thoracic, lumbar, hip, and knee flexion by sitting back on heels, keeping hands forward, and lowering chest to surface. Pelvis tilts posteriorly, with cervical spine maintained in neutral regarding flexion and extension.

| Figure 3-8 | Ankle plantarflexion and dorsiflexion active-assistive or passive range of motion. |

POSITIONING: Patient sitting or lying supine on stable surface with limbs extended. Physical therapist assistant (PTA) standing to side of leg and adjacent to ankle and foot.

PROCEDURE: PTA performs unilateral plantarflexion and dorsiflexion of ankle by stabilizing leg at proximal tibia and pulling foot up and down in sagittal plane. Dorsiflexion motion should be performed by grasping heel while pushing plantar surface of forefoot with PTA's forearm. Dorsiflexion should be performed both with patient's knee extended and with it slightly flexed. Plantarflexion motion should be performed by pushing on dorsal surface of midfoot and forefoot.

NOTE: Same position can be used for active range of motion of ankle. Patient actively performs dorsiflexion and plantarflexion of the ankle, both with the knee extended and with it slightly flexed.

| Figure 3-9 | Toe flexion and extension active-assistive or passive range of motion. |

POSITIONING: Patient sitting or lying supine on stable surface with legs extended. Physical therapist assistant (PTA) standing to side of leg and adjacent to ankle and foot.

PROCEDURE: PTA performs unilateral flexion and extension of one or more toes at metatarsophalangeal joints by grasping entire digit and moving it in sagittal plane while stabilizing metatarsal bones of forefoot.

Figure 3-10 Shoulder abduction and adduction active-assistive or passive range of motion.

POSITIONING: Patient lying supine on stable surface with one arm at side and shoulder in lateral rotation. Physical therapist assistant (PTA) standing at patient's side and adjacent to shoulder.

PROCEDURE: PTA performs unilateral abduction and adduction of shoulder by grasping patient's limb under elbow and at wrist and hand and moving arm toward head and then back to patient's side in frontal plane. Elbow can be positioned in flexion or extension. Patient's scapula should be allowed to move, and shoulder must be positioned in lateral rotation when moving arm overhead to minimize subacromial impingement.

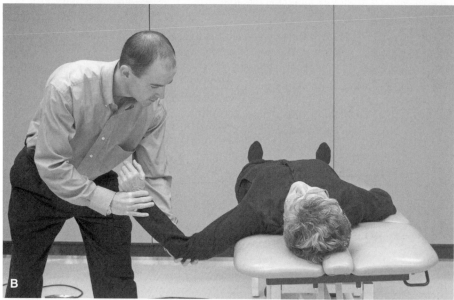

Figure 3-11   Shoulder horizontal adduction and abduction active-assistive or passive range of motion.

POSITIONING: Patient lying supine on stable surface with one arm in 90 degrees of flexion. Physical therapist assistant (PTA) positioned at patient's side adjacent to shoulder.

PROCEDURE: PTA performs horizontal adduction and abduction of shoulder by grasping patient's wrist and elbow and moving upper arm toward opposite shoulder (horizontal adduction) **(A)** and then back to starting position (horizontal abduction) **(B)** in horizontal plane (relative to patient). Patient's scapula should be allowed to move, and elbow can be positioned in flexion or extension.

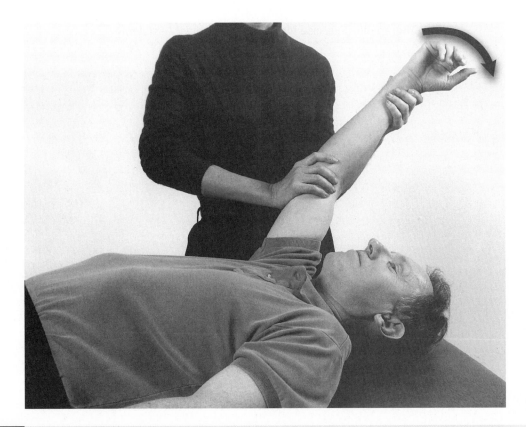

Figure 3-12 Shoulder flexion active-assistive or passive range of motion.

POSITIONING: Patient lying supine on stable surface with one arm at side and shoulder positioned in neutral relative to rotation. Physical therapist assistant (PTA) standing at patient's side and adjacent to shoulder.

PROCEDURE: PTA performs unilateral flexion of shoulder by grasping patient's arm at elbow, crossing over to grasp patient's wrist and hand, and moving arm toward head and then back to patient's side in sagittal plane. Elbow can be positioned in extension, and patient's scapula should be allowed to move.

Figure 3-13 Shoulder abduction and adduction active range of motion (AROM).

POSITIONING: Patient standing or sitting with upper extremities in anatomic position.

PROCEDURE: Patient performs active shoulder abduction and adduction (unilateral or bilateral).

NOTE: Same position can be used for performing AROM for shoulder flexion, extension, horizontal abduction, and horizontal adduction.

Figure 3-14   Shoulder rotation active-assistive or passive range of motion.

POSITIONING: Patient lying supine on stable surface with one arm in 90 degrees of shoulder abduction (neutral rotation) and 90 degrees of elbow flexion. Physical therapist assistant (PTA) standing at patient's side and adjacent to elbow.

PROCEDURE: PTA performs unilateral medial and lateral rotation of shoulder by grasping patient's distal forearm, stabilizing elbow, and moving forearm in swinging motion toward floor in sagittal plane (relative to patient).

NOTE: Rotation motion can also be performed with patient's shoulder in less than 90 degrees of abduction if necessary.

Figure 3-15   Shoulder rotation active range of motion.

POSITIONING: Patient standing or sitting with elbows flexed at 90 degrees.

PROCEDURE: Patient performs active medial **(A)** and lateral **(B)** rotation of shoulder (unilateral or bilateral) by swinging forearms toward and away from abdomen in horizontal plane while keeping upper arms against trunk.

Figure 3-16 Combined shoulder flexion and lateral rotation active range of motion.

POSITIONING: Patient standing or sitting with arms at side.

PROCEDURE: Patient performs active motion of combined shoulder flexion and lateral rotation at one shoulder by performing shoulder flexion with elbow flexed and reaching toward posterior portion of shoulder and scapula on same side.

Figure 3-17 Combined shoulder extension and internal rotation active range of motion.

POSITIONING: Patient standing or sitting with arms at side.

PROCEDURE: Patient performs active motion of combined shoulder extension and medial rotation at one shoulder by performing shoulder extension with elbow flexed while reaching toward inferior angle of scapula on same side.

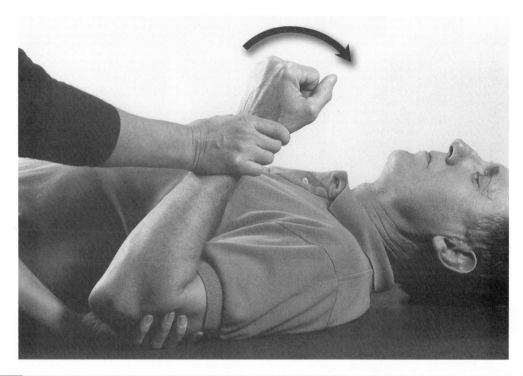

| Figure 3-18 | Elbow flexion and extension active-assistive or passive range of motion. |

POSITIONING: Patient lying supine on stable surface with arms at side. Physical therapist assistant (PTA) standing or sitting at side of patient and adjacent to elbow and forearm.

PROCEDURE: PTA performs unilateral elbow flexion and extension by grasping patient's distal forearm, stabilizing elbow and upper arm, and moving forearm toward and away from upper arm in sagittal plane. Movement should be performed with patient's forearm pronated and supinated.

NOTE: Same position can be used for active range of motion of elbow flexion and extension.

| Figure 3-19 | Forearm pronation and supination active-assistive or passive range of motion. |

POSITIONING: Patient lying supine on stable surface with one arm in 90 degrees of elbow flexion. Physical therapist assistant (PTA) standing or sitting at patient's side and adjacent to elbow.

PROCEDURE: PTA performs unilateral forearm pronation and supination by grasping patient's distal forearm, stabilizing elbow and upper arm, and rotating forearm toward and away from patient in horizontal plane.

NOTE: Same position can be used for active range of motion of forearm pronation and supination. Patient actively rotates forearm.

Figure 3-20   Wrist flexion, extension, and deviation active-assistive or passive range of motion.

POSITIONING: Patient lying supine on stable surface with one arm in 90 degrees of elbow flexion. Physical therapist assistant (PTA) standing or sitting at patient's side and adjacent to forearm.

PROCEDURE: PTA performs unilateral flexion, extension, and deviation of wrist by grasping patient's hand; stabilizing distal forearm in neutral rotation; and moving wrist into flexion, extension, radial deviation, and ulnar deviation.

NOTE: Same position can be used for active range of motion at wrist. Patient actively flexes, extends, and deviates wrist.

Figure 3-21   Finger flexion and extension active-assistive or passive range of motion.

POSITIONING: Patient lying supine on stable surface or sitting in chair with one arm in 90 degrees of elbow flexion. Physical therapist assistant (PTA) standing or sitting at patient's side and adjacent to hand.

PROCEDURE: PTA performs unilateral flexion and extension of one or more digits at metacarpophalangeal and interphalangeal joints by grasping segment distal to joint and moving it in sagittal plane while stabilizing segment proximal to joint.

NOTE: Same position can be used for active range of motion at fingers. Patient actively flexes and extends fingers.

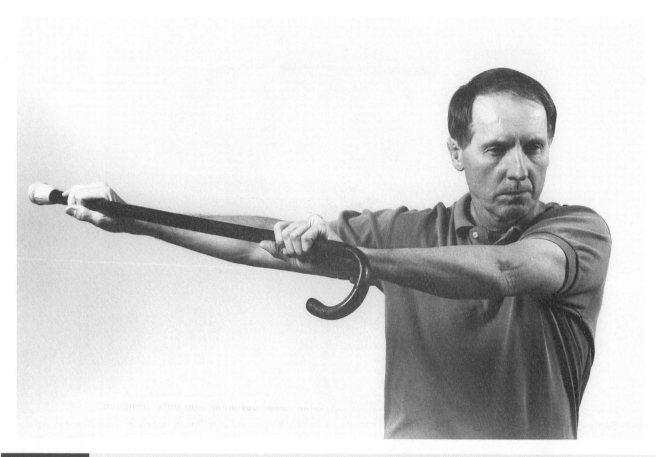

Figure 3-22 Shoulder horizontal adduction and abduction active-assistive range of motion with cane.

POSITIONING: Patient lying supine on stable surface or standing with arms in 90 degrees of shoulder flexion, elbows fairly extended, and wand held in hands.

PROCEDURE: Patient performs unilateral or bilateral horizontal abduction and adduction of shoulder by moving wand and arms back and forth across chest, keeping trunk stable.

Figure 3-23   Shoulder rotation active-assistive range of motion with cane (sitting).

POSITIONING: Patient sitting on stable surface with cane elevated over head with full elbow extension and wand held in hands **(A)**.

PROCEDURE: Patient performs bilateral lateral rotation of shoulders by moving wand and arms back behind the head (lateral rotation) **(B)**. Patient should not flex the cervical spine to achieve this movement.

Figure 3-24 Cervical rotation active-assistive range of motion (AAROM) or passive range of motion (PROM).

POSITIONING: Patient lying supine with head off stable surface. Physical therapist assistant (PTA) sitting or standing at end of stable surface, supporting patient's head with his/her elbows at about 90 degrees.

PROCEDURE: PTA performs cervical rotation motion bilaterally with grasp and support applied to patient's occipital region. Extension and lateral flexion motions are avoided.

NOTE: Similar positioning can be used for AAROM and PROM for cervical flexion, lateral flexion, and extension.

Figure 3-25 Cervical rotation active range of motion (AROM).

POSITIONING: Patient sitting, standing, or lying supine.

PROCEDURE: Patient performs active cervical rotation motion bilaterally; flexion, extension, and lateral flexion motion are avoided.

NOTE: Rotation motion can be self-assisted by patient using one hand to support the mandible and assist with the motion. Similar positioning can be used for AROM for cervical flexion, lateral flexion, and extension.

Figure 3-26   Lumbar rotation active-assistive or passive range of motion.

POSITIONING: Patient lying supine with knees flexed, feet flat on stable surface, and arms relaxed at side (hook-lying). Physical therapist assistant (PTA) standing to one side of patient and adjacent to lumbopelvic region.

PROCEDURE: PTA performs lumbar rotation motion bilaterally by moving knees laterally with one hand and stabilizing thorax with other. Pelvis should raise off stable surface on opposite side during movement.

Figure 3-27   Lumbar rotation active range of motion.

POSITIONING: Patient lying supine with knees flexed, feet flat on stable surface, and arms relaxed at side (hook-lying).

PROCEDURE: Patient performs active lumbar rotation motion bilaterally by moving knees laterally while keeping shoulder girdles and upper back flat on stable surface. One side of pelvis should rise up off stable surface during movement.

| Figure 3-28 | Lumbar flexion active range of motion. |

POSITIONING: Patient sitting upright in sturdy chair with feet flat on floor, pelvis in neutral, and hands in midline.

PROCEDURE: Patient performs active lumbar flexion by slowly lowering head, upper extremities, and trunk toward floor while allowing pelvis to tilt posteriorly and then returns to upright position. Cervical spine should be kept in neutral position relative to flexion and extension.

| Figure 3-29 | Thoracic and lumbar extension active range of motion. |

POSITIONING: Patient standing on stable, level surface with hands placed on iliac crests; pelvis in neutral.

PROCEDURE: Patient performs active thoracic and lumbar extension by slowly leaning trunk backward and allowing pelvis to tilt anteriorly and then returns to upright position.

Figure 3-30   Lumbar and hip flexion active-assistive range of motion (self-assisted).

POSITIONING: Patient lying supine with knees flexed, feet flat on stable surface, and arms relaxed at side (hook-lying).

PROCEDURE: Patient performs self-assisted lumbar and bilateral hip flexion by grasping behind one knee and pulling knee toward chest. **(A)** For slightly more difficult exercise, patient grasps both knees and pulls knees toward chest **(B)**.

NOTE: Allowing pelvis to tilt posteriorly during motion will result in greater range of lumbar flexion; stabilizing pelvis in neutral will result in greater range of hip flexion.

Figure 3-31 Lumbar extension active-assistive range of motion (self-assisted).

POSITIONING: Patient lying prone on stable surface with elbows flexed so that forearms and hands are under shoulder and upper arm.

PROCEDURE: Patient performs self-assisted lumbar extension by raising head and upper back off of surface. Force is provided by elbow extensors straightening elbows. Lumbar extensor muscles should remain relaxed during motion.

Figure 3-32	Shoulder abduction AAROM (with pulley).

POSITIONING: Patient sitting and holding one handle of pulley system in each hand **(A)**.

PROCEDURE: Patient performs unilateral or bilateral abduction of shoulders by pulling rope down on one side, causing other arm to be lifted into abduction **(B)**. Trunk should be kept stable, elbow extended on arm being lifted, and shoulder being lifted must be positioned in lateral rotation when moving arm overhead to minimize subacromial impingement.

Figure 3-33	Continuous passive motion (CPM) for knee flexion and extension.

POSITIONING: Patient lying supine in bed with involved lower extremity stabilized in CPM device (with straps, padding, and an underlying rigid frame). Movement hinge is aligned with knee joint.

PROCEDURE: Range, rate, and duration of motion are programmed. Unilateral flexion and extension of knee are performed continuously by device for hours at a time.

CASE STUDY 1

PATIENT INFORMATION

In an intensive care unit of a hospital, physical therapy was ordered for a 63-year-old woman with a diagnosis of traumatic brain injury as the result of an automobile accident. The patient was in stable condition. Examination performed by the PT at bedside indicated that the patient was comatose and unresponsive. ROM (passive) to all extremities was full, with no limitations present. Strength and functional movements were not examined because the patient was not able to respond. No discoloration or disruption of the integumentary system was noted.

LINK TO
GUIDE TO PHYSICAL THERAPIST PRACTICE

The diagnosis of traumatic brain injury relates to pattern 5I—"Impaired arousal, range of motion, and motor control associated with coma, near coma, or vegetative state" in the *Guide to Physical Therapist Practice*. The disorders grouped into this pattern include intracranial injury. Anticipated goals of intervention within practice pattern 5I include the maintenance of ROM and joint integrity through the use of specific therapeutic exercise of ROM.[21]

INTERVENTION

Short-term goals were for the patient to maintain full ROM in all extremities to prevent contracture. The PT met with the PTA to briefly discuss the patient's diagnosis and intervention. In addition, the PTA was reminded that even though the patient is comatose, the assumption is that the patient can hear and understand; therefore, explanation and continued verbal communication are essential. The PTA was instructed to perform daily gentle PROM to all joints of the upper and lower extremities. If the patient became more lucid, the PTA was instructed to contact the PT. Daily the PTA performed PROM to the hip and knee (Figs. 3-1 through 3-3), ankle (Fig. 3-8), and toes (Fig. 3-9) of the lower extremity and the shoulder (Figs. 3-10 through 3-12, 3-14), elbow (Figs. 3-18 and 3-19), wrist (Fig. 3-20), and fingers (Fig. 3-21) of the upper extremity.

PROGRESSION

Five Days After Initial Examination

Upon entering the patient's room, the PTA was greeted by a patient who was oriented to person, place, and time. The PTA introduced himself and explained the intervention that would be performed that day. The PTA performed the PROM regimen for the patient. During the treatment, the PTA observed that the patient was assisting the therapist during some of the movements and was moving all four extremities actively during the intervention. Upon completion of the intervention, the PTA contacted the PT about the change of status in the patient.

The next day the PT accompanied the PTA to the patient's room and found that the patient was coherent and sitting up in a chair. Upon completion of an upper- and lower-quarter screening examination, the PT determined that the patient had gross muscle strength of 3/5. The PT modified the patient's goals to the achievement of full strength of the upper and lower extremities. The PTA was instructed to progress the patient's exercise program to AROM of the upper and lower extremities. The PTA modified the exercise program. Daily the PTA performed AROM to the hip and knee (Fig. 3-1) of the lower extremity and the shoulder and elbow (Figs. 3-13, 3-15 through 3-17, 3-22, 3-23) of the upper extremity.

OUTCOME

Two days after AROM exercises were initiated to the extremities, the patient was transferred to a rehabilitation facility.

SUMMARY: AN EFFECTIVE PT–PTA TEAM

When the status of the patient drastically improved, the PTA was correct to perform the same treatment that he had been doing and to notify the PT of the change in status. It was not appropriate for the PTA to progress the intervention to AROM without the reassessment of the patient by the PT. Depending on how accessible the PT was to the PTA, the PTA might have been able to page the PT, the PT may have been able to come to the room, and the patient may have been able to be progressed to AROM activities on that same day. In both of these scenarios, the action by the PTA was the correct one.

SUMMARY

- This chapter presented the benefits, applications, and techniques of various forms of ROM exercise as part of a rehabilitation program. The three forms of ROM exercise are passive, active-assistive, and active. All forms offer physiologic benefits such as maintenance of joint movement and nutrition, prevention of connective and muscle tissue shortening, increased circulation, pain inhibition, and promotion of connective tissue remodeling. AAROM and AROM exercises offer added benefits to muscle tissue, aiding motor function, movement performance, and coordination.

- A wide range of benefits are offered by ROM exercises; they play a useful role in the regimen of care for a multi-

tude of pathologic conditions involving the musculoskeletal, neuromuscular, cardiopulmonary, and integumentary systems. Selection of the specific form of ROM exercise by the PT that is appropriate for the client depends on the diagnosis, impairment, and level of function. Performed gently and with caution, ROM activities can be implemented by the PTA quite early after trauma or surgery. Techniques of ROM exercise, regardless of the type, include motion in anatomic body planes, in diagonal or combined patterns, and in functional patterns that simulate those used in daily activities.

- External force used during PROM or AAROM exercises can be applied by the PTA or by the patient. In addition, a wand, pulley, or mechanical device can be used as an external force to increase PROM or AAROM.

GERIATRIC PERSPECTIVES

- Joint ROM and flexibility (like strength) are lost gradually after approximately age 30, with greater losses after age 40.[1] The age-related changes affecting joint flexibility include increases in the viscosity of the synovium, calcification of articular cartilage, and stiffening of the soft tissue (particularly the joint capsule and ligaments).

- Joint movements that are often used in activities of daily living exhibit less decrease in ROM than less frequently used movements. For example, anterior trunk flexion range is less likely to be lost than backward extension, and upper extremities maintain ROM more than lower extremities. In addition, the ankle joint loses ROM with aging. Women tend to lose more ankle range than men do. Between the ages of 55 and 85, women lose as much as 50% in ankle range, but men lose only 35%.[2] Occupational and leisure activities throughout life may lead to osteokinematic limitations because of the development of bone spurs and degenerative changes in the articular surfaces.

- Normative data for ROM in older adults have not been adequately established. ROM for older adults has been found to differ from the general population.[3] Clinicians should consider these differences when examining older adults and setting goals for them.

- Functional ROM refers to the joint range used during performance of functional activities. An understanding of functional ROM assists the clinician in establishing a plan of care that is based on functional need rather than an ideal or normal joint ROM.[4] Functional ranges for some activities of daily living have been established.[5]

- To maximize the benefits achieved through ROM exercises, the new motion should be incorporated into a functional activity or pattern. For example, a gain in shoulder flexion should be reinforced by passive, active-assistive, or active reaching tasks such as retrieving objects from overhead shelves. Research has shown that purposeful, task-oriented activities increase the physiologic gain for the patient.[6]

1. Spirduso WW. *Physical dimensions of aging.* Champaign, IL: Human Kinetics; 1995.
2. Vandervoort AA, Chesworth BM, Cunningham DA, et al. Age and sex effects on mobility of the human ankle. *J Gerontol Med Sci.* 1992;47:M17–M21.
3. Walker JM, Sue D, Miles-Elkovsy N, et al. Active mobility of the extremities in older adults. *Phys Ther.* 1984;64:919–923.
4. Goldstein TS. *Functional rehabilitation in orthopaedics.* Gaithersburg, MD: Aspen; 1995.
5. Young A. Exercise physiology in geriatric practice. *Acta Med Scand.* 1986;711(suppl):227–232.
6. Gliner JA. Purposeful activity in motor learning theory: an event approach to motor skill acquisition. *Am J Occup Ther.* 1985;39:28–34.

PEDIATRIC PERSPECTIVES

■ The developing individual exhibits much greater mobility and flexibility than the adult.[1] Just as it is important to remember that ROM decreases with age secondary to collagen stiffening, clinicians must recognize that a wide range of normal mobility exists in children and adolescents. Because of immature bone and extremely flexible collagen, newborns exhibit patterns of extreme ROM, as evidenced by excessive dorsiflexion in which the dorsum of the foot can be dorsiflexed to such a degree to make contact with the anterior tibia. This hypermobility decreases throughout childhood.

■ Maintenance of ROM is essential for children with juvenile rheumatoid arthritis (JRA). Contractures involving both joint and muscle can be anticipated based on an understanding of typical patterns of restriction associated with JRA. AROM exercises for management of morning stiffness in this population are essential. The soft-tissue flexibility and hypermobility normally present in children suggest the need for intensive therapy for muscle and joint dysfunction in the young patient with JRA.[2] See Chapter 4 for more information on stretching.

1. Kendall HO, Kendall FP, Boynton DA. *Posture and pain.* Melbourne, FL: Krieger; 1971.
2. Wright FV, Smith E. Physical therapy management of the child and adolescent with juvenile rheumatoid arthritis. In: Walker JM, Helewa A, eds. *Physical therapy in arthritis.* Philadelphia: WB Saunders; 1996:211–244.

References

1. Cech D, Martin S. *Functional movement development across the life span.* 2nd ed. Philadelphia: WB Saunders; 2002.
2. Rosse C, Gaddum-Rosse P. *Hollinshead's textbook of anatomy.* 5th ed. Philadelphia: Lippincott-Raven; 1997.
3. Norkin CC, Levangie PK. *Joint structure and function: a comprehensive analysis.* 4th ed. Philadelphia: FA Davis Co; 2005.
4. Prentice WE. *Therapeutic modalities for allied health professionals.* New York: McGraw-Hill; 1998.
5. Smith KL, Weiss EL, Lehmkuhl DL. *Brunnstrom's clinical kinesiology.* 5th ed. Philadelphia: FA Davis Co; 1996.
6. Hall CM, Brody LT. *Therapeutic exercise: moving toward function.* 2nd ed. Philadelphia: Lippincott Williams & Wilkins; 2005: 120–124.
7. O'Toole M. *Miller-Keane encyclopedia & dictionary of medicine, nursing, & allied health.* 7th ed. Philadelphia: WB Saunders; 2003.
8. Norkin CC, White JD. *Measurement of joint motion: a guide to goniometry.* 3rd ed. Philadelphia: FA Davis Co; 2003.
9. Brown ME. *Therapeutic recreation and exercise.* Thorofare, NJ: Slack; 1990.
10. Zachazewski JE. Improving flexibility. In: Scully RM, Barnes MR, eds. *Physical therapy.* Philadelphia: Lippincott; 1989: 698–738.
11. Cornwall MW. Biomechanics of noncontractile tissue. *Phys Ther.* 1984;64:1869–1873.
12. Magee DJ. *Orthopedic physical assessment.* 4th ed. Philadelphia: WB Saunders; 2002.
13. Akeson WH. Effects of immobilization on joints. *Clin Orthop.* 1987;219:28–37.
14. Donatelli R, Owens-Burchhart H. Effects of immobilization on the extensibility of periarticular connective tissue. *J Orthop Sports Phys Ther.* 1981;3:67–72.
15. Cummings GS, Tillman LJ. Remodeling of dense connective tissue in normal adult tissues. In: DP Currier, RM Nelson, eds. *Dynamics of human biologic tissue.* Philadelphia: FA Davis Co; 1992:45–73.
16. Minaire P, Neunier P, Edouard C, et al. Quantitative histological data on disuse osteoporosis: comparison with biological data. *Calcif Tissue Res.* 1974;17:57–73.
17. Uhthoff HK, Jaworski ZF. Bone loss in response to long-term immobilization. *J Bone Joint Surg Br.* 1978;60-B:420–429.
18. Minaire P. Immobilization osteoporosis: a review. *Rheumatology.* 1989;8(suppl):95–103.
19. Neumann DA. *Kinesiology of the musculoskeletal system.* St Louis, MO: Mosby; 2002.
20. Candolin T, Videman T. Surface changes in the articular cartilage of rabbit knee during immobilization: a scanning electron microscopic study of experimental osteoarthritis. *Acta Pathol Microbiol Immunol Scand.* 1980;88:291–297.
21. Videman T. Experimental osteoarthritis in the rabbit: comparison of different periods of repeated immobilization. *Acta Orthop Scand.* 1982;53:339–347.
22. Buckwalter JA. Mechanical injuries of articular cartilage. In: Finerman GA, Noyes FR, eds. *Biology and biomechanics of the traumatized synovial joint.* Rosemont, IL: American Academy of Orthopaedic Surgeons; 1992.
23. Lindboe C, Platou C. Effects of immobilization of short duration on muscle fibre size. *Clin Physiol.* 1984;4:183–188.
24. Lieber RL. *Skeletal muscle structure and function.* Baltimore: Williams & Wilkins; 1992.
25. Garrett W, Tidball J. Myotendinous junction: structure, function, and failure. In: Woo SL-Y, Buckwalter JA, eds. *Injury and repair of the musculoskeletal soft tissues.* Park Ridge, IL: American Academy of Orthopaedic Surgeons; 1988.
26. Frank D. Physiology and therapeutic value of passive joint motion. *Clin Orthop.* 1984;185:113–125.
27. Tomberlin JP, Saunders HD. *Evaluation treatment and prevention of musculoskeletal disorders.* 3rd ed. Chaska, MN: WB Saunders; 2004.

28. Salter RB. The physiologic basis of continuous passive motion for articular cartilage healing and regeneration. *Hand Clin.* 1994;10:211–219.

29. Salter RB. *Textbook of disorders and injuries of the musculoskeletal system.* 3rd ed. Baltimore: Williams & Wilkins; 1999.

30. Salter RB. Clinical application of basic research on continuous passive motion for disorders and injuries of synovial joints. *J Orthop Res.* 1984;1:325–333.

31. American Physical Therapy Association. *Guide to physical therapist practice.* 2nd ed. Alexandria, VA; 2003.

32. Noyes FR, Barber-Westin SD. Reconstruction of the anterior and posterior cruciate ligaments after knee dislocation: use of early protected postoperative motion to decrease arthrofibrosis. *Am J Sports Med.* 1997;25:769–778.

CHAPTER 4

Stretching Activities for Increasing Muscle Flexibility

William D. Bandy, PT, PhD, SCS, ATC

OBJECTIVES

Upon completion of this chapter, the reader will be able to:

- Define muscle flexibility and identify benefits of muscle flexibility.

- Identify autogenic and reciprocal inhibition and the neurophysiologic properties each uses for effectiveness.

- Identify and apply proper use of autogenic and reciprocal inhibition both together and separately in proprioceptive neuromuscular facilitation (PNF) within the established plan of care.

- Identify and apply appropriate clinical guidelines and indications for static, ballistic, and PNF stretching within the established plan of care.

- Apply common static stretching activities for the muscles of the upper and lower extremities and cervical and lumbar spine within the established plan of care.

Muscle flexibility has been defined as "the ability of a muscle to lengthen, allowing one joint (or more than one joint in a series) to move through a range of motion."[1] Loss of flexibility is "a decrease in the ability of the muscle to deform,"[1] resulting in decreased range of motion (ROM) about a joint. Studies have documented the importance of muscle flexibility for normal muscle function and for the prevention of injury. Some of the proposed benefits of enhanced flexibility are reduced risk of injury,[1–6] pain relief,[7] and improved athletic performance.[2–8]

The goal of a flexibility program is to improve the ROM at a given joint by altering the extensibility of the muscles that produce movement at that joint. Exercises that stretch these muscles over a period of time increase the ROM around the given joint. To increase flexibility, three types of stretching exercises have been described in the literature: ballistic stretching, PNF, and static stretching.

SCIENTIFIC BASIS

Neurophysiologic Properties of Muscle

To effectively stretch a muscle, the physical therapist assistant (PTA) must understand the neurophysiologic properties of muscle that can affect its ability to gain increased flexibility. Two sensory organs in the muscle are defined (muscle spindle and Golgi tendon organ [GTO]), and two important neurophysiologic phenomena are described (autogenic inhibition and reciprocal inhibition) below.

Muscle Spindle

The muscle spindle is a specialized receptor consisting of unique muscle fibers, sensory endings, and motor endings that are located within muscles (Fig. 4-1). Inside the muscle spindle are specialized fibers called intrafusal muscle fibers, which are distinct from ordinary skeletal muscle fibers (extrafusal fibers).[9–11]

The sensory endings of the spindle respond to changes in the length of the muscle and the velocity at which the length changes. The ends of the intrafusal fibers connect to the extrafusal fibers, thus stretching the muscle that stretches the intrafusal fibers. Afferent sensory nerves arise from the intrafusal fibers. Type Ia afferent sensory nerves respond to quick and tonic stretch of the muscle, and type II nerves monitor tonic stretch.[9–11]

When the muscle is stretched, the type Ia and II afferent sensory nerves of the intrafusal fibers of the muscle spindle are activated. This activation causes the muscle being stretched to contract, thereby resisting the stretch. For example, if a clinician applies a quick stretch to the hamstring muscles of a patient, the intrafusal muscle fibers within the muscle spindle react by sending impulses (via type Ia nerve

fibers) to the spinal cord to inform the central nervous system (CNS) that the hamstring muscles are being stretched. Nerve impulses return from the CNS to the muscle (specifically to the extrafusal muscle fibers via α motor neurons) to contract the hamstring muscles reflexively, essentially resisting the attempt of the hamstring muscles to elongate.[9–11]

Golgi Tendon Organ

GTOs are encapsulated structures attached in series to the fibers of the tendons at the junction of extrafusal muscle fibers and tendons (Fig. 4-1). Within the capsule, sensory nerve afferent fibers (type Ib) are attached to small bundles of the tendon. The GTO is sensitive to slight changes in the tendon's tension and responds to added tension by both passive stretch of a muscle (especially at the lengthened range) and active muscle contraction.[9–11]

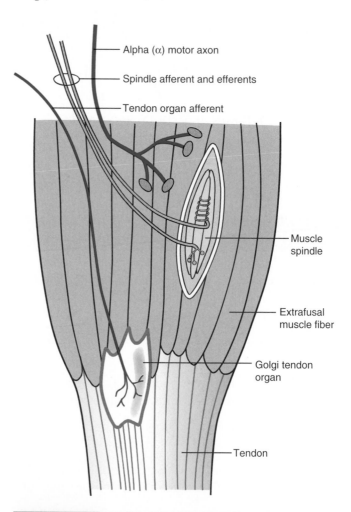

| Figure 4-1 | Muscle spindle and Golgi tendon organ. (Reprinted with permission from Kandel ER, Schwartz JH, Jessell TM. *Principles of neural science*. 3rd ed. New York: Elsevier; 1991.) |

The role of the GTO is to prevent overactivity of the nerve fibers innervating the extrafusal muscle (α motor neurons). In other words, if the muscle is stretched for a prolonged period of time or if an isometric contraction occurs, the GTO fires (via type Ib afferent nerve fibers) and inhibits the tension in that same muscle, allowing the muscle to elongate. For example, if the hamstring muscles are stretched for 15 to 30 seconds in the lengthened range, tension is created in the tendon. The GTO responds to the tension via type Ib nerve fibers. These nerve fibers have the ability to override the impulses coming from the muscle spindle, allowing the hamstring muscles to relax reflexively. Therefore, the hamstring muscles relax and are allowed to elongate.[9–11]

Autogenic Inhibition

Stimulation of a muscle that causes its neurologic relaxation is called autogenic inhibition. Autogenic inhibition can occur when the GTO is activated. For example, a maximal isometric contraction of the hamstring muscles causes an increase in tension of the GTO. Impulses from the GTO protect the hamstring muscles by inhibiting α motor neuron activity, causing the muscles to relax.[9–11] Autogenic inhibition serves as the basis for the PNF stretching techniques discussed later in this chapter.

Reciprocal Inhibition

Reciprocal inhibition is an important neurologic mechanism that inhibits the antagonist muscle as the agonist muscle (the prime mover) moves a limb through the ROM. In any synergistic muscle group, a contraction of the agonist causes a reflexive relaxation of the antagonist muscle. For example, during active flexion of the hip, reciprocal inhibition relaxes the hamstring muscles. This relaxation ensures that the hip flexors are able to move through the ROM without being influenced by contracting hamstring muscles.[9–11] Reciprocal inhibition serves as the basis for a PNF stretching technique discussed later in this chapter.

Static Stretching

Definition

Static stretching is a method by which the muscle is slowly elongated to tolerance (a comfortable stretch, short of pain) and the position is held with the muscle in this greatest tolerated length. In this lengthened position, a mild tension should be felt in the muscle that is being stretched, and pain and discomfort should be avoided.[2,8,9]

A slow, prolonged stretch is used to reduce the reflex contraction from the muscle spindle. More specifically, if the static stretch is held long enough, any effect of the type Ia and II afferent fibers from the muscle spindle may be minimized. In addition, because the static stretch in the lengthened position places tension on the tendon, the GTO may be facilitated to protect the muscle being stretched. This facilitation of the GTO fires type Ib nerve fibers, which inhibit and relax the muscle being stretched (autogenic inhibition). Therefore, the combined neurologic effects that occur during the static stretch are minimizing the influence of the muscle spindle and facilitating the effect of the GTO. This will ultimately allow the muscle being stretched to elongate, increasing muscle flexibility.[10–12]

Most literature documenting the effectiveness of static stretching has been performed on muscles of the lower extremities; little research has been performed on the spine and upper extremities. Gajdosik[13] indicates that using a slow static stretch increases the flexibility of the hamstring muscles, Madding et al[14] report gains in hip abduction ROM after passive stretching, and three studies by Bandy et al[15,16] indicate that static stretching is effective for increasing flexibility of the hamstring muscles. More recently Nelson and Bandy[17] and Davis et al[18] showed gains in hamstring flexibility following static stretch.

Duration

Recommendations for the optimum duration of holding the static stretch vary from as short as 15 seconds to as long as 60 seconds.[13–16] Unfortunately some authors have collected data before and after only one bout of stretching on 1 day and have not provided evidence for the most effective duration for stretching activities that take place for more than 1 day (e.g., weeks).

Bandy et al[15,16] examined different durations of static stretching that were performed 5 days per week for 6 weeks. They examined the effects of hamstring muscle stretching on a relatively young sample across a variety of durations, including comparing groups that stretched for 15, 30, and 60 seconds with a control group that did not stretch. The results indicated that 30 and 60 seconds of static stretching were more effective at increasing hamstring muscle flexibility than stretching for 15 seconds or not stretching at all. No difference was found between 30 and 60 seconds of stretching, indicating that the two durations had equal effect on flexibility. A 30-second static stretch was used by Nelson and Bandy[17] and Davis et al[18] to compare different types of stretching activities, further adding to the evidence that 30 seconds is the optimal time to stretch a muscle.

Examining subjects older than age 65, Feland et al[19] compared a control with groups who stretched the hamstring muscle for 15, 30, and 60 seconds for 10 weeks. Results indicated that the 60-second stretch produced the greatest gain in hamstring flexibility. The results of this one study suggest that the most effective duration of stretch may be effected by age. Further studies are needed to clarify the effect of age on the most effective duration to maintain a static stretch for enhanced flexibility.

Ballistic Stretching

Definition

Ballistic stretching imposes repetitive bouncing or jerking movements on the muscles to be stretched.[1] An example of a ballistic stretch is the sitting toe touch. The individual sits on the ground with the legs straight out in front (long sitting) and reaches the hands forward as far down the legs as possible. Leaning forward by contracting the abdominal muscles, the individual quickly reaches toward the ankles (or, if possible, past the feet) and immediately returns to the original long-sitting position. This movement is repeated 10 to 15 times, with each bounce extending the arms a bit farther.

Although research indicates that ballistic stretching increases muscle flexibility, some clinicians are concerned that the bouncing activity has the potential to cause injury, especially when a previous injury has occurred in the muscle. Theoretically, the quick, jerking ballistic motion can exceed the limits of muscle extensibility in an uncontrolled manner and result in injury.[6,7,20]

In addition, the quick bouncing of the muscle stretches the muscle spindle. As noted earlier, activation of the muscle spindle sends sensory impulses to the spinal cord via type Ia afferent nerves, informing the CNS that the muscle is being stretched. Impulses returning to the muscle via α motor neurons cause the muscle to contract, thereby resisting the stretch.[9-11] Concern exists that the facilitation of the muscle spindle that occurs during ballistic activities may cause microtrauma in the muscle because of the tension created when the muscle is stretched. Thus, ballistic stretching has generally fallen out of favor among most clinicians be-cause of the possibility of injury caused by uncontrolled jerking and bouncing motions and because the activation of the afferent nerve fibers of the muscle spindle causes a contraction of the same muscle that is being stretched.[1,20]

Alternative Perspective

Zachazewski[1] questions whether static stretching has been overemphasized at the expense of ballistic stretching. He argues that the dynamic actions required for high-performance athletic movements require ballistic-type activities (Fig. 4-2). If used appropriately, ballistic stretching may play a vital role in the training of an athlete because so many athletic activities are ballistic in nature.

Zachazewski proposes a "progressive velocity flexibility program," in which the athlete is taken through a series of ballistic stretching activities (Fig. 4-3). The program varies the velocity (slow, fast) and ROM (end range, full range) of the ballistic stretch. He emphasizes that the individual must first perform static stretches. After an unspecified period of training using static stretches, the athletes progress from slow, controlled stretching at the end of the ROM to high-velocity ballistic stretching through the full ROM.

As indicated in Figure 4-3, after a period of performing static stretches, the next step in the progression is slow short end-range activities. This portion of the stretching program incorporates ballistic stretches in a slow, controlled manner with small oscillations at the end of the range. Once the athlete is comfortable with performing the slow oscillations, the program is progressed to slow full-range activities, which are slow ballistic stretches through a much greater range of the length of the muscle. As the program advances over weeks to months, the athlete performs

Figure 4-2 Dynamic activities such as gymnastics incorporate ballistic stretching.

Figure 4-3 Progressive velocity flexibility program. (Reprinted with permission from Zachazewski J. Flexibility for sports. In: Sanders B, ed. *Sports physical therapy.* Norwalk, CT: Appleton & Lange; 1990:201–238.)

a high-velocity ballistic stretch in a small ROM at the end of the ROM, called fast short end-range activities. Finally, a high-velocity ballistic stretch is performed by the athlete through the entire length of the muscle, called fast full-range activities.

Zachazewski emphasizes that two important concepts should be considered before incorporating ballistic activities into a stretching program. First, because sedentary individuals and most geriatric individuals do not frequently use high-velocity, dynamic activities in their daily lives, ballistic stretching may not be appropriate for them. Static stretching appears to be the appropriate means of increasing flexibility of muscle in the nonathletic population. Second, before beginning a ballistic stretching program, the athlete should be properly and extensively trained in static stretching. The proportion of ballistic to static stretching should then be gradually increased as the athletic level of conditioning progresses.

To date, no research has been performed on Zachazewski's progressive velocity flexibility program. Therefore, initiation of the program should be carefully monitored by the PTA to ensure that the athlete is not being overaggressive, creating pain in or damage to the muscle being stretched. In addition, given the aggressive nature of ballistic stretching, it is not appropriate for an injured muscle.

Proprioceptive Neuromuscular Facilitation

According to Knott and Voss,[21] PNF techniques are methods of "promoting or hastening the response of a neuromuscular mechanism through stimulation of the proprioceptor."

Based on these concepts of influencing muscle response, the techniques of PNF can be used to strengthen and increase flexibility of muscle. This chapter focuses on the use of PNF to increase flexibility; Chapter 7 emphasizes the use of PNF to strengthen muscle.

Brief contraction before a brief static stretch of the muscle is the mainstay of the PNF techniques for increasing flexibility of the muscle. The terminology used to describe PNF stretching activities has varied widely, including the use of the following terms: contract–relax, hold–relax, slow reversal hold–relax, agonist contraction, contract–relax with agonist contraction, and hold–relax with agonist contraction. Furthermore, sometimes the same term is used for different PNF stretching techniques. For example, Etnyre and Lee[22] describe contract–relax as involving an isometric contraction, whereas the American Academy of Orthopaedic Surgeons[23] describes contract–relax as using a concentric contraction.

Part of the confusion in the terminology is that in their original description of PNF stretching techniques, Knott and Voss[21] specified diagonal patterns for performing the stretching activity. Today, most clinicians do not perform the techniques using the original diagonal patterns, rather they recommend moving in straight planes. PNF terminology cannot be transferred exactly from diagonal to straight-plane techniques. Thus, there is no consistency in the terminology used to describe PNF stretching techniques.

Three PNF stretching techniques will be defined in this chapter: autogenic inhibition, reciprocal inhibition, and combined.[24] The definitions presented are based on a review of literature[22–27] and on clinical experience.

Figure 4-4 — The lower extremity is passively flexed by the physical therapist assistant to full hip flexion.

Autogenic Inhibition

1. The PTA passively moves the limb to be stretched to the end of the ROM. For example, if the hamstring muscles are to be stretched, the lower extremity (with knee extended) is passively flexed by the PTA to full hip flexion (Fig. 4-4).
2. Once the end ROM of the muscle is attained, the patient applies a 10-second isometric force against the PTA, thereby contracting the muscle. For example, the patient contracts the hamstring muscles by extending the hip against the PTA (Fig 4-5). The isometric contraction of the muscle being stretched (hamstring muscles) causes an increase in tension in that muscle, which stimulates the GTO. The GTO then causes a reflexive relaxation of the muscle (autogenic inhibition) before the muscle is moved to a new stretch position and passively stretched (next step).

3. After the isometric contraction, the patient is instructed to relax and the PTA moves the limb to a new stretch position beyond the original starting point. The patient's leg is then held in the new position for 10 to 15 seconds. For example, the PTA passively and gently moves the leg into more hip flexion, maintaining the position for 10 to 15 seconds (Fig. 4-6).

Figure 4-5 — When the patient isometrically extends the hip against the physical therapist assistant, the hamstring muscles are contracted.

| Figure 4-6 | The physical therapist assistant passively and gently moves the leg into more hip flexion. |

4. Without the patient lowering the leg, the process (steps 2 and 3) may be repeated three to five times. After the last sequence is performed, the leg is lowered.

Reciprocal Inhibition

1. The PTA passively moves the limb to be stretched to the end of the ROM. For example, if the hamstring muscles are to be stretched, the lower extremity (with knee extended) is passively flexed by the PTA to full hip flexion (Fig. 4-4).

2. Once the end ROM is attained, the PTA asks the patient to attempt to perform a concentric contraction of the opposite muscle to the muscle being stretched, causing more of a stretch. For example, the patient is asked to actively flex the hip farther to increase the stretch of the hamstring muscles. This activity is similar to that shown in Figure 4-6, except the increase in hip flexion ROM is not obtained passively by the PTA pushing but is obtained actively by the patient contracting the hip flexors. As described earlier, in any synergistic muscle group, a contraction of the agonist (hip flexor) causes a reflexive relaxation of the antagonist muscle (hamstring), allowing the antagonist muscle to relax for a more effective stretch (reciprocal inhibition).

3. As the patient performs the concentric contraction, causing more of a stretch, the PTA takes up the slack into any ROM that was gained. Keeping the limb in the new stretch position, the PTA asks the patient to relax and holds the position for 10 to 15 seconds. For example, as the patient actively flexes the hip, the PTA maintains hands on the leg and moves with the leg into the hip flexion ROM that is gained and then holds the leg there for 10 to 15 seconds.

4. Without the patient lowering the leg, the process (steps 2 and 3) may be repeated three to five times. After the last sequence is performed, the leg is lowered.

Combination

1. The PTA passively moves the limb to be stretched to the end of the ROM. For example, if the hamstring muscles are to be stretched, the lower extremity (with knee extended) is passively flexed by the PTA to full hip flexion (Fig. 4-4).

2. Once the end ROM of the muscle is attained, the patient applies a 10-second isometric force against the PTA, thereby contracting the muscle to be stretched (autogenic inhibition). For example, the patient contracts the hamstrings by extending the hip against the PTA (Fig. 4-5).

3. After the isometric contraction of the muscle is performed, the PTA asks the patient to attempt to perform a concentric contraction of the opposite muscle, causing more of a stretch (reciprocal inhibition). For example, after the isometric contraction of the hamstring muscles, the patient is asked to actively flex the hip farther.

4. As the patient performs the concentric contraction, causing more of a stretch, the PTA takes up the slack into any ROM that was gained. Keeping the limb in the new stretch position, the PTA asks the patient to relax and holds the position for 10 to 15 seconds. For example, as the patient actively flexes the hip, the PTA maintains hands on the leg and moves with the leg into the

hip flexion ROM that is gained and then holds the leg there for 10 to 15 seconds.

5. Without the patient lowering the leg, the process (steps 2 to 4) may be repeated three to five times. After the last sequence is performed, the leg is lowered.

Research has indicated that PNF stretching techniques are effective in increasing flexibility of muscle. To date, however, no consensus exists as to which single PNF technique is the most effective.[22,26,27]

CLINICAL GUIDELINES

Although several investigations have studied the efficiency of one type of stretching over another, no absolute recommendation for the most appropriate type of stretching activity for increasing muscle flexibility has been made. Research indicates that ballistic stretching, PNF, and static stretching all increase flexibility of muscle.[1,2,18,20] But the greatest potential for trauma appears to be from ballistic stretching because of its jerking motions. In addition, even those who advocate ballistic stretching for advanced training recommend a solid base of static stretching before incorporating ballistic movements into a flexibility program.

Techniques for PNF require the most expertise of the three types of stretching and also require a second individual to perform the techniques. The need for an experienced practitioner makes PNF somewhat cumbersome. The easiest and most common method of stretching used to increase muscle flexibility appears to be static stretching. Therefore, the rest of this chapter emphasizes the static stretch.

Proper static stretching slowly elongates the muscles to a point at which a mild pull or tension is felt by the patient. This elongated position should be held for 30 seconds, during which time the patient should not feel any discomfort. If during the 30-second stretch the mild tension subsides, the patient should change his or her position to achieve a more aggressive stretch of the muscle and to feel a mild pull or tension (but no discomfort or pain). If during the stretch the tension grows in intensity and the patient feels discomfort or pain, he or she should be instructed to ease off the stretch into a more comfortable position while maintaining mild tension. Each stretching activity should be performed at least once per day.[14,15,17]

If possible, attempts should be made to integrate the stretching activity into the client's daily activities. Holding a stretch for 30 seconds can be boring. If the stretch can be performed at the office while talking on the phone, in the car while stopped at a stoplight, or at home while watching television, the patient is more likely to be compliant with the stretching program than if the movements must be performed in a specific place at a specific time. Obviously, not all the techniques presented in this chapter can be performed in all work environments, but the creative PTA can be a great asset to patients who complain that they do not have time to perform a stretching program.

Ideally, stretching to increase flexibility should be performed after a general warmup. The warmup may be a 3- to 5-minute repetitive activity such as walking, slow jogging, stationary bicycling, or active arm exercises. But inability or unwillingness to warm up should not preclude an individual from performing the stretching program. In fact, many stretching programs have failed because of this requirement to start with a warmup. If a warmup is not possible (for whatever reason), following the recommendation of performing the stretch to the point of mild tension should be strictly adhered to.[1,2]

If possible, the muscle to be stretched should be isolated, and the individual should be encouraged to focus on the muscle region that is pulling the body part into the stretch position. Isolating the muscle to be stretched is more effective than performing a general stretch that works two or three muscles (such as bending over and touching the toes). Generally a stretching technique is appropriate if the client feels a mild pull in the muscle that he or she is trying to stretch.

Finally, one point must be reiterated. As noted, the patient should feel only mild tension and no discomfort when stretching. In other words, the patient should not stretch to the point that pain is felt in the muscle or joint. If the patient stretches aggressively and into the painful ROM, the muscle will actually tighten. Aggressive stretching while the muscles are being contracted and tightened may lead to microscopic tears, which in turn may lead to the formation of nonelastic scar tissue. Such scar tissue will not adapt to the normal demands made on the muscle, leading to injury caused by the lack of blood supply and disturbed afferent input.

TECHNIQUES

As noted, most of the techniques described in this chapter focus on the static stretch. In addition, for each technique presented, the suggested duration of stretch is 30 seconds, unless otherwise noted.

Extremities

Figures 4-7 to 4-18 describe common static stretching activities for specific muscles of the lower extremities. Stretching techniques for the upper extremities are more general (i.e.,

Figure 4-7 Sitting hamstring muscle stretch.

PURPOSE: Increase flexibility of hamstring muscles.

POSITION: Patient sitting with leg to be stretched straight out in front of body with knee fully extended.

PROCEDURE: While maintaining the neutral position of the spine and flexing at the hips, the client reaches forward with both hands as far as possible down the leg until a mild tension is felt in the posterior thigh. Patient should lean forward by bringing the chest forward. Flexion of the lumbar spine should be minimal.

not usually specific to any one muscle) and are presented in Figures 4-19 to 4-25.

Spine

When stretching the cervical region, specific muscles can be identified and worked. These static stretches are presented in Figures 4-26 to 4-28. Muscles of the lumbar spine are usually stretched in a general manner, similar to the upper extremities (i.e., the techniques are not specific to any one muscle group). Static stretching techniques for the lumbar spine are presented in Figures 4-29 to 4-32.

Proprioceptive Neuromuscular Facilitation Stretching Techniques

The procedures of PNF stretching can be used for most static stretching procedures identified in Figures 4-7 to 4-32 by having a PTA add a contraction of the stretched muscle at the end of the ROM before the static stretch. Three types of PNF techniques for stretching the hamstring muscles were described earlier in this chapter. Using those basic principles, the PTA should be able to transform most of the static stretching techniques into PNF stretching techniques.

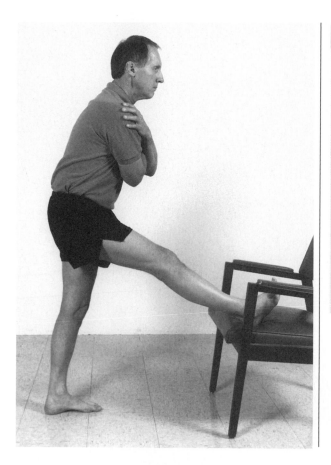

| Figure 4-8 | Standing hamstring muscle stretch. |

PURPOSE: Increase flexibility of hamstring muscles.

POSITION: Patient standing erect with one foot on floor and pointing straight ahead with no rotation of the hip. The heel of the leg to be stretched is placed on an elevated surface with the knee fully extended, toes pointed to ceiling, and no rotation of the hip. The elevated surface should be high enough to cause a gentle stretch in the posterior thigh when the patient leans forward.

NOTE: It is vital that the foot position be maintained. If the weight-bearing foot is allowed to externally rotate, the hamstring muscle will not be effectively stretched.

PROCEDURE: While maintaining a neutral position of the spine and flexion from the hips, the patient leans forward by bringing the chest forward until a mild tension is felt in the posterior thigh. Flexion of the lumbar spine should be minimal.

| Figure 4-9 | Prone quadriceps muscle stretch. |

PURPOSE: Increase flexibility of quadriceps muscles.

POSITION: Patient lying prone. Hips should be placed in neutral and not abducted.

PROCEDURE: Patient reaches back with one hand, grasps the foot, and moves the heel toward the buttock. By pulling on the foot, the patient flexes the knee until a mild tension is felt in the anterior thigh.

NOTE: The figure demonstrates the use of a towel for a patient who cannot reach the foot owing to lack of flexibility in the quadriceps muscle. The patient pulls the towel, which is draped around the foot to flex the knee.

| Figure 4-10 | Standing quadriceps muscle stretch. |

PURPOSE: Increase flexibility of quadriceps muscles.

POSITION: Patient standing and holding on to chair for support, if necessary. Hip remains in neutral and not abducted or flexed.

PROCEDURE: Patient reaches back with hand, grasps the foot, and moves the heel toward the buttock. By pulling on the foot, the patient flexes the knee until a mild tension is felt in the anterior thigh. It is important not to let the hip abduct or flex during the stretch.

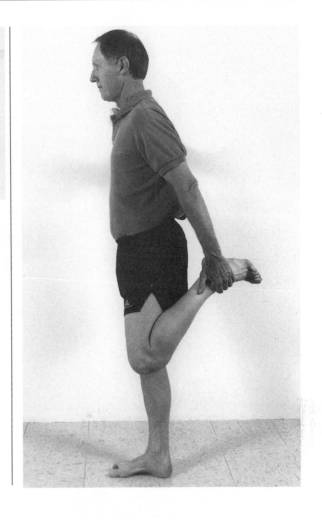

| Figure 4-11 | Modified lotus position. |

PURPOSE: Increase flexibility of adductor muscles.

POSITION: Patient sitting, bending knees, and placing soles of feet together while maintaining neutral position of the spine. The patient grasps both feet with hands.

PROCEDURE: Patient slowly pulls self forward with hands and allows the knees to drop to the floor until a mild tension is felt in the groin. Patient bends forward from the hips, maintaining neutral position of the spine. For increased stretch, the patient can gently push the legs into more abduction by pushing down with the forearms.

Figure 4-12   Forward straddle.

PURPOSE: Increase flexibility of adductor muscles.

POSITION: Patient sitting with knees extended and legs fully spread into abduction.

PROCEDURE: Maintaining neutral position of the spine, patient bends forward from the hips. While bending forward, the hands slide forward in front of the patient until a mild tension is felt in the groin bilaterally.

NOTE: The stretch can be modified by bending the trunk to the left or right and sliding the hands down the leg until a mild tension is felt in the groin unilaterally.

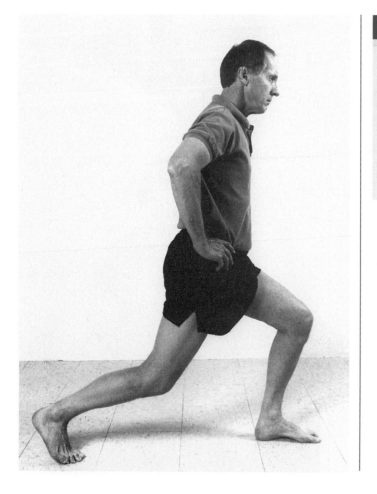

Figure 4-13   Lunge.

PURPOSE: Increase flexibility of hip flexor muscles.

POSITION: Patient standing with one leg forward, similar to taking a giant step.

PROCEDURE: Keeping a neutral spine, patient moves forward into the lunge position until the forward leg is directly over the ankle. The knee of the opposite leg should be resting on the floor. Patient should assume an upright position that allows a mild tension to be felt in the anterior hip of the trailing leg.

| Figure 4-14 | Hip flexor stretch using assistance of chair. |

PURPOSE: Increase flexibility of hip flexor muscles.

POSITION: Patient standing and holding on to chair for support, if necessary. One. leg is firmly planted on the ground and the other leg is placed on chair behind patient.

PROCEDURE: Standing upright, client carefully moves the leg on the ground forward by taking small hops. Once patient finds a position in which a mild tension is felt in the anterior hip of the nonweight-bearing leg, the position is maintained.

Figure 4-15   Standing iliotibial band stretch.

PURPOSE: Increase flexibility of iliotibial band.

POSITION: Patient standing approximately 3 feet away from wall and leaning on wall. Patient places one leg on the ground in front, leaving the other leg straight and behind. Patient internally rotates the hip of the back leg.

PROCEDURE: Patient protrudes the hip of the leg that is back out to the side, as the shoulders are leaned in the opposite direction. Mild tension should be felt at the lateral hip and thigh.

Figure 4-16   Side-lying iliotibial band stretch.

PURPOSE: Increase flexibility of iliotibial band.

POSITION: Patient lying on side. Lower extremity on support surface (iliotibial band not being stretched) flexed to 45-degree hip and knee flexion.

PROCEDURE: Lower extremity to be stretched (iliotibial band not on support surface) is extended in line with trunk and allowed to passively adduct toward support surface. A mild tension should be felt in the lateral thigh.

Figure 4-17	Gastrocnemius muscle stretch.

PURPOSE: Increase flexibility of gastrocnemius muscle.

POSITION: Patient standing with feet shoulder width apart approximately 3 feet from wall with hips internally rotated (toes of feet pointed inward). Knees are extended.

PROCEDURE: Patient leans forward on wall, providing support with forearms. While the patient is leaning forward, the pelvis should be held in and not protruded. The heels should not come off the floor. A mild tension should be felt in the calf area. If it is not felt, patient should stand farther away from wall before leaning forward. If discomfort or pain is felt, patient should move closer to wall before leaning forward.

NOTE: During the procedure, it is important to maintain the original internally rotated position of the hips and flexion of the knees.

Figure 4-18	Soleus muscle stretch.

PURPOSE: Increase flexibility of soleus muscle.

POSITION: Patient standing with feet shoulder width apart approximately 2 feet from wall with hips internally rotated (toes of feet pointed inward). Knees should be flexed to 20 to 30 degrees.

PROCEDURE: While maintaining flexed knees, client leans forward on wall, providing support with forearms. While the patient is leaning forward, the pelvis should be held in and not protruded. The heels should not come off the floor. A mild tension should be felt in the lower third of the posterior leg. If it is not felt, patient should stand farther away from wall before leaning forward. If discomfort or pain is felt, patient should move closer to wall before leaning forward.

NOTE: During the procedure, it is important to maintain the original internally rotated position of the hips and flexion of the knees.

Figure 4-19	Pectoral stretch (with assistance).

PURPOSE: Increase flexibility of pectoralis major muscle.

POSITION: Patient lying supine, grasping hands behind head.

PROCEDURE: While keeping hands grasped behind head, patient relaxes the arms, allowing them to drop down to the support surface. A mild tension should be felt in the anterior shoulder bilaterally. To accentuate this stretch, the physical therapist assistant (PTA) applies a gentle force to the elbows bilaterally to push the elbows down toward the support surface. The force should be gentle, and the PTA must ensure that the patient feels mild tension in the anterior shoulder. The force should not cause pain or discomfort.

Figure 4-20	Horizontal adduction stretch.

PURPOSE: Increase flexibility of muscles of the posterior rotator cuff.

POSITION: Patient sitting or standing. Patient horizontally adducts the shoulder across the chest, with the elbow kept relatively extended. Patient grasps the horizontally adducted shoulder proximal to the elbow.

PROCEDURE: With the grasping hand, patient pulls the shoulder across the chest into more horizontal adduction until a mild tension is felt in the posterior aspect of the shoulder.

Figure 4-21   Internal rotation stretch (with assistance).

PURPOSE: Increase internal rotation flexibility.

POSITION: Patient lying prone with shoulders internally rotated by placing the hand of the shoulder to be stretched behind the back. In most cases, this position will cause winging of the scapula **(A)**.

PROCEDURE: Physical therapist assistant places one hand on patient's winging scapula and applies gentle pressure, pushing it anteriorly against the rib cage until a mild tension is felt by patient in the posterior shoulder **(B)**.

NOTE: The amount of stretch felt by client can be increased or decreased by moving patient's hand farther up or down the spine, respectively.

Figure 4-22   External rotation stretch.

PURPOSE: Increase external rotation flexibility.

POSITION: Patient lying supine with shoulder abducted 90 degrees, holding just the elbow over the edge of the support surface. Patient externally rotates the shoulder.

PROCEDURE: Patient is given a weight to hold while maintaining the initial position. Patient should be encouraged to relax the shoulder muscles completely while grasping the weight, allowing the hand to move toward the floor (external rotation). Physical therapist assistant recommends the amount of weight that allows mild tension to be felt by patient in the anterior shoulder.

NOTE: The amount of shoulder abduction used for this stretch can be varied to stretch the shoulder for different functional activities, especially for athletes involved in overhead activities. Commonly used ranges of abduction in which external rotation stretch is applied are 45 degrees, 90 degrees, and 135 degrees.

Figure 4-23   Towel stretch for rotation.

PURPOSE: Increase flexibility of internal and external rotation.

POSITION: Patient sitting with feet shoulder width apart. For external rotation of the left shoulder, patient grasps towel in the left hand and throws the towel over the left shoulder (placing the left shoulder into external rotation), allowing the towel to hang down to the lumbar spine. Patient places the right arm behind the back and reaches up the spine to grasp towel.

PROCEDURE: By gently pulling inferiorly on the towel with the right hand, patient increases the amount of external rotation in the left arm (which continues to grasp the towel at the shoulder). Patient pulls down with the right hand until a mild tension is felt in the anterior aspect of the left shoulder.

NOTE: The stretch can be reversed to an internal rotation stretch of the right shoulder by using the left arm to pull superiorly. The left hand grasping the towel from above (shoulder) pulls superiorly while the right hand maintains the grasp of the towel from below (lumbar spine), causing an increase in internal rotation of the right shoulder.

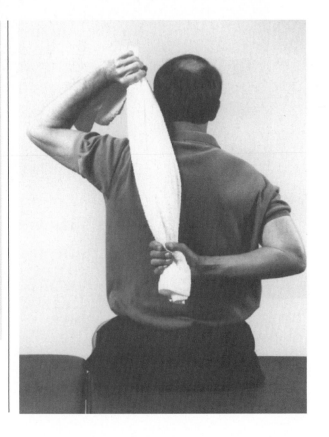

| Figure 4-24 | Biceps brachii muscle stretch (with assistance). |

PURPOSE: Increase flexibility of biceps brachii muscle.

POSITION: Patient standing upright with arms behind body and elbows fully extended. Physical therapist assistant (PTA) standing behind patient.

PROCEDURE: Ensuring that both elbows maintain full extension and the forearms are maintained in neutral position, PTA grasps client's hands with own hands and gently pulls patient's upper extremity into shoulder extension. Patient's upper extremities are pulled into shoulder hyperextension until a gentle tension is felt in the anterior aspect of the upper arm.

| Figure 4-25 | Wrist extension stretch. |

PURPOSE: Increase wrist extension flexibility.

POSITION: Patient standing, facing waist-high support surface.

PROCEDURE: Patient leans forward on waist-high surface, placing hands with palms down on surface, keeping the elbows fully extended. Patient then leans trunk forward over hands, ensuring that elbows are extended, causing hyperextension of wrists. Patient leans forward until a mild tension is felt on anterior aspect of forearms.

NOTE: This procedure can be modified to increase wrist flexion: (a) The dorsal surfaces of the hands are placed on the weight-bearing surface. (b) Patient leans slightly backward until a mild tension is felt in the posterior aspect of the forearms.

Figure 4-26   Trapezius muscle stretch (with assistance).

PURPOSE: Increase flexibility of trapezius muscle.

POSITION: Patient sitting in chair. Physical therapist assistant (PTA) standing behind patient and with one hand at the back of patient's head and the other on the shoulder of the side to be stretched.

PROCEDURE: To stretch the right trapezius muscle, PTA uses the hand on the back of the head to gently push patient's head into flexion, left lateral flexion, and right rotation. The PTA's hand on the right shoulder gently depresses the shoulder to provide a counterforce to cervical movement. Gentle force should be applied by the clinician until a mild tension in the posterolateral aspect on the right side of the cervical spine is reported by patient.

Figure 4-27   Levator scapulae muscle stretch (with assistance).

PURPOSE: Increase flexibility of levator scapulae muscle.

POSITION: Patient sitting in chair. Physical therapist assistant (PTA) standing behind patient with one hand at the back of the head and the other on the shoulder of the side to be stretched.

PROCEDURE: To stretch the right levator scapulae muscle, PTA uses the hand on the back of the head to gently push the patient's head into flexion, left lateral flexion, and left rotation. PTA's hand on the right shoulder gently depresses the shoulder to provide a counterforce to cervical movement. PTA should apply gentle force until a mild tension in the posterolateral aspect on the right side of the cervical spine is reported by patient.

| Figure 4-28 | Scalenes muscle stretch (with assistance). |

PURPOSE: Increase flexibility of scalene muscles.

POSITION: Patient sitting in chair. Physical therapist assistant (PTA) standing behind client with one hand on the back of the head and the other on the shoulder of the side to be stretched.

PROCEDURE: To stretch the right scalene muscle, PTA uses the hand on the back of the head to gently push the patient's head into left lateral flexion and right rotation (no flexion). PTA's hand on the right shoulder gently depresses the shoulder to provide a counterforce to cervical movement. PTA should apply gentle force until a mild tension in the anterolateral aspect on the right side of the cervical spine is reported by patient.

| Figure 4-29 | Prone press up. |

PURPOSE: Increase extension flexibility of lumbar spine.

POSITION: Patient lying prone with hands under shoulders.

PROCEDURE: Patient pushes down with hands, lifting the upper trunk. During the procedure, it is vital that the patient use muscles of the upper extremities and proximal stabilizers of the trunk. The lumbar spine must be relaxed. The pelvis should remain on the supporting surface as much as possible. Once full extension of the lumbar spine is reached, patient pauses at that position for 1 to 2 seconds. This hyperextended position should not be maintained for more than 5 seconds. After the hold, patient lowers himself or herself, with control, to the starting position. The lumbar spine must be relaxed during the entire activity.

| Figure 4-30 | Rotation in side-lying. |

PURPOSE: Increase rotation flexibility of lumbar spine.

POSITION: Patient lying on side with hips and knees flexed. The amount of hip and knee flexion depends on the goal. To increase flexibility of the lower thoracic and upper lumbar spine, the hips and knees should be maximally flexed. To increase flexibility of the lower lumbar spine, the hips and knees should be minimally flexed. A good method is to monitor where patient feels the stretch and adapt the flexion of the hips and knees accordingly.

PROCEDURE: To increase right rotation of the lumbar spine, patient lies on the left side, keeping the left lower extremities on the support surface and rotating the shoulders to the right until a mild tension is felt in the lumbar spine. Patient holds this position from 1 to 2 seconds (cyclic movement) to 30 seconds (prolonged hold) before returning to starting position.

| Figure 4-31 | Rotation in sitting. |

PURPOSE: Increase rotation flexibility of lumbar spine.

POSITION: Patient sitting on support surface.

PROCEDURE: To increase left rotation of the lumbar spine, patient rotates the shoulders to the left until mild tension is felt in the lumbar spine. To accentuate the stretch, patient can place fingers of both hands on the support surface lateral to the left hip. Neutral position of the spine should be maintained.

| Figure 4-32 | Single and double knee to chest. |

PURPOSE: Increase flexion flexibility of lumbar spine.

POSITION: Patient lying supine with bilateral hips and knees flexed so the feet are positioned on the support surface.

PROCEDURE: Patient flexes the hip of one leg, grasps the leg with both hands around the knee, and pulls the leg into more flexion until a mild tension is felt in the lumbar spine. The stretching activity is then repeated with the other leg **(A)**.

NOTE: For a more aggressive stretch, patient flexes both hips, grasps both legs with both hands around the knees, and pulls them into more flexion until a mild tension is felt in the lumbar spine **(B)**.

CASE STUDY 1

PATIENT INFORMATION

The patient was a 45-year-old man who complained of pain in the legs below the knees bilaterally. The patient indicated that for the previous 3 weeks he had been walking 1 mile 4 days per week. He indicated that his lower legs hurt all the time and the pain became worse when he tried to walk at a faster pace.

The examination by the physical therapist (PT) indicated pain with palpation to the anterolateral aspect of the length of the lower legs bilaterally. Passive plantarflexion ROM was full in both legs, but the patient complained of pain with over-pressure at the end of range. Examination of muscle flexibility indicated tightness in the gastrocnemius and soleus muscles. More specifically, left and right passive dorsiflexion with the knee extended (gastrocnemius muscle flexibility) was 0 degrees. Left and right passive dorsiflexion with the knee flexed to 20 degrees (soleus muscle flexibility) was 7 degrees. All resisted movement of the muscles around the ankle was strong and painless.

The patient was diagnosed with inflammation and possible tendonitis of the tibialis anterior muscle, commonly referred to as shin splints. Although shin splints have many origins, it was hypothesized that the pain and inflammation in the lower legs of this patient were caused by a weak tibialis anterior muscle having to dorsiflex against the tight calf muscle in a repetitive fashion.

⊖ LINK TO
GUIDE TO PHYSICAL THERAPIST PRACTICE

Pattern 4E of the *Guide to Physical Therapist Practice*[28] relates to the diagnosis of this patient. This pattern is described as "impaired joint mobility, motor function, muscle performance, and range of motion associated with localized inflammation." Included in the patient diagnostic group of this pattern is tendonitis. The anticipated goals are increasing the quality and quantity of movement between and across body segments through stretching.

INTERVENTION

An initial goal of intervention was to decrease inflammation (pain). Because the patient was complaining of pain in the lower legs all the time and not just when walking or immediately after walking, he was instructed to stop all walking activities. Because of the severe nature of the inflammation that caused the constant pain, it was thought that cessation of the walking was required. The patient reluctantly agreed.

The second goal was to begin to increase the flexibility of the calf muscles gradually in an attempt to decrease the amount of work being performed by the tibialis anterior muscle in pulling against the tight structures of the calf. The PT discussed the goals and plan of care with the PTA. The PT instructed the PTA to perform an autogenic inhibition stretching technique (Figs. 4-4 to 4-6) on the bilateral gastrocnemius muscles to attempt to increase length of the muscle. The PT also instructed the PTA to teach the patient a home program consisting of statically stretching the gastrocnemius muscle using a wall stretch (Fig. 4-17). The patient was also told to perform the exercise two times per day (morning and night), holding the stretch for 30 seconds as discussed in the plan of care by the PT.

PROGRESSION

One Week After Initial Examination

The patient stated that the pain in the lower leg was no longer constant and expressed a desire to begin to walk again. Examination indicated that the patient still had slight pain on palpation to the anterolateral aspect of bilateral lower legs but much less than the initial visit.

Re-examination by the PT indicated that passive dorsiflexion ROM measured with the knee extended (gastrocnemius flexibility) was 3 degrees (3-degree gain since initial examination). Passive dorsiflexion ROM measured with the knee flexed to 20 degrees (soleus flexibility) was 7 degrees (no change). Goals for intervention at this point were to continue to increase flexibility of the calf muscle and to strengthen the tibialis anterior muscle to assist the muscle in repetitive dorsiflexion during the swing phase and the deceleration of the foot after initial contact (heel strike), which occurs during walking.

Again, while in the clinic, following the original plan of care, the PTA performed autogenic inhibition stretching on the bilateral gastrocnemius muscles to attempt to increase length of the muscle. The PT instructed the PTA to progress the home program as follows:

1. Continue static stretching to the gastrocnemius muscle: 30 seconds two times per day.

2. Static stretching to the soleus muscle (Fig. 4-18): 30 seconds two times per day.
3. Isotonic strengthening of the dorsiflexors (Fig. 6-31) using elastic tubing: three sets of 12 repetitions one time per day.
4. Initiate a walking program: limited to a maximum of 0.25 mile three times per week. Ice the lower legs immediately after the walking session.

Two Weeks After Initial Examination

The patient returned to the clinic 2 weeks after the initial examination. The PT, however, was called away to see to another patient. The PTA began the treatment by taking subjective data and objective measurements. The patient indicated that he had no pain during walking. Palpation of the legs bilaterally indicated no pain. Passive dorsiflexion ROM measured with the knee extended (gastrocnemius flexibility) was 5 degrees (5-degree gain since initial examination). Passive dorsiflexion ROM measured with the knee flexed to 20 degrees (soleus flexibility) was 10 degrees (3-degree gain). Goals for the program were not changed because the PT was not available to re-evaluate the patient (continue to increase flexibility of the calf muscle and strengthen the tibialis anterior muscle).

The PTA instructed the patient to continue the home exercise program already established. He was given permission by the PTA to begin walking 0.5 mile three times per week. If no problems occurred after 1 week of walking this distance, the patient was instructed to increase to 1 mile four times per week. He was encouraged to ice after the walking sessions and to return for re-examination and follow-up after 2 weeks.

Five Weeks After Initial Examination

The patient had been scheduled to return 4 weeks after initial examination, but he was unable to return until the fifth week. He complained of being out of shape during his initial walks but reported no discomfort to his lower legs during his weeks of walking 1 mile four times per week. Re-examination by the PT indicated that gastrocnemius flexibility was 10 degrees and soleus flexibility was 15 degrees. Palpation indicated that the lower legs remained pain free.

No treatment was provided. The patient was instructed to continue his training frequency. If no problems occurred with this walking activity, the patient was encouraged to increase his walking distance, if desired. In addition, he was instructed to continue stretching the gastrocnemius and soleus muscles one time per day for 30 seconds. The patient was discharged by the PT and instructed to return if any problems developed.

OUTCOME

The patient sought treatment for bilateral shin splints and presented with tight gastrocnemius and soleus muscles. After a 5-week intervention in which stretching the tight muscles was emphasized along with some strengthening activities, the patient returned to his walking pain-free.

SUMMARY: AN EFFECTIVE PT–PTA TEAM

This case study demonstrates an effective collaborative team effort as well as poor judgment and communication between the PT and PTA. The PTA was able to follow the original plan of care provided by the PT for the first two visits. The PTA was able to treat the patient while in the clinic and instruct him on a home exercise program as requested by the PT. This teamwork allowed the PT to perform other duties while still being aware of the patient's status.

The poor judgment and communication becomes evident on the third visit. Two weeks after the initial examination the patient returned but was not re-examined by the PT. The PTA was able to collect the subjective data and take objective measurements; however, the PTA did not communicate the data to his supervising PT. The PTA did the correct thing by not changing the goals or the home program but used poor judgment by giving the patient permission to increase the walking distance and not return for 2 more weeks. This is not a decision that can be made by the PTA because it is a change to the plan of care. If proper communication was evident, the PTA would have reported the data to the supervising PT and a decision on a plan of care change would have been made by the PT.

Fortunately, upon the patient's return the symptoms decreased and the patient was able to be discharged. The poor judgment and communication did not cause any ill consequences for the patient; however, it probably initiated a lack of trust between the PT and the PTA.

SUMMARY

- The ultimate goal of any stretching program is to increase the ability of the muscle to efficiently elongate through the necessary ROM. This chapter reviewed the three types of stretching activities most frequently referred to in the literature: static stretching, ballistic stretching, and PNF. Although extensive research has been performed on the effectiveness of these three stretching activities, no absolute recommendation can be made for the most appropriate method for increasing flexibility. All three stretching techniques will improve muscle flexibility.

- Static stretching is a technique in which a stationary position is held for a period of time while the muscle is in its elongated position. Static stretching may be the most desirable stretching technique for an individual in terms of results, time, and comfort because once the individual is properly trained, he or she can perform the technique independently.

- Ballistic stretching involves quick bobbing and jerking motions imposed on the muscle. Although some clinicians believe that ballistic stretching may have a role in an advanced stretching program of an athlete, this type of stretching poses the greatest potential for microtrauma to the muscle.

- Using a variety of types of muscle contractions to facilitate the sensory receptors to inhibit and relax the muscle being stretched, PNF has been documented to be an effective stretching technique. However, because PNF requires one-on-one intervention with a clinician, the time and expertise required to perform PNF appropriately make the stretching techniques somewhat cumbersome.

▼ ▼ ▼ GERIATRIC PERSPECTIVES ▼ ▼ ▼

- The age-related effect of connective tissue stiffening is of particular importance for the older adult. A decrease in tissue water content, an increase in collagen bundling, and an increase in elastin crosslinks result in a decrease in the distensibility and tensile strength of muscles, fascia, tendons, skin, and bones. Consequently, ballistic stretching is particularly problematic. Static stretching may potentially be more effective for older adults if applied slowly and held for a slightly longer duration (30 to 60 seconds).[1]

- Modified dynamic flexibility, or functional flexibility, refers to an active type of stretching exercise involving movement of varying degrees and speeds to meet or enhance the ROM typically used during specific activities. It is an important consideration in initiating a stretching program for older adults.[2] Functional flexibility and ROM related to a minimum level of safe performance in activities of daily living have been defined through biomechanics research.[3]

- Stretch weakness is a theoretic phenomenon associated with muscle aging combined with disuse. Stretch weakness is thought to be the result of prolonged stretch applied beyond the physiologic resting length.[4] The phenomenon may be evidenced by altered muscle synergies (e.g., agonist–antagonist imbalances or agonist–antagonist cocontraction). Stretch weakness may also be related to pathologic age-related changes (e.g., postural malalignment and gait changes resulting from the disease process of degenerative joint disease and scoliosis). Stretch weakness should be addressed via a thorough examination of ROM and evaluation of muscle length before initiation of a flexibility or stretching program.

- Static stretching techniques are most effective if used in conjunction with active contraction. Reciprocal inhibition and autogenic inhibition stretching techniques further enhance the therapeutic benefits of static stretching by allowing the agonist to relax. However, the stretch weakness phenomenon may preclude effective use of these PNF techniques. In the presence of agonist stretch weakness, passive stretching of the antagonist is recommended.

- Cognitively impaired patients usually are not candidates for stretching programs because of problems relaxing the muscle to be lengthened.

- A warmup and mild stretching program may be useful in the management of chronic pain and loss of joint range associated with some musculoskeletal and neuromuscular diseases (e.g., arthritis and Parkinson's disease).

- The most effective stretching program should be based on the individual functional needs of the older individual. The primary outcome should be restoration or maintenance of physical independence.

1. Bandy WD, Irion JM, Briggler M. The effect of time and frequency of static stretching on flexibility of the hamstring muscles. *Phys Ther.* 1997;77:1090–1096.

2. Stevens K. A theoretical overview of stretching and flexibility. *Am Fitness.* 1998;16:30–37.

3. Young A. Exercise physiology in geriatric practice. *Acta Med Scand.* 1986;711(suppl):227–232.

4. Kauffman TL. *Geriatric rehabilitation manual.* New York: Churchill Livingstone; 1999.

PEDIATRIC PERSPECTIVES

▲ ▲ ▲   ▲ ▲ ▲

■ The developing individual exhibits much greater mobility and flexibility than the mature individual.[1] Muscle inflexibility, when present, aggravates and predisposes children and adolescents to a variety of overuse injuries, including traction apophysitis.[2] Flexibility deficits that may occur in children and adolescents can be effectively treated using common stretching techniques (as described in this chapter).

■ Ballistic stretching may be the least appropriate stretching technique for children for the same reasons that it is not recommended for sedentary and geriatric individuals. In addition, ballistic stretching may put excessive strain on the apophyses and epiphyses of developing bone.

■ Muscle stretching is imperative for treatment of juvenile rheumatoid arthritis (JRA). The shortening of

muscle and tendon, and the resulting joint contractures, may become a major cause of disability. The greater soft-tissue flexibility and hypermobility in disease-free children younger than 8 years of age suggest the need for early intensive therapy for children with JRA in preventing long-term disability.[3] No evidence exists as to which stretching methods are the most efficacious for children with JRA. Low-load prolonged stretching using splinting methods may be appropriate.[3]

1. Kendall HO, Kendall FP, Boynton DA. *Posture and pain.* Melbourne, FL: Krieger; 1971.
2. Krivickus LS. Anatomical factors associated with overuse sports injuries. *Sports Med.* 1997;24:132–146.
3. Wright FV, Smith E. Physical therapy management of the child and adolescent with juvenile rheumatoid arthritis. In: Walker JM, Helewa A, eds. *Physical therapy in arthritis.* Philadelphia: WB Saunders; 1996:211–244.

References

1. Zachazewski J. Flexibility for sports. In: Sanders B, ed. *Sports physical therapy.* Norwalk, CT: Appleton & Lange; 1990: 201–238.

2. Anderson B, Burke ER. Scientific, medical, and practical aspects of stretching. *Clin Sports Med.* 1991;10:63–86.

3. Jonagen S, Nemeth G, Griksson F. Hamstring injuries in sprinters: the role of concentric and eccentric hamstring muscle strength and flexibility. *Am J Sports Med.* 1994;22:262–266.

4. Worrell TW, Perrin DH, Gansneder B, et al. Comparison of isokinetic strength and flexibility measures between hamstring injured and non-injured athletes. *J Orthop Sports Phys Ther.* 1991;13:118–125.

5. Habertsman JP, VanBolhuis AI, Goeken LN. Sport stretching: effect on passive muscle stiffness of short hamstrings. *Arch Phys Med Rehabil.* 1996;77:658–692.

6. Hurtig DE, Henderson JM. Increasing hamstring flexibility decreases lower extremity overuse injuries in military basic trainees. *Am J Sports Med.* 1999;27:173–176.

7. Henricson AS, Fredriksson K, Persson I, et al. The effect of heat and stretching on the range of hip motion. *J Orthop Sports Phys Ther.* 1984;6:110–115.

8. Worrell TW, Smith TL, Winegardner J. Effect of hamstring stretching on hamstring muscle performance. *J Orthop Sports Phys Ther.* 1994;20:154–159.

9. Hall CM, Brody LT. *Therapeutic exercise: moving toward function.* 2nd ed. Philadelphia: Lippincott Williams & Wilkins; 2005: 125–129.

10. Pearson K, Gordon J. Spinal reflexes. In: Kandel ER, Schwartz JH, eds. *Principles of neural science.* 3rd ed. New York: Elsevier; 2000:713–734.

11. Lundy-Ekman L. *Neuroscience: fundamentals for rehabilitation.* Philadelphia: WB Saunders; 2002:102–106.

12. Waxman SG, deGroot J. *Correlative neuroanatomy.* Norwalk, CT: Appleton & Lange; 1995:58–61.

13. Gajdosik RL. Effects of static stretching on the maximal length and resistance to passive stretch of the hamstring muscles. *J Orthop Sports Phys Ther.* 1991;14:250–255.

14. Madding SW, Wong JG, Hallum A, et al. Effects of duration on passive stretching on hip abduction range of motion. *J Orthop Sports Phys Ther.* 1987;8:409–416.

15. Bandy WD, Irion J. The effect of time of static stretch on the flexibility of the hamstring muscles. *Phys Ther.* 1994;74: 845–850.

16. Bandy WD, Irion JM, Briggler M. The effect of time and frequency of static stretching on flexibility of the hamstring muscles. *Phys Ther.* 1997;77:1090–1096.

17. Nelson RT, Bandy WD. Eccentric training and static stretching improve hamstring flexibility of high school males. *J Athl Train.* 2004;39:31–35.

18. Davis DS, Ashby PE, McCale KL, et al. The effectiveness of 3 stretching techniques on hamstring flexibility using consistent stretching parameters. *J Strength Cond Res.* 2005;19: 27–32.

19. Feland JB, Myrer JW, Schulthies SS, et al. The effect of duration of stretching of the hamstring muscle group for increasing range of motion in people aged 65 years or older. *Phys Ther.* 2001;81:1100–1117.

20. Sady SP, Wortman M, Blanke D. Flexibility training: ballistic, static or proprioceptive neuromuscular facilitation? *Arch Phys Med Rehabil.* 1982;63:261–263.

21. Knott M, Voss DE. *Proprioceptive neuromuscular facilitation: patterns and techniques.* New York: Harper & Row; 1968.

22. Etnyre BR, Lee EJ. Chronic and acute flexibility of men and women using three different stretching techniques. *Res Q Exerc Sport.* 1988;59:222–228.

23. American Academy of Orthopaedic Surgeons. *Athletic training and sports medicine.* 2nd ed. Rosemont, IL: American Academy of Orthopaedic Surgeons; 1991.

24. Davies DS, Hagerman-Hose M, Midkiff M, et al. The effectiveness of 3 proprioceptive neuromuscular facilitation stretching techniques on the flexibility of the hamstring muscle group. *J Orthop Sports Phys Ther.* 2004;34:A33.

25. Allerheiligen WB. Exercise techniques: stretching and warm-up. In: Baechle TR, ed. *Essentials of strength training and conditioning.* Champaign, IL: Human Kinetics; 1994:289–313.

26. Cornelius WL, Ebrahim K, Watson J, et al. The effects of cold application and modified PNF stretching techniques on hip flexibility in college males. *Res Q Exer Sport.* 1992;63:311–314.

27. Osternig LR, Robertson R, Troxel R, et al. Differential response to proprioceptive neuromuscular facilitation (PNF) stretch technique. *Med Sci Sports Exerc.* 1990;22:106–111.

28. American Physical Therapy Association. *Guide to physical therapist practice.* 2nd ed. Alexandria, VA; 2003.

PART

Strength and Power

CHAPTER 5

Principles of Resistance Training

Michael Sanders, EdD, and Barbara Sanders, PT, PhD, SCS

Upon completion of this chapter, the reader will be able to:

- Discuss the physiologic parameters of muscle training related to each of the following: muscle loss, metabolic rate, muscle mass, body composition, bone mineral density, glucose metabolism, gastrointestinal transit time, resting blood pressure, and blood lipid levels.

- Discuss the clinical adaptations of muscle training related to each of the following: muscle loss, metabolic rate, muscle mass, body composition, bone mineral density, glucose metabolism, gastrointestinal transit time, resting blood pressure, and blood lipid levels.

- Identify the roles of motor unit recruitment, cross-sectional area, and force velocity in regulation of muscle contraction.

- Identify the principle elements of exercise training and identify how each element of muscle training affects adaptation of the body.

- Identify symptoms of overtraining and discuss appropriate methods to alleviate overtraining.

- Define periodization and describe how periodization is used in exercise training programs.

The clinician frequently addresses the concepts of strength- and resistance-training, characteristics of muscular performance. Strength is defined as the maximal voluntary force that can be produced by the neuromuscular system, usually demonstrated by the ability to lift a maximal load one time, called the one-repetition maximum (1 RM). Increases in strength occur as a result of resistance training (defined as lifting heavy loads for a relatively few number of repetitions for all types of contractions) and involves a complex set of interactions: neurologic, muscular, and biomechanical.[1] The importance of a strong theoretic background in strength and resistive training allows a common language, standardization of terminology, and practical applications of muscle-training theory. Research has demonstrated that many health and fitness benefits result from engaging in muscle training. Several authors[2,3] have provided copious data on the positive physiologic responses to training programs. The concepts discussed in the following sections provide an important background to the physiologic parameters and practical adaptations of muscle training.

TERMINOLOGY

Muscle performance is usually considered a function of strength; however, strength is only one of three components of muscle performance: strength, power, endurance.

Muscle strength

Muscle strength is the maximum force that a muscle or muscle group can exert during a contraction. Strength is assessed in terms of force, torque, work, and power. Force is that which causes change in an object's motion—mass × acceleration. Torque is the concept of rotational work compared with the idea of force as linear motion. Therefore, it is angular velocity—in other words, the displacement around an axis at the rotational speed. Work is defined as force × distance or the product of the force exerted on an object and the distance the object moves in the direction of the force.

Power

Power is the rate of performing muscle contractions over a distance for a specific amount of time. Power is a critical component of functional activities and is strength with the addition of speed. Power is defined as work/time or force × distance/time. Power is the product of the force exerted on an object and the speed of the object in the direction of the force. The concept of power is generally associated with high speeds of movement, and strength associated with slower speeds; both reflect the ability to exert force at a given speed. Strength is the ability to exert force at any given speed, and power is the mathematical product of force and velocity at whatever speed. Regardless, some functional movements require strength and others power.

Endurance

Muscle endurance is the ability of the muscle or muscle group to sustain contractions repeatedly or over a certain period of time.

Isometric Muscle Action

Isometric action is considered static and is produced when muscle tension is created without a change in muscle length. Static activity is used in therapeutic exercise and in functional activity. Trunk muscles provide a stable base for movement of the upper and lower extremities and thus are functioning in a static or isometric action.

Isotonic Muscle Action

Isotonic activity is dynamic change in muscle length. As the muscle shortens during activity, it is considered concentric muscle action. If the muscle lengthens during activity, it is an eccentric muscle action. Most functional activities require the use of both concentric action and eccentric action. To stand from sitting requires concentric action of the quadriceps muscle group and eccentric contraction of the hamstring muscle group. Eccentric muscle action can produce about 30% more force than concentric actions.[4] Concentric muscle actions take more energy to perform; however, the strength gains between the two types of exercise are similar. Eccentric muscle actions are an important aspect of functional movement, are energy efficient, and can develop the most tension of the various muscle actions. Delayed-onset muscle soreness (DOMS) occurs more often with eccentric exercise.[4]

Isokinetic Muscle Action

Isokinetic muscle action is dynamic activity involving movement. This movement is at a constant velocity throughout the muscle action. The resistance varies during the muscle action. Devices are preset to a constant velocity, which allows the movement to accommodate strength throughout the phase of movement. It is thought that isokinetic exercise provides an opportunity for maximal contraction throughout the movement.

SCIENTIFIC BASIS

Anatomic Considerations of Muscle

Muscle Structure

A muscle is composed of many thousands of cells called muscle fibers. Each muscle fiber has a thin sheathlike covering of connective tissue called the endomysium. Individual muscle fibers are collected into bundles (fasciculi), which are covered with a thicker layer of loose connective tissue (perimysium). The perimysium sends connective tissue partitions (trabeculae) into the bundles to partially subdivide them. A number of fasciculi bundles make up the total belly of the muscle. The muscle belly is covered externally by a loose connective tissue (epimysium or deep fascia), which is continuous with the perimysium of the bundles. At the end of the muscle, the epimysium merges with the connective tissue material of the tendon (Fig. 5-1).[5,6]

Each single muscle fiber does not run through the entire length of the muscle or even through a fasciculus. A muscle fiber can begin in the periosteum and end in the muscle, begin in the tendon and end in the muscle, or begin in the muscle and end in the muscle. Because muscle fibers do not run the length of the whole muscle, the connective tissue sheaths—endomysium around the single fiber, perimysium around the fasciculus, and epimysium around the whole muscle—are necessary to transmit the force of muscle contraction from fiber to fiber to fasciculus and from fasciculus to fasciculus to the tendons, which act on the bones.[5,6]

Muscle Fiber Structure

Each individual muscle fiber is made up of threads of protein molecules called myofibrils, which are enclosed in a special membrane called the sarcolemma. Each myofibril contains smaller threads called myofilaments. These myofilaments are made up of protein molecules called actin (thin filaments) and myosin (thick filaments). The actin and myosin make up the contractile element of the muscle.[5,6] Detailed descriptions of skeletal muscle and muscle fiber, including the sliding filament theory, are available elsewhere.[6,7]

Regulation of Muscle Contraction

Motor Unit

The final pathway by which the nervous system can exert control over motor activity is the motor unit. The motor unit is the functional unit of skeletal muscle and consists of a single motor neuron (with the body contained in the anterior horn of the spinal cord), its axon and terminal branches, and all the individual muscle fibers supplied by the axon. The actual number of muscle fibers in a particular motor unit varies from 5 to more than 100. Muscles involved in delicate movements of the eye have an innervation ratio (the total number of motor axons divided by the total number of muscle fibers in a muscle) of 1:4. Large postural muscles that do not require a fine degree of control have an innervation ratio as large as 1:150. It is important to note that the motor unit functions on an "all or none" principle; thus, all of the fibers within the unit contract and develop force at the same time.[6,8,9]

Motor Unit Recruitment

Motor units can cause an increase in muscle tension through two primary mechanisms. First, the strength of a muscle contraction is affected by the number of motor units recruited. Increased strength of contraction is primarily accomplished by summing the contractions of different numbers of muscle fibers at once. Because all the fibers making up a motor unit contract in unison and to their maximum (if they contract at all), variations in the strength of contractions partly depend on the number of motor units employed. This type of summation, in which different numbers of motor units are brought into play to produce gradations of strength, is called multiple motor unit summation. During this type of summation, only a few motor units are contracted simultaneously when a weak contraction is desired and a great number of motor units are contracted at the same time when a strong contraction is desired. Should all the motor units contract at the same time, the contraction would be maximal. Therefore, the strength of a muscle contraction can be varied by changing the number of motor units contracting at the same time.[6,10]

Second, the strength of a muscle contraction is affected by the frequency of stimulation. When a muscle fiber is stimulated many times in succession with contractions that occur close enough together so that a new contraction starts before the previous one ends, each succeeding contraction adds to the force of the preceding one, increasing the overall strength of the contraction. This type of summation, in which gradations in strength are produced by variations in the frequency of stimulation of the fibers, is called wave summation. Wave summation is characterized by the production of a weak contraction when the fiber is stimulated only a few times per second and a strong contraction when the fiber is stimulated many times per second. A maximum contraction occurs when all the individual muscle twitches become fused into a smooth, continuous contraction called a tetanized contraction.[6,11]

During submaximal efforts, the force of a muscle contraction is obtained by using a combination of multiple motor unit summation and wave summation. The force of a submaximal muscle contraction is obtained by contracting the different motor units of a muscle a few at a time but in rapid succession so that the muscle tension is always of a tetanic nature rather than a twitching one. In a weak

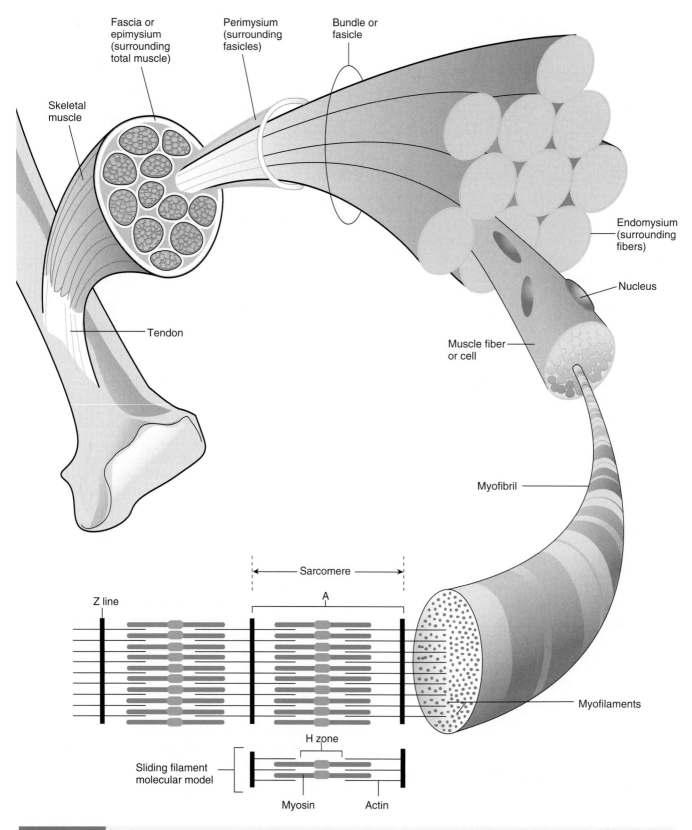

Figure 5-1   The structure of muscle.

contraction, only one or two motor units contract at only two or three times per second, but the contractions are spread one after another among different motor units to achieve a tetanized state. Relatively smooth performances are achieved by low discharge rates of motor units firing asynchronously or out of phase so that when one group of muscles is contracting, another group is resting. When a stronger contraction is desired, a greater number of motor units is recruited simultaneously and fire more frequently. If the majority of the motor units are discharging together at maximal frequency, the force of the muscle will be greater and the motor units are said to be synchronous, or in phase.[6,11]

Cross-sectional Area

Research performed on muscle has shown that the larger the physiologic cross-section of a muscle, the more tension is produced during a maximal contraction.[6,12] This relationship between the strength of a muscle contraction and the cross-sectional area is also influenced by anatomic factors, such as fiber orientation of the muscle. The fibers of most pennate muscles are arranged obliquely to the angle of pull, in contrast to fusiform muscles in which the fibers are typically arranged parallel to a central tendon. Although fusiform muscle contracts through a greater range of motion than pennate muscle, the cross-sectional area of pennate muscle is usually much greater. As a result, pennate muscle fibers have a greater potential for generating more tension during muscle contraction than fusiform muscle fibers (Fig. 5-2).[6]

Force Velocity

The velocity at which a muscle contracts affects the amount of force a muscle can develop. For concentric contractions, muscular tension tends to decrease as the velocity of the shortening contraction increases; as the velocity of the contraction decreases, muscular tension increases. Conversely, during eccentric exercise, the maximal contractile force tends to increase with increasing velocity. It has been theorized that the high stretching force that takes place during lengthening contractions produces an optimal overlap between the actin and myosin filaments, allowing optimal crossbridge formation and increased muscle tension.[6]

Muscle Fiber Type

Human skeletal muscle is composed of different percentages of fiber types. The percentage of fiber-type composition varies widely among muscles and among individuals.[13] Many classifications have been used to differentiate fiber types based on physiologic, histochemical, and biochemical properties.[14,15]

For many years, researchers used physiologic techniques to examine the contractile properties of muscle and the speed

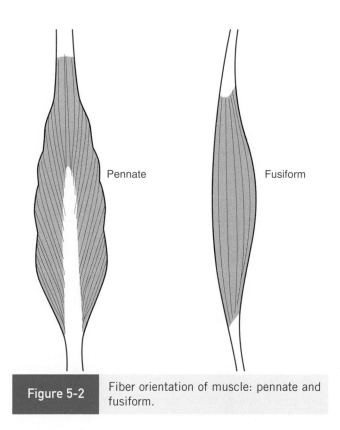

| Figure 5-2 | Fiber orientation of muscle: pennate and fusiform. |

at which a fiber could produce peak tension. Two fiber types were identified: fast twitch (FT) and slow twitch (ST). FT fibers develop high tension quickly but maintain that tension for only a short period of time. ST fibers develop less tension more slowly and are resistant to fatigue. While FT fibers are primarily recruited during short-term, high-intensity work (resistance training), ST fibers are primarily used for long-term, low-intensity work (endurance training).[12–15]

Recent research involving new staining techniques and electron microscopy has led to a classification system that defines three fiber types[14,15]: slow oxidative (or ST), fast oxidative glycolytic (or FT-fatigue resistant), and fast glycolytic (or FT-fast fatigable). Table 5-1 presents the structural and functional characteristics of these fibers.

Adaptation of Muscle in Response to Resistance Training

The increased ability of a muscle to generate increased force after resistance training is the result of two important changes: the adaptation of the muscle and the extent to which the motor unit can activate the muscle. Muscle adaptations include an increase in cross-sectional area, primarily caused by increase in size (hypertrophy) of the muscle fiber. This hypertrophy of the muscle fiber is caused by the increased synthesis of the myofibrillar proteins actin and myosin.[16–18]

TABLE 5-1 Structural and Functional Characteristics of Muscle Fibers

Characteristic	Slow Oxidative	Fast Oxidative Glycolytic	Fast Glycolytic
Diameter	Small	Intermediate	Large
Muscle color	Red	Red	White
Capillary bed	Dense	Dense	Sparse
Myoglobin content	High	Intermediate	Low
Speed of contraction	Slow	Fast	Fast
Rate of fatigue	Slow	Intermediate	Fast
Motor unit size	Small	Intermediate to large	Large
Conduction velocity	Slow	Fast	Fast
Mitochondria	Numerous	Numerous	Few

Improvement in the ability of the motor unit to activate the muscle after resistance training has been inferred on the basis of reports of increases in strength without changes in the cross-section of the muscle. The literature has referred to these "learned" changes in the nervous system as a result of strength training as "neural adaptation."[16,18] One common method for evaluating neural adaptation of muscle is to record the motor unit activity (via electromyography) during a maximal voluntary contraction before and after resistance training. Motor unit activation (via increases in multiple motor unit summation and wave summation) during maximal contraction has been shown to increase after muscle training.[16]

Muscle Loss

Adults who do not strength train lose between 5 and 7 pounds of muscle every decade.[2] Immobilization leads to atrophy as well. Functional loss is greater than the loss of muscle mass.[19] Although endurance exercise improves cardiovascular fitness, it does not prevent the loss of muscle tissue. Only muscle training maintains muscle mass and strength throughout the mid-life years.

Metabolic Rate

Because muscle is active tissue, muscle loss is accompanied by a reduction in resting metabolism rate. Information from Keyes[20] and Evans and Rosenberg[2] indicates that the average adult experiences a 2% to 5% reduction in metabolic rate every decade of life. Regular muscle training prevents muscle loss and the accompanying decrease in resting metabolic rate.

In fact, research reveals that adding 3 pounds of muscle mass increases resting metabolic rate by 7% and daily calorie requirements by 15%.[20] At rest, 1 pound of muscle requires about 35 calories per day for tissue maintenance; during exercise, muscle energy use increases dramatically. Adults who replace muscle through sensible strength training use more calories all day long, thereby reducing the likelihood of fat accumulation.

Muscle Mass

Because most adults do not perform resistance training, they need first to replace the muscle tissue that has been lost through inactivity. Fleg and Lakaha[21] reported that a standard strength-training program can increase total muscle area by 11.4%. This response is typical for men who train at 80% of 1 RM 3 days per week. This increase may result from hypertrophy (increases in fiber size), hyperplasia (increases in fiber number), or a combination.[23,24]

Body Composition

Misner et al[22] reported that after 8 weeks of training; adults who were given a constant diet were able to lower their percent body fat. Weight training with low-repetition, progressive-load activity increased fat-free weight through increased muscular development.

Bone Mineral Density

The effects of progressive-resistance exercise are similar for muscle tissue and bone tissue. The same muscle training stimulates increases in the bone mineral density of the upper femur after 4 months of exercise.[21] Appropriate application of progressive-resistance exercise is the key to increasing bone mineral density and connective tissue strength. Support for this premise comes from several studies that compared bone mineral densities of athletes with those of nonathletes.[25-28] These studies suggest that exercise programs specifically designed to stimulate bone growth should consider specificity of loading, progressive overload, and variation. Exercises should involve many muscle groups, direct the force vectors through the axial skeleton, and allow larger loads to be used. For example, running may be a good stimulus for the femur but would not be effective for the wrist.[29,30]

Glucose Metabolism

Hurley[3] reported a 23% increase in glucose uptake after 4 months of resistance training. Because poor glucose metabolism is associated with type 2 diabetes, improved glucose metabolism is an important benefit of regular-strength exercise. The rates of muscle glycogen use, muscle glucose uptake, and liver glucose output are directly related to the intensity and duration of exercise in combination with diet. Exercise programs alter skeletal muscle carbohydrate metabolism, enhancing insulin action and perhaps accounting for the benefits of exercise in insulin-resistant states.

Gastrointestinal Transit Time

A study by Koffler et al[31] showed a 56% increase in gastrointestinal transit time after 3 months of resistance training. This increase is a significant finding because delayed gastrointestinal transit time is related to a higher risk of colon cancer.

Resting Blood Pressure

Resistance training alone has been shown to significantly reduce resting blood pressure.[32,33] One study revealed that strength plus aerobic exercise is effective for improving blood pressure readings.[32] After 2 months of combined exercise, participants' systolic blood pressures dropped by 5 mm Hg and their diastolic blood pressures by 3 mm Hg.

Blood Lipid Levels

Although the effects of resistance training on blood lipid levels need further research, at least two studies revealed improved profiles after several weeks of strength exercise. Note that improvements in blood lipid levels are similar for both endurance and strength exercise.[34,35]

Exercise Training Principles

Dosage

Exercise dosage can by modified in a multitude of ways. Generally, increasing the intensity or amount of weight is the first adjustment; however, many other changes can be made—increasing sets and repetitions, decreasing rest intervals, and increasing frequency. The parameters are all related and in total are considered the volume of exercise.

Mode

Mode is considered the method of exercise (e.g., the use of free weights or rubber tubing).

Repetitions

Repetition is the number of times the exercise is repeated consistently. The number of repetitions is generally predetermined and make up one set of exercise (e.g., ten repetitions of a biceps curl).

Sets

Sets represent the performance of a particular exercise for a given number of consecutive repetitions, followed by a rest or a different exercise. For example, ten repetitions of an exercise, followed by a 2-minute rest, followed by another ten repetitions, would be considered two sets. Generally most exercise programs include two to three sets of each exercise.

Duration

Duration is considered the number of sets or repetitions of a specific exercise session and the amount of rest between sets.

Frequency

Frequency describes how often the exercises are performed. Frequency of exercise relates to the goal of the exercise program in consideration with the overall program.

Volume

Volume is the total number of repetitions performed during a training session multiplied by the resistance used.

Rest Intervals

The rest interval is another important variable. Generally rest periods vary from 1 minute to 3 minutes depending on the purpose of the exercise program.

Overload

Within the human body, all cells possess the ability to adapt to external stimuli, and general adaptations occur continually. In addition to everyday adjustments, adaptation also occurs more specifically as a result of training. When an increased training load challenges an individual's current level of fitness, a response by the body occurs as an adaptation (such as an increase in muscle strength) to the stimulus of the training load. This increase in training load that leads to an adaptation in muscle is called overload. The initial response is fatigue and adaptation to the training load. Overload causes fatigue, and recovery and adaptation allow the body to overcompensate and reach a higher level of fitness.[17]

Intensity and Volume

The stress placed on the body in training, both physiologic and psychologic, is called the training load or stimulus. The training load is quantified as the intensity and volume of training, which are integrally related and cannot be separated. One depends on the other at all times.[36] Intensity and volume are defined in this section, and their use in a training model (periodization) is presented later in this chapter.

Intensity is the strength of the stimulus or concentration of work per unit of time, often thought of as the quality of effort. Examples of the quantification of intensity include endurance or speed expressed as a percent of maximum oxygen consumption, maximum heart rate speed (in meters per second), frequency of movement (stride rate per activity), strength (kilograms or pounds per lift), or jumping and throwing (height or distance per effort).

Also referred to as the extent of training, volume is the amount (quantity) of training performed or the sum of all repetitions or their duration. Examples of the quantification of volume include kilograms lifted, meters run (sprint training), kilometers or miles run (distance training), number of throws or jumps taken, number of sets and repetitions performed, or minutes or hours of training time.[36]

The beginner or the deconditioned individual should use small loads to avoid too much overload and possible injury. Care must be taken not to recommend too great a volume increase per training session, which can lead to excess fatigue, low efficiency of training, and increased risk of injury. Therefore, if the client requires more training but the volume of training per session is already adequate, the best alternative is to increase the number of training sessions per week, rather than increase the volume per training session. This concept relates to the idea of density of training, which is the number of units of work distributed per time period of training.[36] More information on intensity and volume will be presented later in this chapter.

Specificity

The concept of specificity is that the nature of the training load determines the training effect. To train most effectively, the method must be aimed specifically at developing the type of abilities that are dominant in a given sport. In other words, each type of exercise has its own specific training effect, which results in the specific adaptations to imposed demands principle. The load must be specific to the individual and to the activity for which he or she is training. As a corollary to the law of specificity, general training must always precede specific training.[36,37]

Cross-training

The principle of cross-training suggests that despite the idea of specificity of training, athletes may improve performance in one mode of exercise by training in another mode. Although cross-training occasionally provides some transfer effects, the effects are not as great as those that could be obtained by increasing the specific training by a similar amount.

For example, a factory worker may want to participate in an alternative training session that would continue to help increase her aerobic endurance, and she would like to pursue something different from walking to put variety in her exercise program. This walker may decide to use swimming as a cross-training technique to meet her goals. Although the worker may benefit from swimming, the cross-training activity will not increase her performance in walking as much as if she had spent the same time actually walking. In other words, the cross-training (swimming) of

this individual may have increased her performance to a certain level; however, if she had spent the same amount of time and intensity walking (specific training), she would have realized even more gains.

Although cross-training benefits are sometimes observed, they are usually noted in physiologic measures and rarely in performance. Therefore, cross-training is an inefficient method for increasing performance capacity.[36]

Overtraining

A progressive increase in training stimulus is necessary for improvements in fitness levels. However, in attempts to achieve this increased level of fitness, an individual may not take sufficient time to fully recuperate after chronic bouts of training. Overtraining is thought to be caused by training loads that are too demanding on the individual's ability to adapt, resulting in fatigue, possible substitution patterns, and injury. Overtraining occurs when the body's adaptive mechanisms repetitively fail to cope with chronic training stress, resulting in performance deterioration instead of performance improvement.[38]

Overtraining may lead to physiologic and psychomotor depression, chronic fatigue, depressed appetite, weight loss, insomnia, decreased libido, increased blood pressure, and muscle soreness. In addition, other metabolic, hormonal, muscular, hypothalamic, and cardiovascular changes often accompany the overtrained state. Overtraining can be characterized by negative affective states such as anxiety, depression, anger, lack of self-confidence, and decreased vigor.[37]

Studies have used a variety of terminology to describe overtraining and its affiliated states. For example, Mackinnon and Hooper[39] describe the following progressive stages: staleness, overtraining, and burnout. Mackinnon et al[40] later suggested that overtraining can lead to staleness, but overtraining reflects a process and staleness represents an outcome or product. Despite the continuing debate of semantics, try to keep the terminology simple when speaking to an individual unfamiliar with the subject.

Not surprisingly, rest has been suggested to alleviate many of the symptoms caused by overtraining. After an intense training session, an individual typically recuperates within 24 hours. Other methods to help avoid staleness (which can be caused by overtraining) include mini break periods and occasional changes in routine; furthermore, the client may benefit if the pressure to perform is eased. Severe overtraining and staleness may require a long recovery period, which should be expected to be slow.[39]

Modifications to the workout may help prevent overtraining. Training should include stresses to the metabolic pathways and motor skills needed for the person's particular activity. All cross-training should be secondary. For example, an activity primarily requiring power or speed may compromise training for cardiovascular endurance.

Overtraining should not be considered as an absolute state. In actuality, overtraining and any of its related states should be viewed as a continuum: from optimally recuperated to extremely overtrained. It is conceivable that a person may be slightly overtrained yet still be able to achieve modest gains in performance. Obviously, the more desirable situation would be optimal recuperation and consequently greater gains.[39]

Precautions

The physical therapist (PT) should consider several precautions when developing a muscle-training program. For cardiovascular reasons, the client should not hold his breath during exertion (Valsalva maneuver). This maneuver can be avoided during muscle training by encouraging the client to breathe properly during exercise. Encourage him/her to count, talk, or breathe rhythmically during exercise. The individual can also be instructed to exhale during the lift and inhale during recovery.

Muscle soreness may develop as a result of exercise and should be of relatively short duration. DOMS develops 24 to 48 hours after exercise and resolves within 1 week. Eccentric exercise causes more DOMS than concentric exercise. It can be reduced by the client performing both warmup and cooldown stretching exercises. In addition, the client should be cautioned about potential soreness owing to exercise.

Fatigue and overtraining, described earlier, are important considerations in the design of any exercise program. Adequate recovery should be built into the program.

CLINICAL GUIDELINES

Training Programs

Training programs address all types of muscle action, including static and dynamic activities. More detailed information on isometric, isotonic, and isokinetic exercise (including suggestions for clinical use) is presented in Chapters 6 through 9.

The concept of open- and closed-kinetic–chain exercises has received considerable attention in the scientific literature, particularly in terms of rehabilitation.[41,42] A closed-kinetic–chain (CKC) exercise is one in which the distal segment is fixed and a force is transmitted directly through the foot or the hand in an action, such as a squat or a pushup. An open-kinetic–chain (OKC) exercise is one in which the distal segment is not fixed and the segment can move freely, such as leg extensions. OKC and CKC exercises produce markedly different muscle recruitment and joint motions. Most human movements, such as walking and running, contain a combination of open- and closed-chain aspects.[42] The PT and physical therapist assistant

(PTA) should address both CKC and OKC activities for the rehabilitation of an individual (Chapters 6 through 9).

Exercise Guidelines

To be successful, an exercise program must be effective, safe, and motivating to the participant. To be effective and achieve physiologic benefits, an exercise routine must have the appropriate mode, duration, frequency, and intensity.

In addition to the training period, individuals should be instructed to include 5 to 10 minutes of warmup and cooldown exercises in their routines. Programs should be individually tailored to the needs and interests of participants. Any exercise routine that includes adequate warmup and cooldown periods, incorporates proper stretching exercises, and is designed to progress slowly in intensity is unlikely to result in injuries.

An exercise routine must have some motivational appeal if individuals are to adhere to the program long enough to achieve the desired results. A program with incremental, achievable goals and a mechanism to measure progress is likely to encourage participation. Perhaps of even greater importance is the ongoing examination of the participant's response to exercise, including monitoring for changes in balance, strength, and flexibility.

The American College of Sports Medicine[43] recommendations for resistance training exercise are presented in Table 5-2. Further recommendations for the warmup period are presented in Table 5-3.

TABLE 5-2 American College of Sports Medicine Recommendations for Resistance-Training Exercise

Perform a minimum of eight to 10 exercises that train the major muscle groups.

Workouts should not be too long; programs longer than 1 hour are associated with high dropout rates.

Perform one set of eight to 12 repetitions to the point of volitional fatigue.

More sets may elicit slightly greater strength gains, but additional improvement is relatively small.

Perform exercises at least 2 days per week.

More frequent training may elicit slightly greater strength gains, but additional improvement is relatively small.

Adhere closely to the specific exercise techniques.

Perform exercises through the full range of motion (ROM).

Elderly trainees should perform exercises in the maximum ROM that does not elicit pain or discomfort.

Perform exercises in a controlled manner.

Maintain a normal breathing pattern.

Exercise with a training partner when possible.

A partner can provide feedback, assistance, and motivation.

TABLE 5-3   American College of Sports Medicine
             Recommendations for Warmup Exercises

Perform 12 to 15 repetitions with no weight before the
workout set, with 30 seconds to 4 minutes of rest before
the workout set.
A specific warmup is more effective for weight training than
a general warmup. Example of a general warmup: jumping
jacks.
No warmup set is required for high-repetition exercises,
which are not as intense and serve as a warmup in
themselves. Example: 20–50 repetitions for abdominal
training.
Perform a second warmup if the muscles and joints involved
may be more susceptible to injury. Example: squats and
bench press may require a second warmup.

Periodization—Advanced Resistance Training

Periodization is the gradual cycling of specificity, intensity,
and volume of training to achieve optimal development of
performance capacities; it consists of periodic changes of
the objectives, tasks, and content of training. Periodization
is a high-level concept, most commonly used in training
athletes. Although used primarily with athletes, the concept
of changing volume and intensity can be used for all patients. Periodization can be explained as the division of the
training year to meet specific objectives. The objectives
make up a year-long program for optimal improvement in
performance and preparation for a definitive climax to a
competitive season. The goals are met through systematic
planning of all segments of the training year or season. Periodization prevents a plateau response from occurring
during a prolonged training regimen by providing manipulation of the different variables and continual stimulation to
the client in phases or cycles.[44,45]

The trend has been to increase both the intensity and
volume of training at all levels of development, making the
proper manipulation of these two variables extremely important when avoiding overtraining and breakdown. Increases in both intensity and volume do not necessarily
yield improved performances. To realize meaningful results while observing the law of specificity, exercises should
be performed near the absolute intensity limit only 55% to
60% of the total training time during a preparation period.
The intensity is increased to 80% to 90% during a competitive period.

The level of achievement of the client determines the
proportion and distribution of intensity and volume. For
the beginner, progress is illustrated by a linear increase in
intensity and volume; however, volume should take
precedence. At the elite level, a linear increase will not

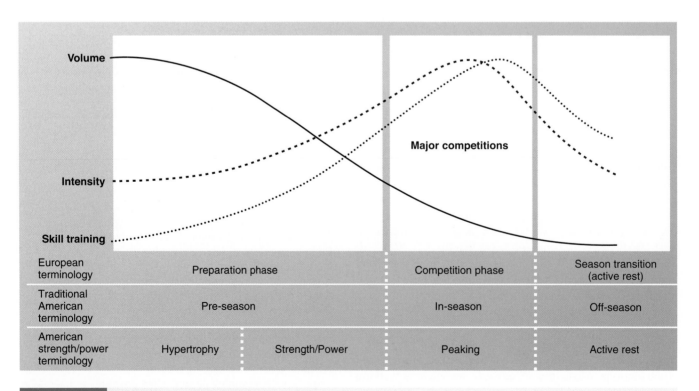

Figure 5-3   Periodization training phases.

yield desired results. At this level, sudden jumps in volume and intensity (load leaping) may be required to simulate further improvement. It is important to understand the relationship of volume and intensity to the major demands of the event. When speed and strength are the main demands, intensity must be emphasized to facilitate improvement; this is especially true during the competitive period of the season. When endurance is the main demand, volume represents the principal stimulus for progress.

Periodized training, in essence, is a training plan that changes the workout sessions at regular time intervals. Figure 5-3 presents the classic interaction of intensity and volume and how these variables can be manipulated to emphasize the different aspects of training by "phasing," or cycling the workouts. The following sections explain Figure 5-3 and present a suggested training program that uses periodization for high-performance athletes.[44,45]

Preparation Phase (Preseason)

Hypertrophy

The goal of the hypertrophy subphase is a major gain in strength to provide the foundation for obtaining power, muscular endurance, speed, and skill in later phases of the periodization cycle. This subphase encourages neuromuscular adaptation by using high repetitions of many exercises (large volume) and therefore demanding maximal neuromuscular recruitment. The training should be performed three times per week. By applying the correct stress level to the muscles being trained and allowing adequate recuperation/regeneration time (2 to 3 minutes), maximum muscular hypertrophy can be achieved. Training parameters used in this phase are outlined in Table 5-4.

Strength/Power

During the strength/power subphase, muscle strength and power are the main training goals. The role of this subphase is to make the difficult transition from the emphasis on volume to an emphasis on intensity and skill. Power refers to the ability of the neuromuscular system to produce the greatest amount of force in the shortest amount of time. Specific power training needs to be incorporated to convert maximum strength gains into explosive, dynamic athletic skill. Careful planning can help enhance power output while maximum strength is maintained.

Several methods exist that can be used to improve power (e.g., free weights, plyometrics). These loads must be performed dynamically to create maximal acceleration. The number of repetitions depends on the training stimulus; the range is six to 20. The PT must be extremely selective when choosing the appropriate exercises for power training. The program should consist of no more than two to four exercises. The rest interval should be 3 to 5 seconds.

TABLE 5-4 Principles of Periodization Training for Athletes

Preparation Phase

Hypertrophy
  Occurs during the early stages of off-season preparation
  Goals are to develop a strength/endurance base for future, more intense training
  Training begins with low-intensity skills at high volume
  Repetitions are gradually decreased and resistance levels are gradually increased
Strength/power
  Intensity level is gradually increased to >70% of the athlete's one-repetition maximum for five to eight repetitions
  Volume of training is decreased and intensity is slowly increased; training for intensity and skill are increased and speed work intensifies to near competition pace

Competition Phase

Early maintenance (early in season)
  Goal is to maintain strength while gradually reducing total volume
  Program becomes sport specific
Peaking (late in season)
  Greater reduction of volume as maximum performance date or season nears
  Reduction of load to ≤70%
  May totally stop resistance training 3 to 5 days before peak competition

Transition Phase
  Goal is to allow body to recover from rigors of competitive season
  Resistance training is stopped to allow muscles, tendons, and ligaments to heal
  Performing other activities (outside of lifting) is preferred over total rest; cross-training

Training parameters used in this subphase of the preparation phase are outlined in Table 5-2.

Competition Phase (In Season, Peaking)

To avoid deleterious detraining effects during the competitive season, the athlete must continue to follow a sport-specific resistance-training program. The resistance-training aspect of the program, however, progresses to a minimum maintenance phase, while the training for specific skills needed to participate in the sport takes priority, increasing in intensity and progressing to a maximum phase. The specific program is based on the dominant physiologic demands of the sport (power or muscular endurance).

The sports-specific maintenance program is performed in conjunction with other tactical and technical skills.

▼ ▼ ▼ GERIATRIC PERSPECTIVES ▼ ▼ ▼

■ The ability to generate an appropriate force of contraction appears to decline by 0.75% to 1.0% per year between the ages of 30 to 50 years, followed by a more accelerated decline in later years (15% per decade between 50 and 70 years; 30% loss between 70 and 80 years).[1,2] Maximum isometric force, contraction time, relaxation time, and fatigability demonstrate different degrees of age-related change.[3–5] The loss of muscle strength with aging is largely associated with the decrease in total muscle mass that is known to occur after age 30 (age of peak performance). This loss of total muscle mass is the result of a combination of physiologic phenomena, including specific decreases in the size and number of muscle fibers, changes in biochemical capacity and sensitivity, changes in soft tissue and fat, and a general loss of water content in connective tissue.[6]

■ Age-related loss of muscle strength is not uniform across muscle groups and types. In general, muscle strength of the lower extremities declines faster than muscle strength of the upper extremities. Isometric strength (force generated against an unyielding resistance) is better maintained than dynamic strength (1 RM contraction). The disproportionate decline in muscle strength may be more related to disuse than to aging.[7]

■ Functionally, the age-related loss of muscle strength results in a general slowing down of muscle contraction and fatigability, which affects the type and duration of muscle training. Training programs that use slow-velocity contractions, repeated low-level resistance, and contractions over a range (from small to large) improve the strength outcome. To avoid an increase in intrathoracic pressure, holding one's breath should be avoided when lifting weight.

■ Males are more able to maintain muscle strength than females. However, when the ratio of lean muscle to fat, weight, and height differences are considered, the sex differences are less obvious.

■ Based on a review of existing literature, Welle[8] recommended that the intensity of muscle training be kept at about 80% of maximum capacity, two to three sets of eight to 12 repetitions for each exercise at this level of intensity with rest periods between sets. This regime should be repeated two to three times a week. As maximum capacity increases, the amount of resistance should be increased accordingly.

■ Increased muscle oxidative capacity, increased use of circulating nutrients, and strength gains from 30% to 100% have been documented in older and frail adults after strength training.[8,9] Risk of late-onset muscle soreness may be increased in older adults secondary to the slowed reabsorption of lactates. In addition, certain medications may affect blood flow to the exercising muscle; therefore, a good history and screen are strongly advised before a muscle training program is initiated for older individuals. Unfortunately, no standardized screening protocol exists to identify which individuals should avoid muscle training. In the current medical system, routine screening using exercise testing equipment is not cost effective. One option is to more closely screen individuals with specific conditions, such as hypertension, using electrocardiogram and blood pressure monitoring during a weight-lifting stress test.[10]

■ Endurance or fatigability of the aged muscle is much greater than in young muscles. Using an animal model, Brooks and Faulkner[11] reported a maximum sustained power of old muscles to 45% of the muscles in young mice. However, if muscle fatigue and endurance are examined relative to strength, older individuals were found to be comparable to younger individuals.[12]

■ Resistance training does result in strength gains in older adults; however, the relationships of increased strength to improvement in physical performance and to the remediation of disabilities have not been clearly defined.[13]

■ Resistive training has been tolerated well by older adults.[14] Judge[15] recommended a strengthening program using moderate velocities of movements with graded resistance, placing emphasis on the following muscle groups: gluteals, hamstrings, quadriceps, ankle dorsiflexors, finger flexors, biceps, triceps, and combined shoulder and elbow musculature.

1. Era P, Lyyra AL, Viitasalo J, et al. Determinants of isometric muscle strength in men of different ages. *Eur J Appl Physiol.* 1992;64:84–91.
2. LaForest S, St-Pierre DMM, Cyr J, et al. Effects of age and regular exercise on muscle strength and endurance. *Eur J Appl Physiol.* 1990;60:104–111.
3. Brooks SV, Faulkner JA. Contractile properties of skeletal muscles from young, adult and aged mice. *J Physiol.* 1988;404:71–82.
4. Frontera WR, Hughes VA, Lutz KJ, et al. A cross-sectional study of muscle strength and mass in 45- to 78-yr-old men and women. *J Appl Physiol.* 1991;71:644–650.
5. Overend TJ, Cunningham DA, Kramer JF, et al. Knee extensor and knee flexor strength: cross-sectional area ratios in young and elderly men. *J Gerontol Med Sci.* 1992;47:M204–M210.
6. Gabbard C. *Life long motor development.* Dubuque, IA: Brown; 1992.

7. Spirduso WW. *Physical dimensions of aging*. Champaign, IL: Human Kinetics; 1995.

8. Welle S. Resistance training in older persons. *Clin Geriatr*. 1998;6:1–9.

9. Fiatarone MA, O'Neill EF, Ryan ND, et al. Exercise training and nutritional supplementation for physical frailty in very frail elderly people. *N Engl J Med*. 1994;330:1769–1775.

10. Evans WJ. Reversing sarcopenia: how weight training can build strength and vitality. *Geriatrics*. 1996;51:46–53.

11. Brooks SV, Faulkner JA. Skeletal muscle weakness in old age: underlying mechanisms. *Med Sci Sports Exerc*. 1994; 26:432–439.

12. Lindström B, Lexell J, Gerdle B, et al. Skeletal muscle fatigue and endurance in young and old men and women. *J Gerontol Bio Sci*. 1997;52A:B59–B66.

13. McClure J. Understanding the relationship between strength and mobility in frail older persons: a review of the literature. *Top Geriatr Rehabil*. 1996;11:20–37.

14. Porter MM, Vandervoort AA. High intensity strength training for the older adult: a review. *Top Geriatr Rehabil*. 1995;10: 61–74.

15. Judge JO. Resistance training. *Top Geriatr Rehabil*. 1993;8: 38–50.

Therefore, the number of exercises must be kept low (two to three) and only two strength-training sessions should be performed each week. The length of the training sessions should be 20 to 30 minutes. The total number of sets performed is kept low, usually one to four, depending on whether power or muscular endurance is being trained. For power and maximum strength, two to four sets should be used. For muscle endurance, one to two sets of higher repetitions (10 to 15) should be performed and the rest intervals should be longer than normally suggested (Table 5-4).

Transition Phase (Off Season, Active Rest)

After a long competitive season, athletes are physiologically and psychologically fatigued. They need to engage in an active rest period for at least 4 weeks. The transition phase bridges the gap between two annual training periodization cycles. During this phase athletes continue to train so they do not lose their overall fitness level. Training should occur two to three times per week at low intensity (40% to 50%). Stress is undesirable during this phase (Table 5-4).

TECHNIQUES

Specific techniques for improving muscular strength are extensive, and no one universal approach has been established as being the best. The components of a resistive-training program include the amount of resistance, number of repetitions, number of sets, and frequency of training. Regardless of the techniques used, the level of the participant must be examined and a satisfactory overload component planned. The amount of resistance and the number of repetitions must be sufficient to challenge the muscle to work at a higher intensity than normal.

Later chapters in this book build on the background presented here. There, the reader will find details, specific techniques and protocols, and case studies that pull all this information together, allowing for a more complete understanding of the effective and efficient management and intervention for the client.

SUMMARY

- Individuals gain many health and fitness benefits from participation in a resistance-training program.

- Connective tissue, called the endomysium, serves as a cover for the single muscle fiber. Muscle fibers are bundled together into fasciculi, which are covered by perimysium. A number of fasciculus bundles make up the belly of the muscle, which is covered by the epimysium.

- The performance of muscle is affected by motor unit activation, cross-sectional area of the muscle, and the force–velocity relationship. Muscle is composed of different fiber types, including slow oxidative, fast glycolytic, and fast oxidative glycolytic. Training allows the muscle to generate more force, which is the result of increased muscle size and neural adaptation.

- Training principles that affect performance include overload, intensity and volume, specificity, cross-training, overtraining, and precautions. A wide variety of training programs lead to increased muscle strength. Such programs use, for example, isometric, isotonic, and isokinetic contractions; open- and closed-chain activities; and periodization. A more complete understanding of the structures and function of muscle combined with a base knowledge of resistance-training principles allows the PTA to guide a client in an effective and efficient muscle-training exercise program.

PEDIATRIC PERSPECTIVES

- Absolute muscular strength increases linearly with chronologic age from early childhood in both sexes until age 13 or 14 years. Total muscle mass increases more than five times in males and 3.5 times in females from childhood to adulthood. Increases in strength relate closely to increases in mass during growth throughout childhood.[1]

- During adolescence a significant acceleration occurs in the development of strength, most notably in boys. In boys, peak growth in muscle mass occurs both during and after peak weight gain, followed by gains in strength. In girls, peak strength development generally occurs before peak weight gain.[1,2]

- Weight training in children has been controversial because of concerns regarding potential injury and questionable efficacy in actual strength improvements, owing to low-circulating androgens.[3] In particular, experts have noted the potential for injuries (epiphyseal fractures, disc injuries, bony injuries to the low back) from heavy muscle overload in children. Therefore, moderate strength training is recommended; maximal resistance training should be avoided because of the sensitivity of joint structures, especially the epiphyses. In fact, most researchers agree that maximal lifts of any kind should be avoided in the prepubescent.[4,5]

- Recommendations from various sources regarding strength training of children are relatively consistent and include the following requirements:[1,2,4–7]

  - Close, trained supervision during training.

  - Employment of concentric muscle actions with high repetitions (eight to 12 repetitions; no less than six to eight) and relatively low resistance.

  - Adequate warmup before training.

  - Emphasis on proper form throughout exercise performance.

  - Inclusion of stretching.

- Furthermore, children should not be allowed to exercise to exhaustion. To avoid injury, it is essential that any strength-training equipment or machinery used during training be adjustable or adaptable to the proper size for children.[1]

- Available evidence indicates that with proper strength training, children can improve muscular strength without adverse effects on bone, muscle, or connective tissues.[4,6,7] Children of both sexes may realize increases in muscle strength as great as 40% as a result of resistance training.[4]

- Resistive training in prepubescents has been shown to increase strength without hypertrophy because hormone levels are not high enough to support hypertrophy.[8] Increases in strength that occur in these children as a result of strength training are hypothesized to be the result of neural adaptation or increased coordination of muscle groups during exercise.[5,8]

- There are many proposed benefits of strength training in children, including increased strength and power, improved local muscular endurance, improved balance and proprioception, prevention of injury, positive influence on sport performance, and enhancement of body image.[6,8] Additionally, training with weights can be fun, safe, and appropriate for a child.[2,6]

Basic Guidelines for Resistance Exercise Progression in Children.[a,b]

Age (years)	Considerations
≤7	Introduce child to basic exercises with little or no weight; develop the concept of a training session; teach exercise techniques; progress from body-weight calisthenics, partner exercises, and lightly resisted exercises; keep volume low
8 to 10	Gradually increase number of exercises; practice exercise technique in all lifts; start gradual progressive loading of exercises; keep exercises simple; gradually increase training volume; carefully monitor toleration to exercise stress
11 to 13	Teach all basic exercise techniques; continue progressive loading of each exercise; emphasize exercise techniques; introduce more advanced exercises with little or no resistance
14 to 15	Progress to more advanced youth programs in resistance exercise; add sport-specific components; emphasize exercise techniques; increase volume
≥16	Move child to entry-level adult programs after all background knowledge has been mastered and a basic level of training experience has been gained

[a]If a child of any age has no previous experience, start the program at previous age level and move the child to more advanced levels as exercise toleration, skills, amount of training time, and understanding permit.

[b]Reprinted with permission from Thein L. The child and adolescent athlete. In: Zachezewski JE, Magee DJ, Quillen WS. *Athletic injuries and rehabilitation.* Philadelphia: WB Saunders; 1996: 933–956.

1. American College of Sports Medicine. *ACSM's guidelines for exercise testing and prescription*. 6th ed. Baltimore: Williams & Wilkins; 2000.

2. American Academy of Pediatrics, Committee on Sports Medicine. Strength, training, weight and power lifting, and body building by children and adolescents. *Pediatrics*. 1990; 86:801–803.

3. Campbell SK. *Physical therapy for children*. Philadelphia: WB Saunders; 1995.

4. Sewall L, Michelli LJ. Strength training for children. *J Pediatr Orthop*. 1986;6:143–146.

5. Thein L. The child and adolescent athlete. In: Zachezewski JE, Magee DJ, Quillen WS. *Athletic injuries and rehabilitation*. Philadelphia: WB Saunders; 1996:933–956.

6. Kraemer WJ, Fleck SJ. *Strength training for young athletes*. Champaign, IL: Human Kinetics; 1993.

7. Rians CB, Weltman A, Janney C, et al. Strength training for pre-pubescent males: is it safe? *Am J Sports Med*. 1987; 15:483–488.

8. Falkel JE, Cipriani DJ. Physiological principles of resistance training and rehabilitation. In: Zachezewski JE, Magee DJ, Quillen WS. *Athletic injuries and rehabilitation*. Philadelphia: WB Saunders, 1996:206–226.

References

1. Vogel JA. Introduction to the symposium: physiological responses and adaptations to resistance exercise. *Med Sci Sports Exerc*. 1988;20:S131–S134.

2. Evans W, Rosenberg I. *Biomarkers*. New York: Simon & Schuster; 1992.

3. Hurley B. Does strength training improve health status? *Strength Cond J*. 1994;16:7–13.

4. Wilmore JH, Costill DC. *Physiology of sport and exercise*. 2nd ed. Champaign, IL: Human Kinetics; 1999.

5. Lehmkuhl D. Local factors in muscle performance. *Phys Ther*. 1966;46:473–484.

6. Irion G. *Physiology: the basis of clinical practice*. Thorofare, NJ: Slack; 2000.

7. American College of Sports Medicine. *ACSM's guidelines for exercise testing and prescription*. 6th ed. Baltimore: Williams & Wilkins; 2000.

8. Freund HJ. Motor unit and muscle activity in voluntary motor control. *Physiol Rev*. 1983;63:387–436.

9. English A, Wolf SL. The motor unit. Anatomy and physiology. *Phys Ther*. 1982;62:1763–1772.

10. Milner-Brown HS, Stein RB, Yemm R. The orderly recruitment of human motor units during voluntary isometric contractions. *J Physiol*. 1973;230:359–370.

11. Kukula CG, Clamann HP. Comparison of the recruitment and discharge properties of motor units in human brachial biceps and adductor pollicis during isometric contractions. *Brain Res*. 1981;219:45–55.

12. Young A, Stokes M, Round JM. The effect of high resistance training of the strength and cross-sectional area of the human quadriceps. *Eur J Clin Invest*. 1983;13:411–417.

13. Gollnick PD, Matoba H. The muscle fiber compositions of skeletal muscle as a predictor of athletic success. *Am J Sports Med*. 1984;12:212–217.

14. Peter JB, Barnard RJ, Edgerton VR, et al. Metabolic profiles of three fiber types of skeletal muscle. *Biochemistry*. 1972;11: 2627–2633.

15. Burke RE, Levine DN, Tsairis P, et al. Physiological types and histochemical profiles in motor units of the cat gastrocnemius. *J Physiol*. 1973;234:723–748.

16. Sale DG. Neural adaptation to resistance training. *Med Sci Sports Exerc*. 1988;20:S135–S145.

17. Fleck SJ, Kraemer WJ. Resistance training: physiological responses and adaptations [Part 2 of 4]. *Phys Sportmed*. 1988;16: 75–107.

18. Fleck SJ, Kraemer WJ. Resistance training: physiological response and adaptations [Part 3 of 4]. *Phys Sportmed*. 1988;16: 108–124.

19. Kannus P, Jozsa L, Natri A, et al. Effects of training, immobilization and remobilization on tendons. *Scan J Med Sci Sports*. 1997;7:67–71.

20. Keyes A. Basal metabolism and age of adult men. *Metabolism*. 1973;22:579–582.

21. Fleg HL, Lakaha EG. Role of muscle loss in the age-associated reduction in VO_2 max. *J Appl Physiol*. 1988;60:1147–1151.

22. Misner JE, Boileau RA, Massey BH, et al. Alterations in the body composition of adult men during selected physical training programs. *J Am Geriatr Soc*. 1974;22:33–37.

23. Antonio J, Gonyea WJ. Skeletal muscle fiber hyperplasia. *Med Sci Sports Exerc* 1993;25:1333–1345.

24. MacDougall DJ. Hypertrophy or hyperplasia. In: Komi PV, ed. *Strength and power in sports*. Oxford: Blackwell Scientific Publications; 1992.

25. Dudley DA, Dyamil R. Incompatibility of endurance and strength modes of exercises [abstract]. *Med Sci Sports Exerc*. 1985:17:184.

26. Fiore CF, Corttini E, Fargetta C, et al. The effects of muscle-building exercise on forearm bone mineral content and osteoblast activity in drug free and anabolic steroids self administering young men. *Bone Miner*. 1991;13:77–83.

27. Granhead H, Johnson R, Hansson T. The loads on the lumbar spine during extreme weight lifting. *Spine*. 1987;12: 146–149.

28. White MK, Martin RB, Yeater RA, et al. The effects of exercise on postmenopausal women. *Int Orthop*. 1984;7:209–214.

29. Lane N, Bevier W, Bouxsein M, et al. Effect of exercise intensity on bone mineral. *Med Sci Sports Exerc*. 1988;20:S51.

30. Duncan CS, Blimkie CJ, Cowell C, et al. Bone mineral density in adolescent female athletes: relationship to exercise type and muscle strength. *Med Sci Sports Exerc*. 2002;34: 286–294.

31. Koffler K, Menkes A, Redmond A, et al. Strength training accelerates gastrointestinal transit in middle-aged and older men. *Med Sci Sports Exerc.* 1992;24:415–419.

32. Harris K, Holly R. Physiological response to circuit weight training in borderline hypertensive subjects. *Med Sci Sports Exerc.* 1987;19:246–252.

33. Fleck SJ. Cardiovascular adaptation to resistance training. *Med Sci Sports Exerc.* 1988;20:S146–S151.

34. Stone M, Blessing D, Byrd R, et al. Physiological effects of a short term resistive training program on middle aged untrained men. *Natl Strength Cond Assoc J.* 1982;4:16–20.

35. Hurley B, Hagberg J, Goldberg A, et al. Resistance training can reduce coronary risk factors without altering VO$_2$ max or percent body fat. *Med Sci Sports Exerc.* 1988;10:150–154.

36. Baechle TR. *Essentials of strength training and conditioning.* Champaign, IL: Human Kinetics; 1994.

37. Kegerreis S. The construction and implementation of functional progression as a component of athletic rehabilitation. *J Orthop Sport Phys Ther.* 1983;5:14–19.

38. Fleck SJ, Kraemer WJ. *Designing resistance training programs.* Champaign, IL: Human Kinetics; 1997.

39. Mackinnon LT, Hooper SL. Plasma glutamine and upper respiratory tract infection during intensified training in swimmers. *Med Sci Sports Exerc.* 1996;28:285–290.

40. Mackinnon LT, Hooper SL, Jones S, et al. Hormonal, immunological and hematological responses to intensified training in swimmers. *Med Sci Sports Exerc.* 1997;29: 1637–1645.

41. Beynnon D, Johnson RJ. Anterior cruciate ligament injury rehabilitation in athletics. *Sports Med.* 1996;22:54–64.

42. Palmitier RA, Kai-Nan A, Scott SG, et al. Kinetic chain exercise in knee rehabilitation. *Sports Med.* 1991;11:402–413.

43. American College of Sports Medicine. *Guidelines for exercise testing and prescription.* 6th ed. Baltimore: Williams & Wilkins; 2000.

44. Bompa TO. *Periodization of strength: the new wave in strength training.* Toronto: Varitas; 1993.

45. Bompa TO. *Theory and of training: the key to athletic performance.* 3rd ed. Dubuque, IA: Kendall/Hunt; 1994.

CHAPTER 6

Open-Chain–Resistance Training

William D. Bandy, PT, PhD, SCS, ATC

OBJECTIVES

Upon completion of this chapter, the reader will be able to:

- Define the three types of muscle contractions for open-chain–resistance training.

- Discuss concentric muscle contractions in delayed-onset muscle soreness (DOMS).

- Discuss the role of eccentric muscle contractions in DOMS.

- Identify appropriate clinical guidelines concerning limitations, advantages, and precautions of isometric, isotonic, and isokinetic exercise.

- Discuss proper clinical technique for isometric, isotonic, and isokinetic exercise of the upper and lower extremities performed with and without clinician assistance.

TABLE 6-1 Types of Muscle Contractions for Open-Chain–Resistance Training

Type of Contraction	Action Possible	Example
Isometric	Tension developed; no movement	Pushing against a fixed object (e.g., another person, another body part, a wall)
Isotonic	Concentric, eccentric	Using resistance (e.g., free weights, dumbbells, elastic tubing, cuff weights, pulleys)
Isokinetic	Concentric, eccentric	Using a dynamometer (e.g., Biodex, Cybex)

The rehabilitation of selected pathologies has been documented in the areas of plyometrics, closed-kinetic–chain activities, and functional rehabilitation.[1] Although quite valuable for selected pathologies, these activities put tremendous stress on the joint structures and surrounding muscles. If they are incorporated into the rehabilitation program too soon, tissue damage and delayed healing can occur. Proper progression to these more aggressive activities is of considerable importance. It has been recommended that "the neuromuscular system . . . be adequately trained to tolerate the imposed stress during functional tasks."[1] Adequate training includes the proper use of a comprehensive, progressive, open-chain resistance-training program.

An integral part of a progressive rehabilitation protocol is the proper implementation of an open-chain resistance-training program. The physical therapist (PT) is frequently responsible for designing, monitoring, and supervising a resistance-training program with the goal of increasing muscular strength. Appropriate use of open-chain–resistance training allows a safe progression to a more aggressive rehabilitation program.

Despite recent excitement about aggressive rehabilitation programs used in the advanced stages of healing, it is imperative that the PT and physical therapist assistant (PTA) remember the basic principles of open-chain–resistance training, including the three primary types of exercise:

isometric, isotonic, and isokinetic (Table 6-1). This chapter presents a brief review of the adaptation of muscle to resistance training and emphasizes the appropriate use of each type of exercise in the clinical setting.

SCIENTIFIC BASIS

Isometric Exercise

The term *isometric* means "same or constant" (*iso*) "length" (*metric*). In other words, a muscle that contracts isometrically is one in which tension is developed but no change occurs in the joint angle and the change in muscle length is minimal. The joint angle does not change because the external resistance against which the muscle is working is equal to or greater than the tension developed by the muscle. In this case, no external movement occurs, but considerable tension develops in the muscle (Fig. 6-1).[2,3]

Gains in Strength

The rate of increase in strength after isometric training was first assessed as 5% per week by Hettinger and Muller[4] in 1953. Later Muller[5] suggested that strength gained during

MM tension

MM tension

Figure 6-1	Isometric contraction. Muscle tension occurs in the biceps (*arrows*), but the forearm does not move.

isometric contractions depends on the state of training of the subjects involved in the research; weekly gains varied from 12% per week for individuals in a poor state of training to 2% per week for those in a high state of training. Strength gains after participation in a variety of other isometric-training programs have been reported at 2% to 19% per week.[6,7]

Magnitude

The ideal magnitude of isometric contraction, measured in terms of percent maximal contraction, was first reported to be 67% (two thirds) because loads above that had no additional effect.[4] Cotton[7] studied daily isometric exercise of the forearm flexors and found a significant increase in strength for groups exercising at 50%, 75%, and 100% maximal contraction but found no increase in strength in groups training at 25% of maximal. In addition, he reported that the strength gains were similar in the groups using 50%, 75%, and 100% maximal contraction, supporting Hettinger and Muller.[4] In contrast, Walters et al[6] noted that isometric training was most effective when each contraction was performed maximally. They found that one 15-second maximal isometric contraction daily produced significantly greater strength gains than the same exercise protocol at two thirds of maximal contraction.

Duration

The optimal duration of an isometric contraction necessary to produce strength gains has not been documented. The duration used in research on isometric training has varied from 3 to 100 seconds.[8,9] The majority of studies reviewed report that strength gains after isometric training used 6-second contractions; however, no investigation has compared this to any other duration.

Frequency

Liberson and Asa[10] compared one 6-second isometric contraction daily to twenty 6-second contractions daily. The exercise program incorporating 20 repetitions produced greater strength gains than the exercise program using just one repetition per session.

Specificity of Isometric Training

Although support exists for the use of isometric training, the literature regarding its correct use in rehabilitation is controversial. Some research indicates that isometric training performed at one angle results in strength gains only at the angle trained (angular specificity),[8] but other reports indicate that it also increases strength at adjacent angles.[11]

Bandy and Hanten[11] compared three experimental groups who isometrically trained the knee extensor muscles, each at a different angle of knee flexion (shortened, medium, and lengthened) with a control group. They reported at least a 30-degree transfer of strength regardless of the length of the muscle and at least a 75-degree transfer of strength after exercise in the lengthened position. Results of this study have some interesting clinical implications concerning isometric exercise. If the goal is to provide general strength increases for rehabilitation from pathology or disuse but pain, effusion, or surgical constraints dictate the use of isometric exercise, an efficient way to increase strength throughout the entire range of motion (ROM) is to exercise the muscles in the lengthened position.

Isotonic Exercise

The term *isotonic* means "same or constant" (*iso*) "tension" (*tonic*). In other words, an isotonic exercise is ideally one that produces the same amount of tension while shortening to overcome a given resistance. In reality, an isotonic contraction is one in which the muscles contract while lifting a constant resistance, and the muscle tension varies somewhat over the full ROM owing to changes in muscle length, the angle of pull as the bony lever is moved, and the horizontal distance from the resistance to the joint axis of movement (Fig. 6-2).[2,3]

The definition of isotonic exercise is further differentiated into concentric (shortening) and eccentric (lengthening) contractions, depending on the magnitude of the muscle force and the resistance applied. Concentric refers to a muscle contraction in which the internal force produced by the muscle exceeds the external force of the resistance, allowing the muscle to shorten and produce movement (Fig. 6-3). Eccentric refers to a muscle contraction in an already shortened muscle to which an external resistance greater than the internal muscle force is added, allowing the muscle to lengthen while continuing to maintain tension (Fig. 6-4).[2,3]

Length and Tension

Measurements of the tension created by stimulated muscle fiber show that isometric tension is maximal when the initial length of the muscle at the time of stimulation is stretched to about 20% beyond the normal resting length (defined as muscle fiber that is not stimulated and has no external forces acting on it). The strength of the active contractile component decreases as the muscle is shortened or lengthened from the optimal muscle length.

The sliding-filament theory was proposed to explain changes in tension as muscle length changes from the resting length. It suggests that the force developed by the active contractile component of the muscle is governed by the relative position of the actin and myosin filaments of each sarcomere. The most efficient length of muscle fiber is the slightly elongated position, when the crossbridges of the actin and myosin seem to couple most effectively and produce the greatest tension. During both lengthening and shortening of the muscle, effective coupling of the crossbridges cannot take place; thus, the tension of the muscle contraction decreases.[12,13]

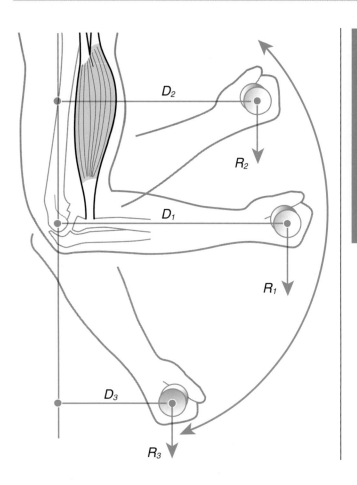

Figure 6-2

Variance of muscle tension during isotonic contraction. Although the resistance (R) is constant, the actual muscle tension varies owing to the changing distance (D) from the resistance to the elbow axis of motion. Specifically, the distance (D_1) from the resistance (R_1) to the axis of motion at 90 degrees of elbow flexion is greater than the distance (D_2) from the resistance (R_2) to the axis of motion in which the elbow is more flexed, and D_1 is greater than the distance (D_3) from the resistance (R_3) to the axis of motion in which the elbow is more extended.

Biomechanical Advantage

The amount of force a muscle is able to generate during a contraction is influenced by the length of the moment arm. The moment arm of the muscle is defined as the perpendicular distance from the axis of motion to the line of action of the muscle. The amount of torque produced by the mus-cle is determined by multiplying the magnitude of the force of the muscle by the moment arm. The farther away from the joint axis the muscle inserts into the bone, the greater the moment arm and therefore the greater the force pro-duced by the muscle contraction (Fig 6-5).[12,13]

The amount of force produced by a muscle contraction is also determined by the angle at which the muscle inserts

Figure 6-3

Concentric contraction, or shortening of muscle against resistance.

Figure 6-4 Eccentric contraction, or lengthening of muscle against resistance.

Slow lowering

A

M_1

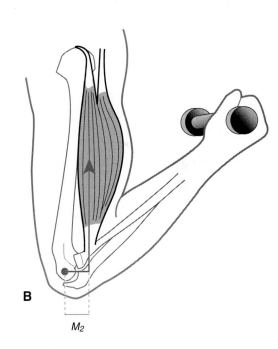

B

M_2

Figure 6-5 Biomechanical advantage.

During elbow flexion the perpendicular distance from the axis of motion to the angle of muscle insertion (moment arm, M) is greater in (A) (M_1) than in (B) (M_2), resulting in a larger biomechanical advantage and a greater potential to produce force in the 90-degree angle of insertion.

into the bone. A 90-degree angle of attachment is optimal for producing a purely rotational force. At angles of attachment greater or less than this optimum angle, the muscle will produce the same amount of force, but some of the rotational force will be lost to distraction or compression forces at the joint. Therefore, the muscle contraction will not be able to exert the same amount of torque.[13] Because of the influence of changing muscle length (length and tension) and the changing leverage of the muscle on the bone (biomechanical advantage), muscle tension during isotonic exercise is less than maximal through the full ROM. Therefore, the ability of the muscle to move a load throughout the ROM is limited by the weakest point in the range.

Eccentric Muscle Contractions

A muscle acting eccentrically responds to the application of an external force with increased tension during physical lengthening of the musculotendinous unit. Instead of the muscle performing work on the resistance, the resistance is said to perform work on the muscle during eccentric loading, a phenomenon referred to as negative work. Examples of the integral nature of eccentric muscle actions in the performance of functional activities are the tibialis anterior controlling foot descent from initial contact to foot-flat during gait, the posterior deltoid slowing the forward movement of the arm during the deceleration phase of throwing, the hamstrings acting as eccentric decelerators of the lower leg during the terminal portion of the swing phase of gait during running, and the eccentric control of forward bending of the trunk into gravity by the spinal extensors. These examples emphasize the importance of including eccentric exercise in resistance training.[14]

Delayed-Onset Muscle Soreness

DOMS is a common occurrence after exercise. Postexercise soreness is more pronounced after eccentric than after concentric exercise. Symptoms associated with DOMS include dull, diffuse pain; stiffness; and tenderness to direct pressure. These symptoms may last up to 1 week, although most cases resolve in 72 hours. Symptom intensity generally peaks at 48 hours. Signs associated with eccentrically mediated DOMS include edema formation in muscle, loss of active ROM, and decreased ability to produce force by the muscle for up to 1 week after intense exercise.[15,16]

Eccentric muscular contractions result in mechanical microtrauma to participating tissues, including direct myofibril and connective tissue damage. This finding has significant implications in the clinical use of resistance training. One important clinical consideration is that DOMS poses a potential threat to unimpeded progression through a therapeutic exercise continuum. Inappropriate implementation of eccentric training may result in an inflammatory microtraumatic response, potentially compromising the patient's function and ability to participate maximally in therapeutic exercise until the inflammatory response subsides.

The deleterious effects of DOMS can be minimized by controlling the frequency of significant eccentric work performed by the patient. Given the recovery period of 3 to 7 days after eccentric exercise, it is proposed that individuals perform maximal eccentric exercise no more than two times per week. Studies that incorporated four eccentric training sessions per week demonstrated either minimal strength gains (2.9%) or actual decreases in force production. Allowing 3 days of recovery between sessions may allow tissue healing and repair to occur.[17,18]

Isokinetic Exercise

Isokinetic exercise involves muscle contractions in which the speed of movement is controlled mechanically so that the limb moves at a predetermined, constant velocity. Electromechanical machinery maintains the preselected speed of movement during activity; once the limb is accelerated to that velocity, a sufficient amount of resistance is applied to prohibit the limb from accelerating beyond the target speed. This accommodating resistance varies as the muscle force varies as a result of changing muscle length and angle of pull, allowing for maximal dynamic loading of the muscles throughout the full ROM. Therefore, isokinetic exercise devices stimulate maximal contraction of the muscle throughout the complete ROM.[19] The use of isokinetic exercise in rehabilitation has received great attention because of its accommodating resistance and its allowance of exercise at higher speeds of contraction, more closely mimicking functional speed. Isokinetic exercise can involve a dynamic shortening contraction of the muscle with the velocity of movement held constant (concentric isokinetic loading) or involve lengthening contractions at controlled angular velocities (eccentric isokinetic loading).

Although an interesting and exciting adjunct to the area of open-chain–resistance training, isokinetic exercise is not a panacea. No research to date has indicated that one type of exercise (isometric, isotonic, or isokinetic) is better than another; instead, all forms of muscular activity are needed to provide the patient with an integrated and progressive resistance-training program.

Quantification

Modern isokinetic equipment contains computer-assisted dynamometers designed to provide the clinician or researcher with a plethora of quantitative information regarding muscle function. Before the design of isokinetic technology, such objective information was not easily obtainable. Among the most commonly used isokinetic parameters are peak torque, work, and power.[20]

Limitations

Isokinetic exercise is, of course, not without its limitations. Human muscle function is not characterized by a constant speed of movement but rather by a continuous interplay of acceleration and deceleration. Also, work is most often performed against a fixed (rather than accommodating) resistance. Functionally, muscle groups work together synergistically with particular activation patterns, which vary from task to task and are not simulated by isokinetic exercise. Therefore, isokinetic training does not simulate normal muscle function. An additional and considerable limitation in the clinical use of isokinetic exercise is the cost of the equipment, which, relative to other types of therapeutic exercise, may be prohibitive.

CLINICAL GUIDELINES

Isometric Exercise

Generally isometric exercises are used in the early stages of a rehabilitation program for an acute injury or immediately after surgery when open-chain–resistance exercises through full ROM are contraindicated because of pain, effusion, crepitus, or insufficient healing. An isometric program may be best until the condition has healed. The exercise program can then be progressed to the point at which the resistance training can occur through the full ROM.[2,3]

Some studies report that isometric contractions do not necessarily need to be maximally performed to achieve strength gains.[7] The use of submaximal isometric training to increase strength may be important for a patient early in the rehabilitation program, when maximal contractions may be painful. Submaximal isometric contractions can be used to increase strength until the patient can be progressed to maximal contractions, as the condition and tolerance to pain allows.

As noted, no research defines the optimal duration for performing an isometric contraction, although some reports suggest that strength gains are achieved after isometric contractions of 6 to 10 seconds, which is the currently suggested duration. In addition, the literature[20] suggests multiple repetitions of the 6- to 10-second contractions with the muscle in the lengthened position. If no increase in symptoms occurs after the exercise sessions, the isometric program can probably be performed by the patient every day. If an increase in symptoms occurs or new problems arise, the isometric program should be performed on alternate days.

Isotonic Exercise

Isotonic exercise is probably the most common type of resistance training because of its ease of performance and low cost.

A number of isotonic programs have been proposed for incorporating the optimal amount of resistance and repetitions to produce maximal gains in muscular strength. These programs vary from the classic progressive-resistance exercise protocol using three sets of 10 repetitions (proposed by Delorme[21] in 1945) to an extremely aggressive program for advanced stages of rehabilitation using more weight and four to six repetitions (proposed by Stone and Kroll[22] in 1982). The Delorme system incorporates progression from light to heavy resistance, adding resistance with each set. There are many variations in the progression; however, the classic Delorme was 50% of ten-repetition maximum (10 RM) for the first set, 75% of 10 RM for the second set, and 100% of 10 RM for the third set. The Oxford system is the opposite of Delorme with progression from heavy to light, and it reverses the resistance levels.[23] The Daily Adjusted Progressive-resistance–exercise (DAPRE) technique was proposed to modify the Delorme and Oxford progressions as a more easily modified progression. DAPRE is used with both free weights and weight machines. The increases in weight are based on a 5 RM or 7 RM and are designed to take previous performance into account.[24] Tables 6-2 through 6-6 present suggested training protocols reported in the literature.[21-25]

Although each program in the tables has documentation showing that strength gains occur when overloading the muscle using that method, no literature exists indicating that any one of these programs is better than the others. In other words, no single combination of sets and repetitions has been documented to be the optimal resistance program for increasing strength for everyone. If the basic principles of overloading the muscle to a higher level than it is accustomed are understood (Chapter 5) and if continued adjustments are made to ensure that the overload principle is progressed as the individual accommodates to the given load, then a wide range of isotonic-resistance programs can be incorporated into the treatment of patients.

Caution should be used when progressing a patient through an isotonic-resistance program. Frequent examination of the patient is necessary to ensure that the exercise program does not lead to an increase in pain, crepitus, and swelling. Although many resistance-training programs

---

TABLE 6-2 Delorme's Progressive-resistance Exercise

Set	Weight[a]	Repetitions
1	50% of 10 RM	10
2	75% of 10 RM	10
3	100% of 10 RM	10

[a]10 RM, maximum amount of weight that can be lifted ten times. For example, if the maximum amount of weight that can lifted ten times is 50 pounds, the first set is 25 pounds for ten repetitions, the second set is 37.5 pounds for ten repetitions, and the final set is 50 pounds for ten repetitions.

TABLE 6-3 The Daily Adjustable Progressive-resistance–exercise Technique

Set	Weight	Repetitions
1	50% of working weight	10
2	75% of working weight	6
3	Full working weight	Maximum[a]
4	Adjusted working weight[a]	Maximum[b]

[a]Used to determine the weight for the fourth set (see Table 6-4).
[b]Used to determine the weight for the third set of the next session (see Table 6-5).

have been shown to increase strength in normal individuals, using a relatively low number of repetitions with high resistance may cause problems in the patient with musculoskeletal pathology. The critical factor in the success of an exercise program is to avoid causing swelling and discomfort while having the patient work to his or her maximum of exercise tolerance. To this end, high repetitions and relatively low resistance should be used early in the isotonic phase of intervention. Two to three sets of ten to 12 repetitions are recommended for the initial stages when using an isotonic protocol.

In addition, when using isotonic-exercise programs, the PTA must be aware of the healing constraints of the pathology and progress the patient along open-chain resistance-training programs in a way that is consistent with fibrous healing. To ensure safety, the patient should not be introduced to maximal stress immediately but be guided in a sequence of resistance exercises involving submaximal work. The proper progression should incorporate limited ROM exercise first, progressing to full ROM while still using a submaximum workload, and finally culminating in unrestricted ROM with maximum effort.

Isokinetic Exercise

The PT and PTA must be aware of the unique advantages and limitations when considering the implementation of isokinetic exercise for optimizing outcomes of intervention.

TABLE 6-4 Guidelines for Determining Adjusted Working Weight for the Daily Adjustable Progressive-resistance–exercise Technique

Number of Repetitions Performed for Set 3	Adjusted Working Weight for Set 4
0–2	Decrease 5–10 pounds
3–4	Decrease 0–5 pounds
5–6	No change
7–10	Increase 5–10 pounds
≥11	Increase 10–15 pounds

TABLE 6-5 Guidelines for Determining Full Working Weight for the Daily Adjustable Progressive-resistance–exercise Technique

Number of Repetitions Performed for Set 4	Full Working Weight for Set 3 of Next Session
0–2	Decrease 5–10 pounds
3–4	No change
5–6	Increase 5–10 pounds
7–10	Increase 5–15 pounds
≥11	Increase 10–20 pounds

The clinical advantages of isokinetic exercise include the ability to control the velocity of movement of the exercising limb segment, the accommodating resistance that allows for maximal muscle loading throughout the ROM, and the quantitative nature of performance assessment afforded by computer interfacing. However, isokinetic training differs significantly from normal function in a number of ways, a deficiency that underscores the importance of integrating all means of open-chain–resistance training in rehabilitation.

When isokinetic exercise is implemented, certain clinical considerations must be addressed. The clinician must select the speed at which the patient will be exercising the involved muscle, keeping in mind that the best approach is for the individuals to train at speeds as close as possible to those encountered functionally. One suggested protocol is for the patient to exercise across a variety of speeds (sometimes referred to as a velocity spectrum) such as eight repetitions at a relatively slow speed (e.g., 60 degrees/second), ten repetitions at a moderate speed (e.g., 180 degrees/second), and 12 repetitions at a fast speed (e.g., 300 degrees/second).

The most appropriate ROM should be selected, factoring in soft-tissue healing constraints and the range in which pain occurs. If preferential recruitment of fast-twitch muscle fibers is desired, maximal isokinetic exercise should be considered because of the allowance for optimal recruitment

TABLE 6-6 Aggressive-Resistance–Training Program

Set	Weight[a]	Repetitions
1	50% of 4 RM	8
2	80% of 4 RM	8
3	90% of 4 RM	6
4	95% of 4 RM	4
5	100% of 4 RM	4

[a]4 RM, maximum amount of weight that can be lifted four times. For example, if the maximum amount of weight that can lifted four times is 100 pounds, the first set is 50 pounds for eight repetitions, the second set is 80 pounds for eight repetitions, the third set is 90 pounds for six repetitions, the fourth set is 95 pounds for four repetitions, and the fifth set is 100 pounds for 4 repetitions.

of fast-twitch fibers through the full ROM. Another protocol uses the concept of multiple-angle isometrics. Isometrics are performed every 20 degrees through the patient's available ROM. Generally the patient performs using the rule of ten—10-second contraction, 10-second rest, ten repetitions, ten sets, ten angles.[26] While initially developed using isokinetic equipment, the concept can be carried into any resistance program. Isokinetic training should incorporate both concentric and eccentric exercise, if possible.

TECHNIQUES

Isometric Exercises

Early in the resistance-training program, the patient may exercise by doing simple isometric exercises called muscle

sets, especially in the lower extremity. The most common of these muscle sets are gluteal sets, quadriceps sets, and hamstring sets. The gluteal set is performed by the patient tightening the gluteal muscles by pinching the muscles of the buttocks together and holding in an isometric contraction for 6 to 10 seconds. The quadriceps set, most easily performed in a supine position, consists of tightening the quadriceps muscle by straightening the knee and holding the contraction isometrically. The hamstring set is also most easily performed in a supine position by pushing the heel of the foot into the surface under the heel, thereby causing an isometric hip extension activity.

The patient can be assisted by the PTA or, with imagination, can use his or her own body for resistance. Figures 6-6 through 6-10 depict a few isometric exercises that can be performed early in the intervention phase for a patient requiring initial strengthening activities.

Figure 6-6   Isometric elbow flexion with physical therapist assistant (PTA) assistance.

PURPOSE: Strengthening biceps muscle of the elbow in two parts of the range of motion.
POSITION: Patient sitting with hips and knees flexed to 90 degrees. PTA places distal hand on client's wrist and proximal hand on client's shoulder. **A.** Exercise at 90 degrees of elbow flexion. **B.** Exercise at 45 degrees of elbow flexion.

PROCEDURE: Client flexes arm as PTA provides isometric resistance to the movement with distal hand. Resistance should be held for 6 to 10 seconds per repetition.

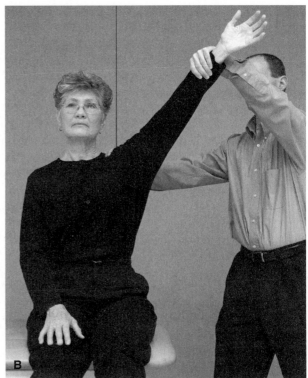

| Figure 6-7 | Isometric shoulder abduction in the plane of the scapula with physical therapist assistant (PTA) assistance. |

PURPOSE: Strengthening abductor muscles of the shoulder in the plane of the scapula in two parts of the range of motion.

POSITION: Patient sitting with hips and knees flexed to 90 degrees. PTA places distal hand on client's wrist and proximal hand on client's shoulder. **A.** Exercise at 45 degrees of shoulder abduction. **B.** Exercise at 120 degrees of shoulder abduction. Shoulder is held in abduction in the plane of the scapula (30 degrees horizontally adducted from the frontal plane).

PROCEDURE: Client abducts arm as PTA provides isometric resistance to the movement with distal hand. Resistance should be held for 6 to 10 seconds per repetition.

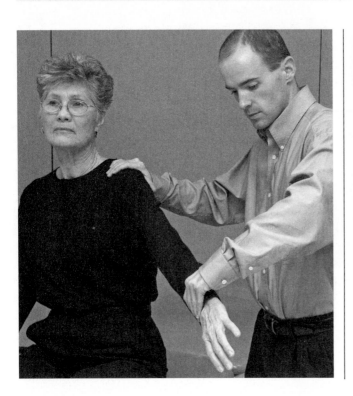

| Figure 6-8 | Isometric exercise applied in empty-can position with physical therapist assistant (PTA) assistance. |

PURPOSE: Strengthening supraspinatus muscle of the shoulder.

POSITION: Patient sitting with hips and knees flexed to 90 degrees. PTA places distal hand on client's wrist and proximal hand on client's shoulder. Client holds arm in empty-can position of abduction, internal rotation, and slightly forward horizontal adduction.

PROCEDURE: Client abducts arm as PTA provides isometric resistance to the movement with distal hand. Resistance should be held for 6 to 10 seconds per repetition.

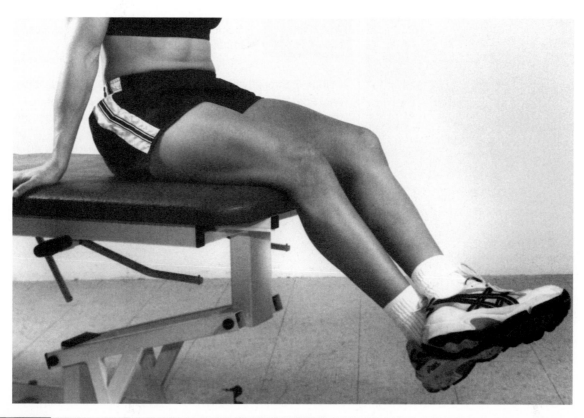

Figure 6-9	Isometric knee extension exercise for independent home program.

PURPOSE: Strengthening quadriceps muscles.

POSITION: Client sitting with both legs flexed to 45 degrees. The left leg placed on the anterior surface of the right leg.

PROCEDURE: The client uses left leg to flex and provides isometric resistance against anterior surface of right leg. Right leg attempts to extend against resistance of left leg. Resistance should be held for 6 to 10 seconds per repetition.

Figure 6-10	Isometric ankle dorsiflexion exercise for independent home program.

PURPOSE: Strengthening tibialis anterior muscle of the ankle.

POSITION: Patient sitting with hip and knee flexed at 90 degrees. Client places right foot on anterior surface of left foot.

PROCEDURE: The client uses right foot to plantarflex and provide resistance against anterior surface of left foot. Left foot attempts to dorsiflex against resistance of right foot. Resistance should be held for 6 to 10 sec per repetition.

| Figure 6-11 | Isotonic exercise applied in empty-can position with dumbbell. |

PURPOSE: Strengthening supraspinatus muscle of the shoulder.

POSITION: Client standing with arm at side, internally rotated, and in the plane of the scapula (30 degrees horizontally adducted from the frontal plane) holding dumbbell.

PROCEDURE: Client abducts arm (concentric) to less than 90 degrees in the plane of the scapula while maintaining upper extremity in internal rotation and elbow extended. It is important that arm stay below the horizontal and not be elevated above 90 degrees to avoid impingement of the shoulder. Following a brief pause at 90 degrees, shoulder is slowly lowered to original position (eccentric).

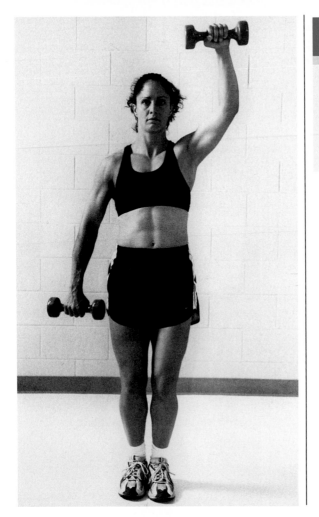

| Figure 6-12 | Stabilization with reciprocal upper-extremity movement. |

PURPOSE: Stabilize spine; strengthen bilateral shoulder girdle.

POSITION: Client standing with trunk in neutral, stable position. Dumbbells may be used.

PROCEDURE: Client alternately raises one extremity while lowering the other.

Isotonic Exercises

Isotonic exercise can be performed by using cuff weights, elastic tubing, dumbbells, and a variety of machines. In addition, the creative PTA will be able to work with the patient to develop resistive devices that do not cost as much as high-tech exercise equipment. Creative devices include purses or backpacks filled with soup cans or books (weighed on a home scale to check that the correct total weight is used). This chapter emphasizes economic and efficient techniques that can be used by the patient at home or in the office. Figures 6-11 through 6-34 present a wide range

Figure 6-13   Stabilization while strengthening upper trapezius muscles.

PURPOSE: Stabilize spine; strengthen upper trapezius muscles.

POSITION: Client standing with trunk in neutral, stable position. Dumbbells may be used.

PROCEDURE: Client abducts both upper extremities simultaneously.

| Figure 6-14 | Isotonic exercise for shoulder external rotation with dumbbell. |

PURPOSE: Strengthening external rotator muscles of the rotator cuff of the shoulder (infraspinatus, teres minor).

POSITION: Client lying prone with upper arm (shoulder to elbow) stabilized on table and forearm (elbow to hand) hanging off table and holding dumbbell. Hand is allowed to hang from the table.

PROCEDURE: Client externally rotates shoulder (concentric), pauses at end range of external rotation, and then slowly lowers arm back to original position (eccentric).

A

B

| Figure 16-15 | Isotonic exercise of shoulder external rotation with elastic tubing. |

PURPOSE: Strengthening external rotator muscles of the rotator cuff of the shoulder (infraspinatus, teres minor) in two different positions of shoulder abduction.

POSITION: Client positions shoulder in conservative position of adduction next to the body **(A)** or a more aggressive position of the shoulder in external rotation at 90 degrees of abduction **(B)**. Client grasps elastic tubing.

PROCEDURE: From an internally rotated position, client externally rotates shoulder against resistance of the elastic tubing (concentric), pauses at end range of external rotation. Then, slowly and with control, the client allows the arm to return to the starting position (eccentric).

Figure 6-16 Pull to chest.

PURPOSE: Stabilize spine; strengthen posterior shoulder girdle and scapular-stabilizing musculature.

POSITION: Client lying supine with hips and knees flexed. Shoulders flexed to allow for grasping of pulley bar.

PROCEDURE: Client pulls bar toward chest by flexing elbows, extending shoulders, and retracting scapulae.

Figure 6-17 Pull to chest.

PURPOSE: Stabilize spine; strengthen biceps and scapular-stabilizing musculature.

POSITION: Client sitting; hips and knees flexed to 90 degrees; feet firmly on floor. Upper extremities in 90 degrees of shoulder flexion to allow grasping of pulley bar.

PROCEDURE: Client pulls bar toward chest by flexing elbows, extending shoulders, and retracting scapulae.

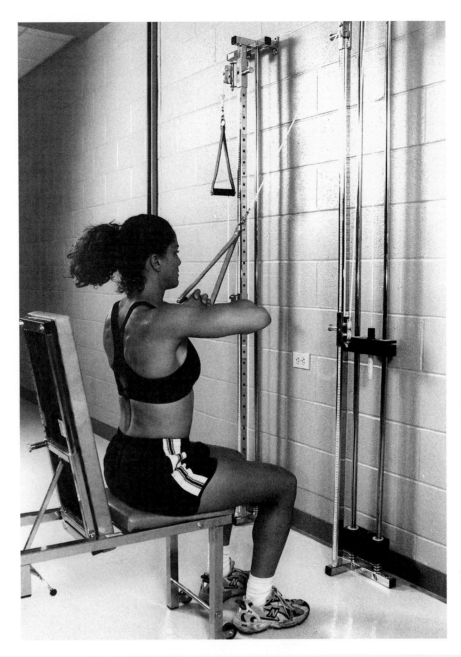

Figure 6-18   Pull to chest from above.

PURPOSE: Stabilize spine; strengthen teres major, latissimus dorsi, and scapular-stabilizing musculature.

POSITION: Client sitting; hips and knees flexed; feet firmly on floor. Upper extremities in about 150 degrees of shoulder flexion to allow grasping of pulley handle.

PROCEDURE: Client pulls pulley handle toward chest by flexing elbows, extending shoulders, and retracting scapulae.

Figure 6-19	Bar raise.

PURPOSE: Stabilize spine; strengthen shoulder flexors, abductors, and external rotators.

POSITION: Client sitting; hips and knees flexed; feet firmly on floor. Arms at side with elbows flexed, grasping pulley bar.

PROCEDURE: Client lifts pulley bar overhead by flexing shoulders.

Figure 6-20   Stabilization while strengthening upper extremity.

PURPOSE: Stabilize spine; strengthen scapular retractors, shoulder flexors, abductors, and external rotators.

POSITION: Client sitting with hips and knees flexed; feet firmly on floor **(A)**. Arms in position to allow for grasping of contralateral pulley handles.

PROCEDURE: Client lifts pulley handles overhead by elevating arms **(B)**.

Figure 6-21	Shoulder abduction.

PURPOSE: Stabilize spine; strengthen shoulder abductors.

POSITION: Client standing with arms at side, grasping pulley handle.

PROCEDURE: Client abducts arm to shoulder height in plane of scapula.

Figure 6-22 Triceps exercise.

PURPOSE: Stabilize spine; strengthen elbow extensors and scapular-stabilizing musculature.

POSITION: Client standing; arms at side with elbows flexed to grasp pulley bar.

PROCEDURE: Client extends elbows.

Figure 6-23	Bar pull.

PURPOSE: Stabilize spine; strengthen scapular retractors and shoulder abductors.

POSITION: Client standing; knees slightly bent; arms in front of body to allow grasping of pulley bar.

PROCEDURE: Client lifts pulley to chin by abducting shoulders and scapular retractors.

A

B

| Figure 6-24 | Stabilization while performing diagonal movement patterns. |

PURPOSE: Stabilize spine; perform functional diagonal movement pattern.

POSITION: A. Client standing with feet staggered, weight on left leg, facing pulley. Client flexes, bends to left side, and rotates spine to left, allowing client to grasp pulley handle with both hands.

PROCEDURE: B. Weight is transferred to right leg. Client extends, bends to right side, and rotates spine to right while lifting pulley handle in diagonal pattern.

Figure 6-25	Horizontal adduction.

PURPOSE: Strengthen trapezius and scapular-stabilizing musculature.

POSITION: Client lying prone on bench; arms hanging off edge of support surface. Dumbbells may be used.

PROCEDURE: Client horizontally abducts arms and retracts scapulae.

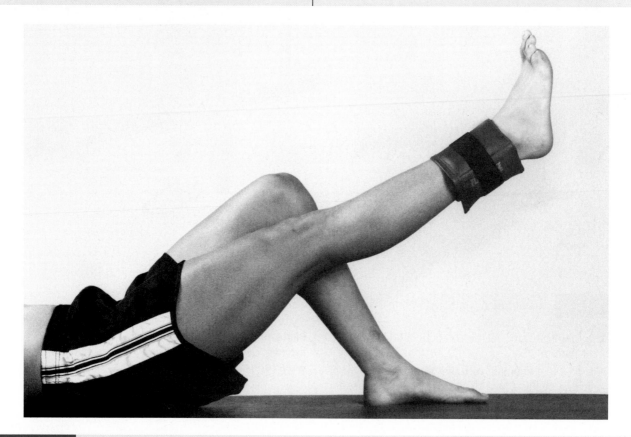

Figure 6-26	Isotonic straight-leg raise with cuff weight.

PURPOSE: Strengthening hip flexors using straight-leg raise.

POSITION: Client lying supine with cuff weight strapped around ankle. Opposite leg may be flexed for comfort of client.

PROCEDURE: Client raises leg (concentric), holds briefly in flexed position, and slowly lowers (eccentric) leg to starting position.

| Figure 6-27 | Isotonic exercise of hip abduction with cuff weight. |

PURPOSE: Strengthening hip abductor muscles.

POSITION: Client lying on side with cuff weight strapped around ankle of leg closest to ceiling. Opposite leg may be flexed for comfort of client.

PROCEDURE: Client raises leg (concentric), holds briefly in abducted position, and slowly lowers (eccentric) the leg to starting position.

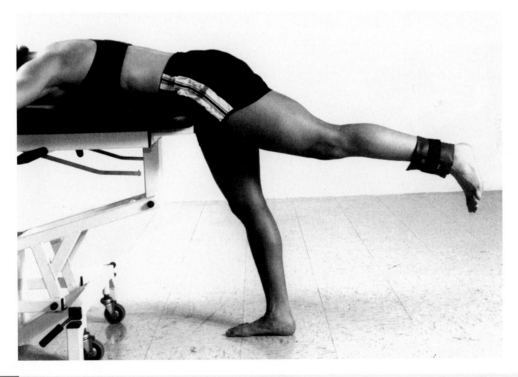

| Figure 6-28 | Isotonic exercise for hip extension with cuff weight. |

PURPOSE: Strengthening hamstring muscles.

POSITION: Client lying prone with leg held over edge of plinth. Cuff weight strapped around ankle.

PROCEDURE: Client slowly lowers leg to the floor (eccentric). After a brief pause client lifts leg into hip extension (concentric).

Figure 6-29   Isotonic knee extension exercise through limited range of motion (ROM) with cuff weight.

PURPOSE: Strengthening quadriceps muscles of the knee in a limited or protected ROM.

POSITION: Client lying supine with cuff weight strapped around ankle. A bolster or towel roll is placed under client's knee allowing a limited ROM (30 degrees of full extension is shown).

PROCEDURE: Client extends knee (concentric) through partial ROM (30 degrees to full extension is shown). Once fully extended, client pauses briefly, holding knee in extended position, and then slowly lowers leg with control from full extension (eccentric).

Figure 6-30   Isotonic knee extension exercise through full range of motion (ROM) with cuff weight.

PURPOSE: Strengthening quadriceps muscles of the knee in full ROM.

POSITION: Client sitting with cuff weight strapped around ankle.

PROCEDURE: Client extends knee through the full ROM (concentric). Once fully extended, client pauses briefly, holding knee in extended position, and then slowly lowers leg with control from full extension (eccentric).

Figure 6-31 Isotonic exercise of ankle dorsiflexion with physical therapist assistant (PTA) assistance and elastic tubing.

PURPOSE: Strengthening tibialis anterior muscle.

POSITION: Client long-sitting with one end of elastic across dorsum of foot. PTA holds other end of elastic tubing.

PROCEDURE: From the plantarflexed position, client dorsiflexes ankle (concentric), pauses at end range of dorsiflexion, and then slowly allows foot to return to starting position (eccentric).

Figure 6-32 Knee flexor muscle strengthening.

PURPOSE: Strengthen knee flexor musculature.

POSITION: Client sitting on end of bench with ankle strapped to pulley.

PROCEDURE: Client flexes knee against resistance of pulley.

Figure 6-33   Knee extensor muscle strengthening.

PURPOSE: Strengthen knee extensor musculature.

POSITION: Client sitting with knee flexed at end of bench with ankle strapped to pulley.

PROCEDURE: Client extends knee against resistance of pulley.

Figure 6-34	Unloaded mini-squats.

PURPOSE: Lower-extremity strengthening and stabilization training with reduced weight bearing.

POSITION: Client standing; holding overhead pulley bar at mid-torso; elbows extended.

PROCEDURE: Keeping elbows extended, client performs mini-squat by flexing hips and knees and lowering body in direction of floor.

of isotonic exercises that can be effectively used for rehabilitation of upper- and lower-extremity dysfunctions.

Isokinetic Exercise

Since the 1970s no other mode of resistance training has received more attention among researchers and clinicians than isokinetic exercise. To determine if isokinetic exercise is appropriate for a patient, the clinician must have a proper understanding of the scientific rationale underlying the method and the clinical rationale for its use. Figure 6-35 shows a common isokinetic dynamometer used in the treatment of patients today. The isokinetic dynamometer shown has the ability to exercise upper and lower extremities.

Figure 6-35   Isokinetic exercise for the lower extremity with Biodex dynamometer.

PURPOSE: Isokinetic strengthening of knee extensors.

POSITION: Client sitting on chair of dynamometer with stabilization straps placed around chest, pelvis, and thigh. Lower part of leg (near ankle) is also stabilized to the isokinetic device.

PROCEDURE: Client extends knee as fast and as hard as possible against accommodating resistance provided by device (concentric). At end of full knee extension, client immediately flexes knee as fast and as hard as possible against accommodating resistance (concentric contraction of reciprocal muscle) or client immediately resists lever arm as it pushes leg into flexion (eccentric contraction of the ipsilateral muscle).

NOTE: The exact nature of the type of contraction depends on how the isokinetic dynamometer is programmed. The example given here is one of many options available with a computer-generated isokinetic dynamometer. (Courtesy of Biodex Medical Systems, Shirley, NY.)

CASE STUDY 1

PATIENT INFORMATION

A 21-year-old college football player (linebacker) presented to the clinic complaining of pain and weakness in the right arm near the cubital fossa. He described the injury as occurring in the third quarter of a football game 2 days earlier when he made an arm tackle of an opposing ball carrier. During the tackle, his right arm was forcibly horizontally abducted behind his back while he pulled the ball carrier to the ground by flexing his elbow. Immediately he felt severe pain in his upper arm, which subsided to a dull pain after 5 minutes. The patient indicated that he was able to complete the game with minimal pain. The following day (1 day before coming into the clinic) he complained of upper arm pain and an inability to extend the elbow without pain.

Examination by the PT indicated acute inflammation, including pain and palpable heat at the anterior surface of the upper arm. In addition, swelling was present at the anterior aspect of the elbow joint. Passive ROM was full but painful at full elbow extension. Resisted elbow flexion was painful and weak (manual muscle testing grade 3/5); resisted shoulder flexion was strong (5/5) but with slight pain. All other examination procedures were pain free. Based on the examination, the patient was diagnosed with a strain to the biceps brachii muscle.

LINK TO
GUIDE TO PHYSICAL THERAPIST PRACTICE

Pattern 4D of the *Guide to Physical Therapist Practice*[27] relates to the diagnosis of this patient. The pattern is described as "impaired joint mobility, motor function, muscle performance, and range of motion associated with connective tissue dysfunction." Included in this diagnostic group is muscle strain, and anticipated goals include increasing strength using resistive exercises (including concentric, dynamic/isotonic, eccentric, isokinetic, and isometric).

INTERVENTION

The PT's initial goals of intervention were to decrease inflammation (swelling, pain), maintain full ROM, and diminish loss of strength during healing. The PT discussed the goals and plan of care with the PTA. The PTA, under the direction and supervision of the PT, instructed the patient in a home program consisting of:

1. Ice before treatment.
2. Active flexion and extension ROM exercises to the elbow: 15 repetitions in the morning and in the evening (Fig. 3-18).
3. Isometric exercises to elbow flexors in two parts of the range (45 degrees and 90 degrees) using submaximal (pain-free) contractions: 20 repetitions in the morning and in the evening (Fig. 6-6).
4. Ice after treatment.
5. Return to clinic in 1 week.

The PTA was to report back to the supervising PT about the ability of the patient to tolerate and perform the home exercise program.

PROGRESSION

One Week After Initial Examination

Upon re-evaluation by the PT, the patient reported no pain with passive ROM of the elbow, decreased pain with resisted elbow flexion, no swelling at the elbow, and no pain with resisted shoulder flexion. Given that inflammation was decreased, the goals of intervention were updated by the PT to promote healing (influence proper collagen deposition, increase blood flow) and to increase strength of the biceps brachii. The PT instructed the PTA to progress the home program as follows:

1. Isotonic elbow flexion exercises using a 2-pound cuff weight: three sets of 12 repetitions twice a day.
2. Isotonic shoulder flexion exercise using a 5-pound weight: two sets of 12 repetitions twice a day (Fig. 6-12).
3. Ice after treatment.

Two Weeks After Initial Examination

The examination by the PT indicated no pain with any resisted movements but a slight loss of strength with elbow flexion (4+/5). The goals of intervention at this point were to aggressively strengthen the biceps brachii.

In the clinic, directed by the PT, the PTA exercised the patient isokinetically by performing eight repetitions of concentric elbow flexion and elbow extension at 60 degrees/second, 10 repetitions at 180 degrees/second, and 12 repetitions at 300 degrees/second. The program was repeated three times (three sets at each speed). The patient was able to perform these exercises without any pain or complaints of any kind. The PTA reported the exercise tolerance of the patient back to the PT and was instructed by the PT to apply ice to the patient following the exercise session. After the intervention session, the PTA, under the direction of the PT, instructed the patient to perform a daily home exercise program of three sets of 15 repetitions of isotonic elbow flexion using elastic tubing.

OUTCOME

Three weeks after the initial examination the patient was pain free for all movements and the strength of elbow flexion on the right was equal to the left, as indicated by manual muscle testing (5/5). The patient was discharged from care by the PT with instructions to call or return if problems developed.

SUMMARY—AN EFFECTIVE PT-PTA TEAM

This case study demonstrates an effective collaborative effort between the PT and the PTA. The PTA is able to follow the instructions of the PT after their re-examination of the patient, perform isokinetic exercises with the patient, and instruct the patient about the home exercise program. The PT is aware of the patient's status and ability to advance the home exercise program due to the good communication between the PT and the PTA after the instruction. The PT expects that the PTA fully understands the interventions included in the clinic exercise and the home exercise program. The PT also expects that the PTA can instruct the patient independently, reporting any adverse effects of the session. This type of working relationship allows the PT to be aware of the athlete's status but at the same time allows him/her to perform examinations on other patients in the clinic, demonstrating effective and efficient teamwork while still providing quality care.

SUMMARY

- The three common modes of exercise (isometric, isotonic, and isokinetic) were defined, and research was presented as a review of the exercise types and to enhance the understanding of their use in clinical intervention.

- Isometric exercises are used most commonly early in the rehabilitation program to avoid open-chain–resistance exercises through the full ROM, which may cause increased pain, effusion, or crepitus. Isometric exercises can also be used at various points in the ROM to enhance more effective strengthening in that part of the range and therefore can be used throughout the entire rehabilitation program, rather than only during the acute or inflammatory phase.

- Isotonic-resistance programs are common, and their effectiveness in increasing strength is well docu-

mented. Isotonic exercise should be performed both concentrically and eccentrically for the most functional result. A potential disadvantage to isotonic exercise is that the actual tension developed varies as the muscle changes length and maximal resistance is not achieved throughout the full ROM.

- Isokinetic exercise is performed at a fixed speed against accommodating resistance. Electromechanical mechanisms vary the resistance to accommodate the fluctuations in muscle force owing to changing muscle length and angle of pull. Therefore, isokinetic exercise devices stimulate maximal contraction of the muscle throughout the complete ROM.

- The PT and PTA must be aware of potential adverse responses of the patient to the open-chain resistance-training program (pain, crepitus, swelling) and of healing constraints that may affect the program. The specific program must be individualized to each patient.

▼ ▼ ▼ GERIATRIC PERSPECTIVES ▼ ▼ ▼

- Open-chain–resistance activities are appropriate for all age groups, even the oldest-old, with few modifications. These activities for senior adults may be exemplified by functional tasks, such as carrying a plate of food or a bag of groceries.

- Open-chain activities are associated with shearing forces across the joint. Of particular importance are the shearing forces that occur parallel to the tibiofemoral joint during open-chain activities. The use of such exercises with added resistance may be problematic after some surgeries, such as total knee replacement.

- Although open-chain–resistance training is not particularly functional, the training provides a means of isolating muscle groups. For example, quadriceps strength is known to decrease with aging. The strength loss has been associated with increased chair rise time and difficulty climbing stairs.

- With aging, the peak force generated during a single maximal contraction against a constant force (isometric strength) and the peak force generated as the muscle is shortening (concentric strength) decrease and the muscle fatigues more quickly.[1–3] Furthermore, the speed of the response to stimuli (reaction time and contraction response) slows progressively with aging.[3]

- In designing a training program that uses open-chain activities for older individuals, a taxonomy of exercise is the recommended choice. The progression should begin with holding muscle contractions (isometric), proceed to control during muscle lengthening (eccentric), and finally progress to a shortening contraction (concentric). Within each level of training, the amount of resistance, duration, and frequency may be progressed.

- Submaximal isometric training (up to 75% of the maximum amount of weight that can be lifted once) for 3 months has been shown to significantly increase strength and cross-sectional area of muscle in older individuals.[4] Use of techniques such as proprioceptive neuromuscular facilitation and task-specific strengthening (Chapter 7) may improve functional carryover to open-chain–resistance training and thus may increase the effect performance.

1. Spirduso WW. *Physical dimensions of aging*. Champaign, IL: Human Kinetics; 1995.
2. Overend TJ, Cunningham DA, Kramer JF, et al. Knee extensor and knee flexor strength: cross-sectional area ratios in young and elderly men. *J Gerontol Med Sci*. 1992; 47:M204–M210.
3. Shephard RJ. *Aging, physical activity, and health*. Champaign, IL: Human Kinetics; 1997.
4. Pyka G, Lindenberger E, Charette S, et al. Muscle strength and fiber adaptations to a year-long resistance training program in elderly men and women. *J Gerontol Med Sci*. 1994;49:B22–B27.

▲ ▲ ▲ PEDIATRIC PERSPECTIVES ▲ ▲ ▲

- Open-chain exercises are appropriate and often a first option for strengthening in children. Open-chain activities provide isolation of muscle groups and are simple to teach. These activities are common in many upper- and lower-extremity movements used by children, such as reaching, throwing, and kicking.

- It is common to use both open- and closed-kinetic–chain modes of exercise in a therapeutic exercise program designed for children. Both are used for improvement of overall strength and function. Open-chain training may be the superior activity in young children for some upper-extremity tasks because children may lack the proximal strength (scapular stabilizers) and alignment to safely support closed-kinetic–chain exercises. An example of this is the scapular prominence that diminishes with age.[1]

- The same concern applies to some lower-extremity and trunk movements, for which open-chain training may be superior to closed chain. Very young children may lack the trunk strength needed to correctly perform some lower-extremity closed-kinetic–chain activities. An example of this is the sway-back posture of toddlers and youth.[1]

1. Kendall FP, McCreary EK et al. *Muscles: testing and function, with posture and pain*. 5th ed. Baltimore: Williams & Wilkins; 2005.

References

1. Bandy WD. Functional rehabilitation of the athlete. *Orthop Phys Ther Clin North Am.* 1992;1:1–13.

2. Falkel J, Cipriani D. Physiological principles of resistance training and rehabilitation. In: Zachazewski JE, Magee DJ, Quillen WS, eds. *Athletic injuries and rehabilitation.* Philadelphia: WB Saunders; 1996:206–228.

3. Arnheim D, Prentice W. *Principles of athletic training.* 8th ed. Baltimore: Mosby–Year Book; 1993:32–73.

4. Hettinger T, Muller EA. Muskelleisting and muskeltraining. *Arbeitphysiologic.* 1953;15:111–126 [Cited in Hislop HJ. Quantitative changes in human muscular strength during isometric exercise. *Phys Ther.* 1963;43:21–38.]

5. Muller EA. Influence of training and of inactivity on muscle strength. *Arch Phys Med Rehabil* 1970;51:449–462.

6. Walters L, Steward CC, LeClaire JF. Effort of short bouts of isometric and isotonic contractions on muscular strength and endurance. *Am J Phys Med.* 1960;39:131–141.

7. Cotton D. Relationship of duration of sustained voluntary isometric contraction to changes in endurance and strength. *Res Q Exerc Sport.* 1967;38:366–374.

8. Belka D. Comparison of dynamic, static, and combination training on dominant wrist flexor muscles. *Res Q Exerc Sport.* 1966;49:245–250.

9. Knapik JA, Mawdsley RH, Ramos MU. Angular specificity and test mode specificity of isometric and isokinetic strength training. *J Orthop Sports Phys Ther.* 1983;5:58–65.

10. Liberson WT, Asa MM. F urther studies on brief isometric exercises. *Arch Phys Med Rehabil* 1959;40:330–333.

11. Bandy WD, Hanten WP. Changes in torque and electromyographic activity of the quadriceps femoris muscles - following isometric training. *Phys Ther* 1993;73:455–467.

12. Norkin C, Levangie, P. *Joint structure and function: a comprehensive analysis.* 4th ed. Philadelphia: FA Davis Co; 2005:92–124.

13. Soderberg G. *Kinesiology. Application to pathological motion.* 2nd ed. Baltimore: Williams & Wilkins; 1997:29–57.

14. Albert M. *Eccentric muscle training in sports and orthopaedics.* New York: Churchill Livingstone; 1991.

15. Smith LL. Acute inflammation: the underlying mechanism in delayed-onset muscle soreness? *Med Sci Sports Exerc.* 1991;23:542–551.

16. Stauber WT, Clarkson PM, Fritz VK, et al. Extracellular matrix disruption and pain after eccentric muscle action. *J Appl Physiol.* 1990;69:868–874.

17. Howell JN, Chelboun G, Conaster R. Muscle stiffness, strength loss, swelling and soreness following exercise-induced injury in humans. *J Physiol.* 1993;464:183–196.

18. Ebbling CB, Clarkson PM. Muscle adaptation prior to recovery following eccentric exercises. *Eur J Appl Physiol.* 1990; 60:26–31.

19. American Academy of Orthopaedic Surgeons. *Athletic training and sports medicine.* 2nd ed. Park Ridge, IL: American Academy of Orthopaedic Surgeons; 1991.

20. Bandy WD, Lovelace-Chandler V. Relationship of peak torque to peak work and peak power of the quadriceps and hamstrings muscles in a normal sample using an accommodating resistance measurement device. *Isok Exerc Sci.* 1991;1: 87–91.

21. Delorme TL. Restoration of muscle power by heavy resistance exercise. *J Bone Joint Surg Am.* 1945;27:645–667.

22. Stone WJ, Kroll WA. *Sports conditioning and weight training: programs for athletic conditioning.* Boston: Allyn & Bacon; 1982.

23. Escamilla R, Wickham R. Exercise based conditioning and rehabilitation. In: Kolt GS, Snyder-Mackler L. *Physical therapies in sport and exercise.* London: Churchill Livingstone; 2003.

24. Hall C, Brody LT. Functional approach to therapeutic exercise for physiologic impairments. In: Hall C, Brody LT. *Therapeutic exercise.* 2nd ed. Philadelphia: Lippincott Williams & Wilkins; 2005.

25. Knight K. Knee rehabilitation by the daily adjustable progressive resistance exercise technique. *Am J Sports Med.* 1979; 7:336–337.

26. Davies GJ. *A compendium of isokinetics in clinical usage.* 4th ed. La Crosse, WI: S&S Publishers; 1992.

27. American Physical Therapy Association. *Guide to physical therapist practice.* 2nd ed. Alexandria, VA; 2003.

Proprioceptive Neuromuscular Facilitation

Marcia H. Stalvey, PT, MS, NCS

OBJECTIVES

Upon completion of this chapter, the reader will be able to:

- Demonstrate an understanding of diagonal patterns used in proprioceptive neuromuscular facilitation (PNF).

- Demonstrate an understanding of the integrated roles of flexion/extension, unilateral/bilateral movement, and distal to proximal timing in PNF.

- Apply techniques for upper-extremity diagonal patterns including scapular patterns, unilateral upper-extremity patterns, bilateral symmetric upper-extremity patterns, and bilateral asymmetric trunk patterns with and without equipment within the established plan of care.

- Apply techniques for lower-extremity diagonal patterns including unilateral lower-extremity patterns and bilateral symmetric lower-extremity patterns with and without equipment within the established plan of care.

- Apply correctly proper PNF-strengthening techniques using slow reversals, repeated contractions, timing for emphasis, and agonist reversal within the established plan of care.

- Apply correctly proper PNF-stability techniques using alternating isometric contractions and rhythmic stabilization within the established plan of care.

PNF is a philosophy of treatment developed in the 1950s by Kabat[1,2] and expanded under the vision of physical therapists Knott and Voss.[3] The basic principles of PNF emphasize the need for maximal demands to achieve maximal potential. The strong segments are used to facilitate the weak; improvement in specific functional activities is always the goal. Traditionally used for individuals with neurologic diagnoses,[4,5] PNF has wide applications for the rehabilitation of individuals with musculoskeletal dysfunctions. It is widely accepted that the central nervous system (CNS), through neural adaptation, plays a part in the strength gains beyond those attributable to increases in muscle hypertrophy.[6,7] PNF can be used effectively as part of an overall progressive rehabilitation program to hasten that neural adaptation through motor relearning, to improve strength and flexibility, and to promote a functional progression. The purposes of this chapter are to:

Review the philosophy, principles, and neurophysiologic basis of PNF.

Review and illustrate the more commonly used PNF diagonal patterns.

Describe and illustrate applications of selected PNF techniques.

Provide specific examples of the clinical application of PNF.

SCIENTIFIC BASIS

PNF is one of the traditional neurophysiologic approaches to therapeutic exercise, based on the classic work of Sherrington[8] and a hierarchic concept of the nervous system.[1,2] We now know that motor control is far more complex than just a muscle spindle and "top-down" organization,[9,10] and the use of PNF for CNS deficits has been somewhat controversial in light of more contemporary models of motor control. However, the literature substantiates the basic principles of PNF and their application to a wide variety of diagnoses, including the injured athlete.[11-17] PNF is most commonly used to restore range of motion (ROM), decrease pain, increase strength and endurance, hasten motor learning, improve coordination, facilitate proximal stability, and begin functional progression.[11,12,15,18]

Kabat[1,2] based his concepts of facilitation on the neurophysiology of the muscle spindle, applying Sherrington's laws of reciprocal innervation and successive induction to a therapeutic exercise technique. Reciprocal innervation states that contraction of the agonist produces simultaneous relaxation (inhibition) of the antagonist.[10] Successive induction suggests that voluntary motion of one muscle can be facilitated by the action of another.[10] For example, contraction of the biceps (the agonist), followed by contraction of the triceps (antagonist) results in increased response of biceps (the agonist). Additional neurophysiologic rationale is provided when specific techniques and applications are described.

CLINICAL GUIDELINES

One of the most easily and widely modified approaches to therapeutic exercise, PNF is readily applied to all stages of rehabilitation of the injured individual. In the acute stages of injury, isometric contractions, manual contacts, and an indirect approach are used to help guide and teach movements to the patient when swelling and pain interfere. PNF provides the physical therapist (PT) and the physical therapist assistant (PTA) with a means of manually grading an activity, giving precise feedback tailored to the patient's needs, activities, and level of rehabilitation. Techniques and patterns can be modified to avoid pain and to protect the integrity of a surgical procedure and/or joint. Ultimately, PNF patterns and techniques can be used to provide isometric, concentric, and eccentric strengthening using high-tech devices (e.g., pulleys, elastic bands, and isokinetic devices) and low-tech procedures (manual contact).

Basic Procedures

PNF uses specific proprioceptive and other sensory inputs to facilitate motor responses and motor learning. These inputs (or procedures) include tactile stimulation through the PTA's manual contacts or grip, resistance, stretch, irradiation (overflow), traction, approximation, verbal commands, and visual cues.[3,19,20]

Manual Contact

The PTA should touch only the surface of the area being facilitated. This manual contact gives the PTA a means of controlling the direction of motion and eliminating, correcting, or minimizing substitution. The contact also applies a demand (referred to as the appropriate resistance) and gives specific cutaneous and pressure stimulation. Usually one manual contact is placed distally and the other proximally to incorporate both distal movement and proximal stabilization of the musculature in the trunk, scapula, or pelvis. Precise placement depends on the relative strength of the patient.

Resistance

One of the hallmarks of PNF and the cornerstone of many of its techniques is resistance. Resistance is a means of guiding movement, securing maximal effort, and aiding motor relearning. Optimal resistance is defined as resistance that is graded appropriately for the intention of the movement. Simply put, maximal resistance is the most resistance that can be applied by the PTA and still result in a smooth, co-ordinated motion for a particular activity performed by the client. Therefore, it is essential not to over-resist the movements being facilitated and to allow the motion to occur.

If the task requires concentric or eccentric muscle contractions, the intention is either a shortening or a lengthening movement. Optimal resistance can change constantly throughout the ROM, depending on strength, joint stability, pain, and ability of the patient. Examples include eccentric resistance for the glenohumeral rotators and scapular stabilizers for the throwing athlete and concentric control for the jumper or sprinter. The intention of isometric muscle work is not motion but rather postural stability. Resistance to isometric contractions is therefore built up gradually so that no motion occurs. PNF is especially suited for use with a functional injury because of the emphasis on varying the type and speed of control needed, especially eccentric control.[15]

Manually resisted diagonal patterns and selected techniques allow the PTA to closely monitor the patient, finely grade the feedback, and change the challenge of the activity to meet the individual's needs. Patterns can be incorporated into independent and home programs using pulleys, weights, rubber tubing, and equipment, which are particularly necessary for muscle strength greater than 4/5 (as tested via manual muscle test).

Quick Stretch

Quick stretch is one of the most powerful neurophysiologic tools available.[2,3,9,10] When followed by resistance, quick stretch facilitates the muscle stretched. The stretch reflex is elicited by a gentle, quick "nudge" or "tap" to the muscles under tension, either from a fully elongated starting position or superimposed on an active muscle contraction. Quick stretch is contraindicated with pain, fracture, or recent surgical procedure.[6,7]

Irradiation

Used together, quick stretch and resistance can result in irradiation (or overflow) from the stronger segments to the weaker. Overflow, as defined by Sherrington,[8] occurs at the level of the anterior horn cell and is the "spread of facilitation with increased effort." Typically, overflow proceeds into muscles that are synergistic to the prime mover or to the muscles needed to stabilize that motion. This facilitation is directly proportional to the amount of strength in the resisted muscle groups and the amount of resistance applied. Irradiation is the key to using a strong motion to reinforce a weaker motion, such as facilitating ankle dorsiflexion through overflow from resistance applied to strong hip and knee flexion. Similarly, overflow may be used to promote

proximal stabilization, such as strengthening trunk flexion through overflow from the resistance of strong bilateral lower-extremity flexion. Irradiation can be especially helpful in re-establishing early active motion when pain is a factor. Because the patterns of irradiation are only partly predictable, closely monitoring the results and modifying the resistance are essential for best results.

Traction and Approximation

Manual traction and approximation are powerful facilitatory techniques that must be carefully modified in patients with pain or instability and after surgery.[11,12,20] Both procedures are contraindicated when joint instability, pain, or a recent surgical procedure is present. Use of traction and approximation can be gradually and cautiously reinstated as motor control and structural stability improve.

Traction is an elongating vector force applied along the long axis of the limb, slightly separating the joint surfaces. Traction is generally used to promote isotonic movement in phasic muscle groups, such as with pulling or antigravity motions (e.g., breast stroke in swimming).

Approximation is a compressive force applied through the long axis of the trunk or limb that facilitates stabilization, extension, and tonic muscle responses, especially in the lower extremities and trunk. For example, heel strike in gait provides a type of quick approximation that is followed by sustained approximation as the body weight progresses over the foot and extended hip. Closed-chain weight bearing on an aligned, extended arm facilitates scapular stabilization and control, in part, through the effects of approximation.

Verbal Commands

Verbal commands instruct the client what to do, when and how to perform a task, and how to correct a task.[19,20] These commands need to be simple, direct, and timed to coordinate the effort and motion. Softly spoken commands tend to be soothing and useful in the indirect approach with the patient with pain. Firm commands (louder) usually elicit stronger effort from the patient.

Visual Cues

Visual cues provide additional feedback for directional and postural control, assisting in the incorporation of appropriate head and trunk motions. Initially vision can be substituted for proprioceptive loss, but care must be exercised to avoid visual dependence.

Diagonal Patterns

PNF is perhaps best known for the spiral and diagonal movement patterns identified by Kabat.[1,2] These patterns of synergistic muscle combinations offer a mechanical lever arm to therapeutic exercise because they combine all planes of movement, cross midline, and are similar to normal functional movement. A narrow groove of motion exists, delineated by the shoulder in the upper extremity and the hip in the lower extremity, in which maximum power is achieved. Optimally both the client and the PTA move in that groove. Each pattern has motion in flexion or extension, abduction or adduction, and external or internal rotation. The largest ROM occurs in flexion and extension, the least in rotation. However, Kabat considers rotation to be the most important factor in eliciting strength and endurance changes.

Definition

The patterns of movement can be named two different ways: either by diagonal 1 (D1) or diagonal 2 (D2) or more simply for the motion occurring at the proximal joint. For example, shoulder flexion-abduction-external rotation (D2 flexion) or hip extension-adduction-external rotation (D2 extension). In this chapter, the motion of the proximal joint will be emphasized when describing patterns; reference to D1 and D2 will be secondary.

Tables 7-1 and 7-2 describe the components of the two upper- and lower-extremity diagonals, each consisting of two antagonistic patterns. In the extremity patterns, certain combinations of motions occur together consistently. Rotation of the shoulder and forearm occur in the same direction: supination with external rotation and pronation with internal rotation. When the shoulder abducts, the hand and wrist extend; hand and wrist flexion occur with shoulder adduction. In the lower extremity, ankle dorsiflexion

TABLE 7-2 Lower-extremity Diagonal Patterns

Pelvis	Anterior elevation	Posterior elevation
Hip	Flexion	Flexion
	Adduction	Abduction
	External rotation	Internal rotation
Knee	Varies	Varies
Ankle	Dorsiflexion	Dorsiflexion
Foot	Inversion	Eversion
Toes	Extension	Extension
	D1 FLEXION	**D2 FLEXION**
	Hip	
	D2 EXTENSION	**D1 EXTENSION**
Pelvis	Anterior depression	Posterior depression
Hip	Extension	Extension
	Adduction	Abduction
	External rotation	Internal rotation
Knee	Varies	Varies
Ankle	Plantarflexion	Plantarflexion
Foot	Inversion	Eversion
Toes	Flexion	Flexion

combines with hip flexion and plantarflexion with hip extension. Ankle eversion occurs with hip abduction; ankle inversion occurs with hip adduction. Internal hip rotation coincides with abduction motions; external rotation with adduction motions. Therefore, memorizing every component of the pattern is not necessary.

The intermediate joint (elbow, knee) may remain straight, flexed, or extended, depending on the function required. Varying the elbow position changes the muscle activity at the shoulder, in part because of the change in lever arm for the PTA.

Unilateral Versus Bilateral

Patterns may be performed unilaterally or bilaterally. Unilateral patterns focus on a specific motion of the joint. Bilateral patterns emphasize the proximal limb movement and the trunk by combining two extremities moving at the same time, either symmetrically (same diagonals, like the butterfly stroke), or asymmetrically (opposite diagonals, going toward the same side, as in throwing the hammer). Bilateral patterns permit the PTA to elicit overflow from a strong segment to facilitate weaker motions in the ipsilateral or contralateral extremity. Unilateral and bilateral patterns will be described in detail later in this chapter.

Normal Timing

The normal timing of the PNF patterns is distal to proximal, with the foot or hand leading the motion. For example, when performing a unilateral flexion adduction pattern (D1 flexion), the forearm and wrist supinate, flex first, and then

TABLE 7-1 Upper-extremity Diagonal Patterns

Scapula	Anterior elevation	Posterior elevation
Shoulder	Flexion	Flexion
	Adduction	Abduction
	External rotation	External rotation
Elbow	Varies	Varies
Forearm	Supination	Supination
Wrist	Radial flexion	Radial extension
Fingers	Flexion	Extension
	D1 FLEXION	**D2 FLEXION**
	Shoulder	
	D2 EXTENSION	**D1 EXTENSION**
Scapula	Anterior depression	Posterior depression
Shoulder	Extension	Extension
	Adduction	Abduction
	Internal rotation	Internal rotation
Elbow	Varies	Varies
Forearm	Pronation	Pronation
Wrist	Ulnar flexion	Ulnar extension
Fingers	Flexion	Extension

hold while the shoulder flexes and adducts. Shoulder external rotation initiates simultaneously with the distal wrist motion and completes as the shoulder approaches end range. Even when the ankle or hand has adequate strength, the recruitment pattern may be faulty, particularly in a normally functioning or highly trained individual. Correct sequencing or normal timing can be facilitated by manually restraining the proximal segments until the distal component is activated. This normal timing promotes motor learning.

General Treatment Design

In keeping with the PNF philosophy of using the strong to facilitate the weak, the PT first identifies the individual's strength, which is usually an extremity or quadrant that is pain free, strong, and demonstrates controlled and coordinated motion. Impairments in ROM, strength, and control are noted next. Functional limitations, such as inability to jump without pain, are identified next; then specific goals are set.

The PTA must also understand the biomechanics of the specific functional movement pattern, the key muscle components, the types or range of muscle contractions, and the stage of motor control needed. Depending on the activity, upper extremity demands may be for closed-chain movements (as in parallel bar work in gymnastics) or open-chain movements (as in throwing a baseball). Most activities, however, require both open- and closed-chain activities. The PT can then select appropriate PNF techniques and the corresponding PNF patterns to meet the functional goal.

Biomechanical considerations—such as the size of the base of support, the height of the center of gravity, the length of the lever arm, open- versus closed-chain activity, and the number of joints involved in the activity—can be varied to advance a therapeutic exercise program. PNF can also be effectively combined with the use of modalities, soft-tissue techniques, and mobilization. It is not necessary to do diagonal patterns to "do PNF," although the diagonal patterns are useful. Rather, the basic philosophy, principles, and techniques of PNF can be applied to functional activities to achieve a wide range of goals.

Clinical Application

Table 7-3 presents PNF diagonal pattern "helpers" that assist the PT and PTA in applying PNF patterns effectively. These helpers emphasize the PTA's body position and preparation of the client and remind the PTA of key cues for PNF principles.

For clarity, most of the patterns in this chapter are shown in supine. However, all of the PNF patterns and techniques may be applied in any posture and should not be limited to supine. The hip flexion-abduction pattern in side-lying emphasizes antigravity strengthening of the hip

TABLE 7-3	Proprioceptive Neuromuscular Facilitation Diagonal Pattern Helpers

The physical therapist assistant (PTA)'s position
Face the direction of motion
Shoulders and pelvis face the line of movement
Take up all the slack in all components of motion

Patient's position
Close to the PTA
Starting position is one of optimal elongation

Manual contacts
Combinations of proximal and distal

Quick stretch to initiate
Use body weight, not arm strength
Nudge

Move with the patient
The PTA's center of gravity *must* move
Distal component initiates motion

When performing reversals
Change distal manual contact first

abductors. Lower-extremity patterns should be progressed so the patient is able to perform them in an upright position, often with a narrowed base of postural support. Upper-extremity patterns combined with weight bearing in standing facilitate stability and controlled mobility essential to the development of skilled motion.[21] Bilateral-extremity patterns can be used in sitting to facilitate trunk control. Performance of these patterns in a functional posture can help achieve more complex movements.

The diagonal movement patterns are similar to the motions used in activities of daily living as well as in sports. For example, kicking a soccer ball is similar to the lower-extremity flexion-adduction pattern (D1 flexion). Opening an overhead cabinet is a widened version of upper-extremity extension-abduction and internal rotation with the elbow flexing pattern (D1 extension). Holding a tennis racket overhead for a serve corresponds to the flexion-abduction of the upper-extremity pattern (D2 flexion); release, deceleration, and follow-through are similar to extension-adduction with internal rotation patterns (D2 extension).

Selected commonly used limb and trunk patterns are described in the following sections. It is beyond the scope of this chapter to detail all patterns and possible combinations. For further information on any other patterns or techniques, see the texts by Adler et al[19] and Knott and Voss.[3]

Upper-extremity Diagonal Patterns

Scapular Patterns

Perhaps the most underused but most helpful of all the PNF patterns are the patterns for the scapula. Both stability and mobility of the scapulae are required if the upper extremity is to function normally and pain free. Most individuals presenting with shoulder dysfunction benefit from retraining of scapular stabilizers.[21] Scapular patterns can be initially performed in side-lying and progressed to sitting or standing. Similarly, activities can begin in a closed-chain context and move to an open-chain context as control improves.

There are four scapular patterns, two in each of the corresponding upper-extremity patterns. Scapular elevation patterns work with upper-extremity flexion, and scapular depression patterns with upper-extremity extension (Figs. 7-1 to 7-4).

Unilateral Upper-extremity Patterns

Unilateral upper-extremity patterns offer the PTA a long lever arm from which to facilitate the extremity and trunk (Table 7-1). When upper-extremity patterns are performed, care must be exercised in those individuals with anterior glenohumeral laxity or those who have just had surgery. Motions should not exceed 90-degree flexion, abduction, or rotation in early treatment to avoid stressing unstable structures. Similarly, weight bearing on an extended arm, in quadruped or modified plantigrade, should be closely monitored in individuals with posterior instability. The key concept is to start with the pattern that is strongest, most stable, or least painful (Figs. 7-5 to 7-8).

Bilateral Symmetric Upper-extremity Patterns

Any time two-extremity patterns are combined, the emphasis shifts to the trunk and proximal-extremity components. Symmetric patterns eliminate the trunk rotation component of the movement and, as such, are ideal for the patient who cannot tolerate much trunk rotation. In general, full ROM in distal motions are sacrificed to facilitate proximal control. Although any combination of patterns is possible, the more commonly used patterns are shown in Figures 7-9 to 7-11. Bilateral symmetric upper-extremity patterns are particularly easy and effective when performed with pulleys.

Bilateral Asymmetric Trunk Patterns

A strong trunk is essential for normal function and successful performance of many activities. Trunk patterns for PNF, including upper-extremity chops and lifts and bilateral symmetric lower-extremity patterns (described later in this chapter), can be used to strengthen trunk musculature or to irradiate into the neck, scapula, and extremities. Chops and lifts are bilateral asymmetric patterns that can be done in supine, sitting, prone, or any other position in

the biomechanical progression that challenges the individual. Because they are asymmetric patterns, significant trunk rotation and crossing of midline occurs, which may need to be moderated for some individuals.

Chops are a combination of extension-abduction (D1 extension) in the lead arm and extension-adduction (D2 extension) in the grasping arm. Chops can also facilitate functional activities such as rolling or coming to sit (Fig. 7-12).

Lifts are a bilateral asymmetric pattern combining flexion-abduction (D2 flexion) in one arm with flexion-adduction (D1 flexion) in the other. Lifts are an effective tool for facilitating upper trunk extension and scapular stabilization at the end range (Fig. 7-13).

Lower-extremity Diagonal Patterns

Unilateral Lower-extremity Patterns

The two lower-extremity diagonals are shown in Table 7-2. As in the upper extremity, the intermediate joint (knee) may flex, extend, or stay straight. Again, the starting position for each pattern is at the end of the antagonistic pattern. Common patterns are presented in Figures 7-14 to 7-17.

Bilateral Symmetric Lower-extremity Patterns

Bilateral symmetric lower-extremity patterns involve the combination of both extremities working together. Holding the feet bilaterally while performing the bilateral pattern places the emphasis on the lower trunk moving on the upper trunk. These patterns emphasize irradiation from stronger to weaker segments or limbs. The patterns are usually initiated in sitting (Fig 7-18), but can be performed in prone to facilitate knee flexion activities.

Bilateral lower-extremity patterns are not used as frequently for musculoskeletal dysfunction as are bilateral upper-extremity patterns and thus are not emphasized. For more information on bilateral patterns, see the texts by Adler et al[19] and Knott and Voss.[3]

Progression and Integration with Equipment

All of the patterns described so far can be performed as part of an equipment-based program, most easily with a pulley. The patterns can be adapted to more elaborate isokinetic equipment, with the rotational components greatly reduced. Braces may be worn during the pulley program to limit range and protect stability of grafts as needed. Anything done with pulleys in the clinic can be performed with elastic tubing in the home. Examples of setups are shown in Figures 7-19 and 7-20.

| Figure 7-1 | Scapular anterior elevation. |

PURPOSE: Strengthening of levator scapula, serratus anterior, and scalene muscles in diagonal plane of the scapula.

POSITION: Client lying on side. The physical therapist assistant standing behind client's hips in the line of motion, facing the client's head. Both hands overlapping on the anterior glenohumeral joint and acromion **(A)**.

PROCEDURE: Client anteriorly elevates scapula against appropriate resistance. Movement is in a diagonal arc up toward client's nose **(B)**.

A

B

| Figure 7-2 | Scapular posterior depression. |

PURPOSE: Strengthening of rhomboids and latissimus dorsi muscles in diagonal plane of the scapula.

POSITION: Client lying on side. The physical therapist assistant standing behind the client's hips in the line of motion, facing the client's head. Both hands are flat-palmed on the middle to lower scapula, along the vertebral border **(A)**.

PROCEDURE: Movement is down to the ipsilateral ischial tuberosity **(B)**.

Figure 7-3 Scapular posterior elevation.

PURPOSE: Strengthening of trapezius and levator scapulae muscles in diagonal plane of the scapula.

POSITION: Client lying on side. The physical therapist assistant standing at client's head, facing the hips. Manual contacts on the distal edge of the upper trapezius, close to the acromion **(A)**.

PROCEDURE: Movement is in an arc as the client shrugs up toward the ear **(B)**.

| Figure 7-4 | Scapular anterior depression. |

PURPOSE: Strengthening of rhomboids and pectoralis minor and major muscles in diagonal plane of the scapula.

POSITION: Client lying on side. The physical therapist assistant standing at client's head, facing the hips. Manual contacts on the pectoral muscle and coracoid process anteriorly and on the lateral border of the scapula posteriorly **(A)**.

PROCEDURE: Client pulls shoulder down toward umbilicus **(B)**.

Figure 7-5	Upper extremity: flexion-adduction-external rotation (D1 flexion).

PURPOSE: Strengthening, range of motion (ROM), or control of shoulder flexion and adduction, scapular anterior elevation, and wrist flexion. Pattern of choice for initiating rotator cuff activities because of reduced external rotation and abduction ROM components.

POSITION: Client lying supine. Begins with client's shoulder in slight extension with hand near hip. The physical therapist assistant (PTA) standing at client's elbow, facing feet. Distal manual contact on the palm provides most of the traction and rotatory control. Proximal contact can be on the biceps or onto the pectorals **(A)**.

PROCEDURE: Client told to "turn and squeeze my hand," then "pull up and across your nose." The PTA pivots toward client's head as the arm moves past. Ends with client's elbow crossing midline around the nose **(B)**.

Figure 7-6

Upper extremity: extension-abduction-internal rotation (D1 extension).

PURPOSE: Strengthening, range of motion (ROM), or control of shoulder extension and abduction, scapular depression, internal rotation, and wrist extension.

POSITION: Client lying supine. The physical therapist assistant (PTA) standing at client's side near head. Client's arm flexed and adducted. Manual contacts on dorsal surface of the hand (distal) and on posterior surface of the humerus or scapula (proximal) **(A)**.

PROCEDURE: Quick stretch, especially in the form of traction, applied simultaneously to the hand and shoulder. Client told to "pull wrist up and push your arm down to your side." As arm moves past the PTA, traction can be switched to approximation to increase proximal recruitment. Ends with wrist extended and arm at client's hip **(B)**.

| Figure 7-7 | Upper extremity: flexion-abduction-external rotation (D2 flexion). |

PURPOSE: Strengthening, range of motion, or control of shoulder flexion and abduction, scapular anterior elevation, and wrist extension.

POSITION: Client lying supine. The physical therapist assistant (PTA) standing at client's shoulder facing client's feet with a wide base of support in the diagonal of movement. Client's extremity starts from across body, in an elongated, extended position, with elbow crossing the body near hip. Distal manual contact on dorsal hand; proximal contact either on proximal humerus or on scapula to emphasize shoulder and scapular motions **(A)**.

PROCEDURE: The PTA takes limb to a fully elongated position, taking up all slack in the muscle groups, and gently applies quick stretch; client told to "pull wrist up and reach." Wrist completes extension before the other components **(B)**.

Figure 7-8   Upper extremity: extension-adduction-internal rotation (D2 extension).

PURPOSE: Strengthening, range of motion, or control of shoulder extension and adduction, scapular depression, and wrist flexion.

POSITION: Client lying supine. The physical therapist assistant (PTA) standing near the client's shoulder. Distal manual contact palm to palm with client **(A)**. Proximal contact on pectoral muscles to emphasize recruitment of trunk and scapula or on proximal humerus.

PROCEDURE: Elongation and quick stretch applied; client told to "squeeze and turn your wrist, then pull down and across." The PTA pivots slightly as the limb passes the PTA's center of gravity. Ends in shoulder extension, forearm in pronation, elbow across midline **(B)**.

<table>
<tr><td>**Figure 7-9**</td><td>Upper extremity: bilateral symmetric flexion-abduction.</td></tr>
</table>

PURPOSE: Strengthening of shoulder flexion, trunk extension, and control using two strong upper extremities.

POSITION: Client lying supine. The physical therapist assistant standing at the client's head, arms crossed. Manual contacts on dorsum of wrists **(A)**.

PROCEDURE: Client lifts both arms straight overhead against resistance **(B)**.

151

| Figure 7-10 | Upper extremity: bilateral symmetric extension-adduction. |

PURPOSE: Strengthening shoulder extension and adduction, upper trunk flexion, and control using two strong upper extremities.

POSITION: Client lying supine. Manual contacts at wrists **(A)**.

PROCEDURE: Client told to "squeeze and pull down and across" **(B)**.

Figure 7-11 Upper extremity: bilateral symmetric extension-abduction (with pulleys).

PURPOSE: Strengthening, range of motion, or control of shoulder extension, trunk extension, and stabilization.

POSITION: Sitting in chair, client grasps pulley handles with arms crossed, in a position of shoulder adduction, flexion, and external rotation; wrists in flexion and radial deviation **(A)**.

PROCEDURE: Client told to "straighten your wrists and pull your arms down to your sides" **(B)**.

| Figure 7-12 | Upper extremity: chops. |

PURPOSE: Strengthening of trunk flexion; overflow to extremity extensor musculature.

POSITION: Client lying supine. The physical therapist assistant (PTA) standing at the end of pattern so that client chops down to the PTA. Client grasping one arm at the wrist. Manual contacts placed distally on dorsal wrist and proximally on scapula or proximal humerus of the abducting (free, nongrasping) arm **(A)**.

PROCEDURE: Client told to "tuck your chin and chop down and across to your knees." Head and neck flex, following the leading straight (abducting) arm. Neck motions can be cued with verbal reminders or light, guiding resistance on the forehead. The PTA restrains arm motion until trunk musculature has been activated **(B)**.

| Figure 7-13 | Upper extremity: lifts. |

PURPOSE: Facilitate trunk extension, rotation, and lateral bending toward the leading (abducting) arm.

POSITION: Client lying supine. The physical therapist assistant (PTA) standing at end of the pattern so client lifts up to the PTA. Lead, abducting arm straight; following limb grasping opposite forearm. Distal manual contact on dorsum of abducting arm; proximal contact on occiput to emphasize neck extension or on scapula **(A)**.

PROCEDURE: Client told to "look up and lift your arms up to me" **(B)**.

Figure 7-14 Lower extremity: flexion-adduction-external rotation (D1 flexion).

PURPOSE: Strengthening, range of motion, or control of hip flexion, abduction, external rotation, and ankle dorsiflexion and inversion.

POSITION: Client lying supine. Begins with the physical therapist assistant (PTA) moving limb into an elongated position of hip and knee extension (slightly off the plinth), internal rotation, and ankle plantarflexion with eversion. Manual contacts placed proximally on anterior distal femur and distally on dorsum of foot **(A)**.

PROCEDURE: Corkscrew-like elongation given to entire pattern. Ankle dorsiflexion with inversion initiates motion and provides the PTA a handle for traction. As limb moves into flexion, knee and heel cross midline. Knee and ankle both must finish in line, at or slightly across midline **(B)**.

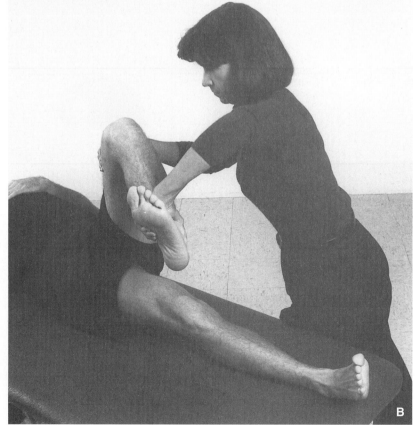

| Figure 7-15 | Lower extremity: extension-abduction-internal rotation (D1 extension). |

PURPOSE: Strengthening, range of motion, or control of hip extension, abduction, internal rotation, and ankle plantarflexion and eversion.

POSITION: Client lying supine. The physical therapist assistant (PTA) standing with a wide base of support facing client in line of movement. Client's extremity in a position of hip and knee flexion, full dorsiflexion, and inversion; knee and heel at or slightly across midline. The PTA cupping ball of foot distally and providing proximal contact on hamstrings **(A)**.

PROCEDURE: Quick stretch applied simultaneously to hip, knee, and ankle as client told to "point your foot down and kick down and out to me." Ankle plantarflexion and eversion initiate motion, with full hip and knee extension concluding simultaneously **(B)**.

| Figure 7-16 | Lower extremity: flexion-abduction-internal rotation (D2 flexion). |

PURPOSE: Strengthening, range of motion, or control of motion of hip flexion, abduction, internal rotation, and ankle dorsiflexion and eversion.

POSITION: Client lying supine. The physical therapist assistant (PTA) standing at client's hip, facing feet. Both legs positioned slightly away from the PTA so limb in question begins in an abducted, extended, and externally rotated position. Proximal manual contact on dorsum of foot; distal contact on anterior distal femur just above knee **(A)**.

PROCEDURE: Client told to "bring your toes up and out; swing your heel out to me." Ends with heel close to lateral buttock and hip and knee aligned with each other **(B)**.

Figure 7-17 Lower extremity: extension-adduction-external rotation (D2 extension).

PURPOSE: Strengthening, range of motion, or control of hip extension, adduction, external rotation, and ankle plantarflexion and inversion.

POSITION: Client lying supine. The physical therapist assistant (PTA) standing in groove, facing client's feet. Manual contacts distally on instep of foot and proximally on medial femur **(A)**.

PROCEDURE: Distal motion must come in first, facilitated by quick stretch into flexion. Limb extends with knee finishing across midline **(B)**. The PTA may elect to stand at end of pattern to better manually resist extension and adduction.

Figure 7-18　Lower extremity: bilateral flexion with knee extension in sitting position.

PURPOSE: Strengthening, range of motion (ROM), or control of knee flexion and extension using advanced lower-extremity pattern in sitting.

POSITION: Client sitting with knees flexed and ankles plantarflexed. The physical therapist assistant (PTA) standing in front of client centered in middle of both grooves. Manual contacts at dorsal aspect of both feet **(A)**.

PROCEDURE: Quick stretch and traction into knee flexion and ankle plantarflexion initiates motion. Ankle dorsiflexion must occur first as client extends both knees. Client told to "lift your toes up and straighten your knees together" **(B)**. At end of ROM, the PTA switches manual contacts to balls of feet; gentle quick stretch into knee extension initiates motion as client plantarflexes ankle and flexes knees against appropriate resistance.

| Figure 7-19 | Elastic tubing for lower extremity (D1 flexion). |

PURPOSE: Strengthening, range of motion, or control of flexion.

POSITION: Client standing, leg extended and in slight abduction while holding on to chair for balance. End of tubing is hooked around dorsum of flexing extremity **(A)**.

PROCEDURE: Client dorsiflexes ankle and flexes extremity up and across body, keeping knee straight **(B)**. Eccentric control may be emphasized as client slowly returns extremity to start position against pull of tubing. Pattern simulates kicking a ball.

A

B

161

| **Figure 7-20** | Elastic tubing for upper extremity (D2 flexion). |

PURPOSE: Strengthening, range of motion, or control of flexion, adduction, and internal rotation in a functional standing position.

POSITION: Standing; client's extremity across body, grasping tubing with shoulder extended, adducted, and internally rotated; elbow pronated and wrist flexed.

PROCEDURE: Client told to "pull wrist up and reach." Pattern simulates throwing a ball.

TECHNIQUES

All of the PNF patterns and functional movement progressions can be combined with specific techniques to facilitate the stages of movement control: mobility, strength, stability, and skill.[20] The injured individual may require improvement at any or all of these stages. The goal is to combine facilitation, inhibition, strengthening, and relaxation with different types of muscle contractions to achieve specific functional goals. Table 7-4 shows the most common uses for the different techniques. Note that many of the techniques have multiple and overlapping functions.

Mobility Techniques

Often the first challenge for the injured patient is to appropriately contract the muscle(s) again. *Rhythmic initiation* can help overcome pain, anxiety, and decreased control and is an effective technique for assisting the initiation of motion. The patient is taken through the complete motion passively, then asked to gradually actively participate with the motion. Eventually, the individual is progressed into a slow reversal technique with the application of guiding and facilitating resistance.

Strengthening Techniques

Strengthening is the major focus of most rehabilitation programs. There are distinct advantages of PNF over the use

---

TABLE 7-4 Summary of Proprioceptive Neuromuscular Facilitation Techniques

Mobility
Reciprocal inhibition[a]
Autogenic inhibition[a]
Rhythmic initiation

Strengthening
Slow reversals
Repeated contractions
Timing for emphasis
Agonist reversal

Stability
Alternating isometrics
Rhythmic stabilization

Skill
Timing for emphasis
Resisted progression

Endurance
Slow reversals
Agonist reversals

[a]See Chapter 4.

---

of traditional weight training for strengthening. Manually resisted PNF patterns and activities allow the PTA to more precisely monitor and correct substitutions. The use of normal movement patterns, the emphasis on eccentric control and functional progression, and the ability to vary the speed are additional advantages of PNF over traditional progressive-resistive programs. Nelson et al[15] noted better carryover to functional performance measures, including vertical leap and throwing distance, with PNF-strengthening activities than with traditional progressive-resistive–exercise programs. Furthermore, PNF patterns and principles can be applied to use with equipment. Specific PNF techniques, which can be used to facilitate strengthening, include slow reversals, repeated contractions, timing for emphasis, and agonist reversals.

Slow reversals of reciprocal movement is a high-use technique for applying resistance to increase strength and endurance, teach reversal of movement, and increase coordination. Both directions of a diagonal pattern are performed in a smooth, rhythmic fashion with changes of direction occurring without pause or relaxation. Generally slow reversals begin with the stronger pattern first to take advantage of the principle of successive induction. To eliminate lag time when switching directions, the PTA changes the distal manual contact first, provides a new quick stretch, and resists the motion into the opposite direction. The speed, ROM, and quickness of change of direction can be varied to emphasize specific portions of a range or control. Similarly, isometric and eccentric contractions can be superimposed anywhere in the range at any time. Isometric contractions at the weak point in the range have been shown to increase motor neuron recruitment and increase muscle spindle sensitivity, which may be important for enhancing postural stabilizers that may have been overstretched.

Slow reversals are particularly helpful for the patient who is beginning to work on timing and reversals of motion in preparation for sport-specific training, such as throwing or cutting motions. Reversals are rarely slow in daily activities or in sports. The speed of change and type of contraction can be altered constantly in the session to work on neuromuscular control. When focusing on control drills, verbal commands should be kept to a minimum, forcing the individual to rely on tactile and proprioceptive input alone.

Repeated contractions of the weak muscle help facilitate initiation of motion, enhance recruitment, increase active ROM and strength, and offset fatigue. To apply repeated contractions, the PTA fully elongates all the muscles in the pattern, then gives a quick nudge to stretch the muscle further. The patient is told to keep pulling as repeated stretches and resistance are applied, and the limb moves farther toward the end range. Because repeated contractions use quick stretch, their use is contraindicated with joint instability, pain, fracture, or recent surgical procedure.

Timing for emphasis, or *pivots*, blocks the normal timing of muscular contraction to focus on the recruitment, strength, or coordination of a specific muscle group, often in a particular portion of the range. To use this technique effectively, the client must have three things: (a) a strong, stabilizing muscle group; (b) a "handle" or segment onto which the clinician may hold; and (c) a pivot point, or the movement being emphasized. Commonly the distal or intermediate component is pivoted, but any motion is possible.

For example, consider the use of timing for emphasis for ankle dorsiflexors. Lower-extremity flexion against resistance is initiated against manual resistance. At the strongest part of the range, the patient performs an isometric hold of the entire pattern. The PTA applies quick stretch to the dorsiflexors, allowing movement of the dorsiflexors while holding the isometric contraction elsewhere. The pivot on the ankle is repeated two to three times. The activity is finished with quick stretch to the entire pattern to facilitate movement through the entire pattern. This activity can be used in an upright position or in a more functional posture.

The technique of *agonist reversal* is the use of eccentric muscle contractions within a pattern or resisted functional activity to enhance control and strength. The patient is told to keep pulling as the PTA takes the limb back (overpowering the patient) to the original starting position (causing an eccentric contraction). Because the vast majority of high-skill activities have deceleration components, eccentric work is part of essential preparation for functional activities. A common example is the overhead worker who must control the deceleration of the arm to avoid excessive stress on supporting noncontractile structures. Agonist reversals can be particularly beneficial for treating tendonitis and patellar tracking disorders.

Stability Techniques

Stability includes both nonweight-bearing isometric muscle stability and dynamic postural activities while weight bearing in proper biomechanical alignment. Techniques frequently used to promote stability include alternating isometrics and rhythmic stabilization.

Alternating isometric contractions is the simplest of these techniques. The clinician provides isometric resistance to the patient in one direction (usually the stronger), telling the patient to "hold, don't let me move you." Resistance is gradually switched to the other direction by moving one hand at a time to the opposite side and telling the patient to switch and hold. No movement of the individual or of the joint should occur (Fig 7-21).

Alternating isometric contractions progress to *rhythmic stabilization*, in which an isometric cocontraction for stability is generated around the joint or trunk. This is a bidirectional, rotational technique, with smooth co-contraction in all three planes occurring simultaneously. Manual contacts are placed

Figure 7-21 Alternating isometrics to trunk flexors in sitting.

PURPOSE: Activation and strengthening of trunk flexors; overflow and facilitation of hip, knee, and ankle flexor muscles.

POSITION: Client sitting with no back support. The physical therapist assistant (PTA) sitting in front of client. Manual contacts with flat hand just inferior to bilateral clavicles.

PROCEDURE: The PTA gradually applies resistance, matching client's effort, so there is little trunk movement. Overflow may result in active movement into hip, knee, and ankle flexor musculature as resistance is built up. Resistance is applied first to one side of trunk (anterior) and then to the other side (posterior).

Figure 7-22 Rhythmic stabilization to trunk.

PURPOSE: Stabilization and control of trunk through cocontraction of musculature on both sides of trunk.

POSITION: Client sitting upright with no back support. The physical therapist assistant (PTA) sitting in front or behind client with hands on opposite aspects of trunk at inferior clavicle and mid-scapula.

PROCEDURE: Client told to "hold" or "match me" against manual resistance, which attempts to rotate trunk. Resistance is built up slowly over 5 to 10 seconds, then held and gradually reduced. To change direction of rotary force, the PTA approximates through shoulders, gradually sliding manual contacts from anterior to posterior and vice versa.

on opposite sides of the limb or trunk (Figs. 7-22 and 7-23). Isometric rotational resistance is gradually built up, held, and then gradually switched to go the other direction. The key to accomplishing smooth change of direction is the use of approximation and the firm, maintained sliding input provided around the joint surface during the transition. The resistance can change directions as many times as is necessary. Most easily used to promote proximal trunk control, rhythmic stabilization can be applied to bilateral or even unilateral extremity patterns.

Skill

An individual performs a variety of activities with consistent and proper timing, sequencing, speed, and coordinated con-

trol. PNF uses the techniques of resisted progression, normal timing, and timing for emphasis to promote skilled movement. In addition, the techniques of agonist reversals (eccentric contractions) and slow reversals can be used effectively to vary the muscular contractions required within a single exercise session, progressing from isometric to eccentric.

Timing for emphasis enhances the distal to proximal sequence of motions. Stronger, proximal motions are resisted and held back until the desired distal motion is elicited with quick stretch and resistance. The timing may first be enhanced in nonweight-bearing postures and then progressed to upright postures. Skilled performance of movement may also be facilitated by manual resistance, pulleys, or elastic tubing. Examples include resisted gait, braiding, or cutting motions.

| Figure 7-23 | Rhythmic stabilization to bilateral upper extremity. |

PURPOSE: Promote cocontraction and stabilization about upper trunk and shoulders; relaxation and range of motion (ROM).

POSITION: Client lying supine. The physical therapist assistant (PTA) standing at head of client. Generally started in mid-ROM or where control is best; may be progressed to other parts of ROM as intervention progresses. Manual contacts on opposite sides of wrist.

PROCEDURE: Client told to "hold" or "match me" against manual resistance, which attempts to flex one arm up and extend the other. Resistance is gradually built up slowly over 5 to 10 seconds, then held and gradually reduced. To change direction of force, the PTA approximates through extended arms, gradually sliding manual contacts from anterior to posterior and vice versa

CASE STUDY 1

PATIENT INFORMATION

A 37-year-old female competitive recreational soccer player presented on referral from her orthopedist with a diagnosis of patellar tendonitis and patellofemoral dysfunction. She reported that the morning after the previous week's game she had pain in her left knee accompanied by mild swelling, difficulty ascending and descending stairs, and occasional buckling of the knee when trying to run. She could recall no specific incident or onset of the pain during the game. She also reported occasional crepitus and increased stiffness in the knee after sitting for long periods. She did report a previous medial collateral ligament injury to the same knee in college, which was treated conservatively with good success and return to unbraced competitive play. She was eager to return to her sport.

Examination by the PT revealed mild swelling on the inferior-lateral aspect of the patellar tendon region and tenderness to palpation at the inferior pole of the patella. The patellar position was slightly laterally and posteriorly tilted. The range of motion at the knee was limited to 0 to 100 degrees owing to rectus femoris tightness. The hamstrings were tight bilaterally (0- to 70-degree straight-leg raise). Strength testing indicated left quadriceps strength at 3/5 with a 20-degree extensor lag; hamstrings were measured at 4/5. Recruitment of the left vastus medialis oblique (VMO) was poor. The strengths of all other muscles tested were 5/5. All ligamentous stability testing noted intact ligaments with no instability present. The examination confirmed the diagnosis made by the physician of patellar tendonitis and patellofemoral syndrome.

LINK TO
GUIDE TO PHYSICAL THERAPIST PRACTICE

The patient's diagnosis is consistent with pattern 4E of the *Guide*[22]: "impaired joint mobility, motor function, muscle performance, and range of motion associated with localized inflammation." Included in this diagnostic group is tendonitis, and direct intervention involves "strengthening using resistive exercises."

INTERVENTION

The PT's initial intervention was directed at reducing inflammation, regaining full ROM, reducing pain with activity, and independence in a home program. The PT instructed the PTA to perform the following treatment and report the patient's response to the treatment in the post-treatment session.

1. Ice the affected knee before treatment.
2. Manually resisted reciprocal-inhibition stretching technique to the hamstrings bilaterally in supine (Figs. 4-4 thru 4-6)
3. Bilateral lower-extremity extension (Fig. 7-18), combined with isometric holds and timing for emphasis at the end range of knee extension (to improve recruitment of VMO and achieve active terminal knee extension).
4. Patellar taping and biofeedback to assist patellar alignment during PNF.
5. Home program: hamstring stretching on an elevated surface using modified contract relax and isometric quad sets.
6. Ice at the end of treatment.

PROGRESSION

One Week After Initial Treatment

At the time of re-examination by the PT, the patient presented with pain-free knee flexion (0 to 115 degrees) with mild complaints of "catching" at the end of active full extension. The straight-leg raise increased to 0 to 85 degrees. Quad lag improved to 0 to 10 degrees. The patient reported continued difficulty ascending and descending stairs.

The PT directed the PTA to continue with clinic treatment of manually resisted PNF patterns, progressing to unilateral flexion-adduction pattern (D1 flexion) in supine (Fig. 7-14), using slow reversals to increase recruitment and delay fatigue. The PTA was also instructed by the PT to introduce standing activities, including alternating isometrics and rhythmic stabilization to quadriceps and hamstrings using manual resistance. The home program was progressed, under the direction of the PT, as follows:

1. Standing lower-extremity flexion-adduction with elastic tubing (Fig. 7-19).
2. Partial-range wall squats and slides with knees flexed to a maximum of 20 degrees; emphasis on isometric holds and eccentrics in the closed-chain position.
3. Continue hamstring stretching and patellar taping.
4. Ice after treatment.

Two Weeks After Initial Examination

After 2 weeks of intervention the PT's examination indicated full knee flexion and straight-leg range to 95 degrees. No active quadriceps lag was present, and the quadriceps strength tested at 4+/5. The patient reported that she was able to ascend stairs with minimal discomfort and had only mild discomfort with descent. The goal at this time was to continue to strengthen the VMO and begin progression to resistive exercise with increasing knee motion to prepare for kicking activities and return to play.

The PT instructed the PTA to continue with clinic treatment of unilateral flexion-adduction pattern with knee extending, using slow reversals and progressing to timing for emphasis on left knee extension, pivoting off the stronger right lower extremity. In addition, the patient performed standing resisted flexion with knee extension to simulate striking a soccer ball, first emphasizing standing on the involved limb and then striking with it.

The PTA, under the direction and supervision of the PT, progressed the home program to include jogging. If no pain occurred with jogging, the patient was instructed to begin cutting activities. She was told to continue with stretching, strengthening, and ice as needed.

OUTCOMES

Three weeks after initial intervention the patient called to cancel the next appointment. She reported resolution of pain and return to play without complication.

SUMMARY—AN EFFECTIVE PT-PTA TEAM

This case study demonstrates an effective and trusting relationship between the PT and PTA. In this scenario the PTA must be knowledgeable of advanced treatment techniques regarding PNF patterns, neuromuscular re-education, and patellar taping techniques. The PT expects the PTA to fully understand the treatment techniques and be able to reciprocate the plan of care requested by the PT. It is also expected that good communication exists between the PTA and supervising PT so that any adverse effects of the treatment are reported. This type of situation usually requires the PT and the PTA to have a long-time working relationship in which there is ongoing education and a good comfort level with the PTA's skills in advanced techniques.

GERIATRIC PERSPECTIVES

- The specific techniques of PNF, combining diagonal patterns with facilitatory stimuli (tactile contact, resistance, irradiation, approximation, verbal commands, and vision), make the approach useful for promoting strengthening, motor learning, and restoration of motor control in older adults with musculoskeletal and neuromuscular deficits. Research has demonstrated that older adults have decreased response to proprioceptive stimuli, especially if the movement is passive and with small changes in the joint angle.[1] Tactile contact and approximation may promote a better feel of the movement pattern for older adults.

- Detection of joint angular movement (the angular threshold) appears to improve with increasing magnitude and speed.[1] Use of PNF diagonals with verbal commands to increase awareness of joint angular movement is an effective intervention for decreasing the angular threshold and promoting motor learning.

- The synergistic recruitment of agonist–antagonist is an appropriate means of incorporating more functional-based strengthening in the rehabilitation for subacute and chronic joint problems. As outlined by Hertling and Kessler,[2] a gradual progression from isometric to eccentric to isotonic muscle strengthening is more likely to demonstrate functional carryover than is rote strengthening. Use of this progression is analogous to promoting stability (holding cocontraction), then grading the stability to allow muscle lengthening, and finally inhibiting the antagonist to allow selective contraction in agonist (controlled mobility). The goal is for the older adult to develop automatic controlled mobility during functional performance.

- Patterns and techniques of PNF are effective for improving isometric, eccentric, and isotonic control in movements requiring control at varied joint angles (small to large ranges). An example of such movement is coming from sit to stand and the control that is needed in flexion to extension of the hip and knee. D1 flexion and D2 extension diagonals combined with techniques such as alternating isometrics and rhythmic stabilization and progressing to agonist reversal and then to slow reversals and repeated contractions is suggested for assisting the older adult to gain skill in performance of synergistic movements.

- Resistance may be applied using dumbbells, cuff weights, rubber tubing, or items available in the home (cans of soup, bags of dried beans). As suggested for children, clear, precise verbal and written instruction may be necessary and helpful for promoting compliance and understanding in older adults.

1. Schultz AB, Ashton-Miller JA, Alexander NB. Biomechanics of mobility in older adults. In: Hazzard WR, Blass JP, Ettinger WH, et al, eds. *Principles of geriatric medicine and gerontology.* 4th ed. New York: McGraw-Hill; 1998: 131–142.
2. Hertling D. *Management of common musculoskeletal disorders: physical therapy principles and methods.* 3rd ed. Philadelphia: Lippincott-Raven; 2005.

SUMMARY

- PNF is a philosophy of treatment that uses normal diagonal movement patterns, variable resistance, and a variety of specific techniques to meet the patient's goals. Basic principles of PNF include the use of specific manual contacts, resistance, and proprioceptive techniques. Optimal resistance is defined as the amount that challenges the patient while still allowing the desired smooth, coordinated movement.

- PNF diagonal patterns cross the midline, incorporating all planes of movement, and are similar to many sport-specific movements. Diagonal patterns should be modified according to the structural stability of the joint and extremity. Although primarily a manual technique, PNF patterns and principles are readily applied to the use of equipment for home programs and increased challenge.

- PNF includes methods to increase the ROM, teach the initiation of movement (rhythmic initiation), increase strength (slow reversals, repeated contractions, timing for emphasis), improve stability (agonist reversals, rhythmic stabilization), and improve skill (resisted progression, normal timing).

- Although an understanding of the philosophy, principles, and techniques of PNF can be gained by reading, skilled application to treatment is best achieved through supervised practice. To best use the information presented here, it is important to practice the techniques and receive feedback from a skilled PNF practitioner.

PEDIATRIC PERSPECTIVES

▲ ▲ ▲   ▲ ▲ ▲

■ The principles and patterns of PNF can be, and often are, incorporated into rehabilitation of children with both neuromuscular and musculoskeletal impairments and functional limitations. PNF diagonal patterns may be used during development and rehabilitation of athletic skills because these patterns are similar to the patterns used during sporting motions.

■ Interventions of PNF closely parallel the normal sequence of motor behavior acquisition that occurs in children: proximal to distal, stability to mobility. Improvement in all types of motor ability depends on motor learning. Motor learning is enhanced through sensory inputs from multiple systems, including visual, verbal, tactile, and proprioceptive.[1]

■ PNF techniques use multiple forms of sensory input. Remember that throughout childhood sensory systems are developing and do not demonstrate the

same responses as in the adult. Children may not respond like adults in development or rehabilitation of motor ability.

■ In younger children, expect less independence for performing complex motor patterns with multiple components (diagonal patterns). This may be due to attention span or memory and emotional maturity issues. More time may be needed for active-assisted or manual-resistance treatments for children than for adults. Children may have difficulty adapting an exercise to include tubing, weights, or pulleys. Instruction and feedback in several forms may be necessary (verbal, written, pictorial).

1. Horak FB. Assumptions underlying motor control for neurologic rehabilitation. In: Lister MJ, ed. *Contemporary management of motor control problems; proceedings of the II Step conference.* Alexandria, VA: Foundation for Physical Therapy; 1991:11–28.

References

1. Kabat H. Central mechanisms for recovery of neuromuscular function. *Science.* 1950;112:23–24.

2. Kabat H. The role of central facilitation in restoration of motor function paralysis. *Arch Phys Med.* 1953;33:521–533.

3. Knott M, Voss DE. *Proprioceptive neuromuscular facilitation.* New York: Harper & Row; 1968.

4. Trueblood PR, Walker JM, Gronley JK. Pelvic exercise and gait in hemiplegia. *Phys Ther.* 1989;69:32–40.

5. Wang RP. Effect of proprioceptive neuromuscular facilitation on the gait of athletes with hemiplegia of long and short duration. *Phys Ther.* 1994;74:1108–1115.

6. Sale DG. Neural adaptation to resistance training. *Med Sci Sports Exerc.* 1988;20(suppl):S135–S145.

7. Bandy WD, Dunleavy K. Adaptability of skeletal muscle: response to increased and decreased use. In: Zachazewski JE, Magee DJ, Quillen WS, eds. *Athletic injures and rehabilitation.* Philadelphia: WB Saunders; 1996:55–91.

8. Sherrington C. *Integrative activity of the nervous system.* New Haven, CT: Yale University Press; 1960.

9. Loeb GE, Ghez C. The motor unit and muscle action. In: Kandel E, Schwartz JH, Jessel TM. *Principles of neural science.* 4th ed. McGraw-Hill; 2000:674–694.

10. Pearson K, Gordon J. Spinal reflexes. In: Kandel E, Schwartz JH, Jessel TM. *Principles of neural science.* 4th ed. McGraw-Hill; 2000:713–736.

11. Engle R. Knee ligament rehabilitation. *Clin Manage.* 1990;10:36–39.

12. Engle RP, Canner GG. Proprioceptive neuromuscular facilitation (PNF) and modified procedure for anterior

cruciate ligament (ACL) instability. *J Orthop Sports Phys Ther.* 1989;11:230–236.

13. Macefield G, Hagbarth KE, Gorman R, et al. Decline in spindle support to alpha motor neurons during sustained voluntary contractions. *J Physiol.* 1991;440:497–512.

14. Moore MA, Kulkulka CG. Depression of Hoffman reflexes following voluntary contraction and implications for proprioceptive neuromuscular facilitation therapy. *Phys Ther.* 1991;71:321–329.

15. Nelson AG, Chambers RS, McGowan CM, et al. Proprioceptive neuromuscular facilitation versus weight training for enhancement of muscular strength and athletic performance. *J Orthop Sports Phys Ther.* 1986;7:250–253.

16. Osterling LR, Robertson RN, Troxel RK, et al. Differential responses to proprioceptive neuromuscular (PNF) stretch techniques. *Med Sci Sport Exerc.* 1990;22:106–111.

17. Roy MA, Sylvestre, Katch FI, et al. Proprioceptive facilitation of muscle tension during unilateral and bilateral extension. *Int J Sports Med.* 1990;11:289–292.

18. Anderson MA, Foreman TL. Return to competition: functional rehabilitation. In: Zachazewski JE, Magee DJ, Quillen WS, eds. *Athletic injures and rehabilitation.* Philadelphia: WB Saunders; 1996:229–261.

19. Adler SS, Beckers D, Buck M. *PNF in practice: an illustrated guide.* London: Springer-Verlag; 1993.

20. Sullivan PE, Marcos PD. *Clinical decision making in therapeutic exercise.* Norwalk, CT: Appleton & Lange; 1995.

21. Paine RM, Voight M. The role of the scapula. *J Orthop Sports Phys Ther.* 1993;18:386–391.

22. American Physical Therapy Association. *Guide to physical therapist practice.* 2nd ed. Alexandria, VA; 2003.

Closed-Kinetic–Chain Exercise

Kevin E. Wilk, PT, DPT, and Michael M. Reinold, PT, DPT, ATC

OBJECTIVES

Upon completion of this chapter, the reader will be able to:

- Define closed-kinetic–chain (CKC) and open-kinetic–chain (OKC) exercise.

- Describe the benefits of CKC exercise.

- Identify and apply general, appropriate clinical guidelines, indications, and limitations of CKC exercise.

- Identify appropriate goals for CKC techniques for the glenohumeral and scapulohumeral joints and for the lower extremity.

- Apply appropriate CKC techniques for upper- and lower-extremity exercise within the established plan of care.

In this chapter the physiologic rationale and clinical application for CKC exercises is discussed. In addition, specific exercise drills and their application to patients are presented.

SCIENTIFIC BASIS

Terminology

In the past there has been confusion concerning the clinical use of OKC and CKC exercises for rehabilitation. Questions regarding function and safety are frequently brought up when clinicians are deciding which type of exercise to incorporate into a rehabilitation program for a patient. The common assumption that CKC offers a safer, more functional approach to returning the patient to premorbid levels has helped CKC exercises gain popularity in sports medicine. Although incorporation of both OKC and CKC exercises in rehabilitation protocols may be beneficial to the injured patient, CKC exercises offer the patient a dynamic method for increasing neuromuscular joint stability using sport-specific drills. Unfortunately, many clinicians do not have a clear sense of the exact definitions of CKC and OKC exercises.

Originally kinetic-chain terminology was used to describe linkage analysis in mechanical engineering. In 1955 Steindler[1] suggested that the human body could be thought of as a chain consisting of the rigid overlapping segments of the limbs connected by a series of joints. He defined a kinetic chain as a combination of several successfully arranged joints constituting a complex motor unit. Furthermore, he observed that when a foot or hand meets considerable resistance, muscular recruitment and joint motion are different from that observed when the foot or hand is free to move without restriction. Today most individuals believe CKC exercise takes place when the terminal segment of an appendage is fixed, such as during a squat, leg press, or push-up exercise. Conversely, OKC exercise occurs when the terminal segment is free to move, such as during a seated knee extension exercise or biceps curl maneuver.

Others have defined the open- and closed-chain activities differently. Panariello[2] defined CKC activity of the extremity as an activity in which the foot or hand is in contact with the ground or a surface. He emphasized that the body weight must be supported for a CKC to exist.

Although the definitions of OKC and CKC are widely applied in sports medicine, there are numerous exercises and functional activities that do not fall within these concrete delineations. In addition, few exercises can be absolutely classified as an OKC or CKC. In fact, most exercises and functional activities, such as running and jumping, involve some combination of OKC and CKC succession. In addition, activities in which the distal segment is fixed on an object but the object is moving (e.g., skiing and ice skating) cannot be classified absolutely as CKC. Therefore, limited situations occur when a true CKC effect takes place. Most exercises fall somewhere between a truly fixed CKC and OKC exercise, especially those that involve the upper-extremity kinetic chain.

The conditions that apply to the lower extremity (such as weight-bearing forces) that create a CKC effect do not routinely occur in the upper extremity. However, because of the unique anatomic configuration of the glenohumeral joint, when the stabilizing muscles contract, a joint compression force is produced that stabilizes the joint, producing much the same effect as a CKC exercise for the lower extremity. Thus, the principles of CKC exercise as explained for the lower extremity may not apply for upper-extremity exercises.[2,3] Lephart and Henry[4] developed a scheme of OKC and CKC exercises for a clinical progression of drills for the shoulder that they termed a "functional classification system" (Tables 8-1 and 8-2).*

Tables 8-1 and 8-2 offer suggestions of OKC and CKC exercises as presented by Lephart and Henry[4] and are supported by the authors of this chapter. The editors respectively disagree with the classification of isometric strengthening and PNF (slow reversals) as CKC activities and suggest that they are OKC exercises. But, as appropriately stated by the authors of this chapter, few exercises can be absolutely classified as open or closed, and disagreement will occur.

TABLE 8-1 Open- and Closed-kinetic–chain Exercises for the Glenohumeral Joint

Phase	Closed-kinetic Chain	Open-kinetic Chain
Acute	Isometric press-up, push-up, and strengthening; weight-bearing shift; axial compression against wall	
Subacute	Resisted wall circles and wall abduction/adduction; sliding board; push-ups; PNF[a] slow reversals	Isotonic and isokinetic strengthening
Advanced	Push-ups on balance board; lateral step-ups; shuttle walking; StairMaster; unilateral weight bearing; plyometric push-ups	Isotonic and isokinetic strengthening; plyometrics; sport-specific training

[a]PNF, proprioceptive neuromuscular facilitation.

TABLE 8-2 Open- and Closed-kinetic–chain Exercises for the Scapulothoracic Joint

Phase	Closed-kinetic Chain	Open-kinetic Chain
Acute	Isometric punches, strengthening, press-ups	Isotonic strengthening
Subacute	Push-ups, military presses, press-ups	Isotonic and isokinetic strengthening; rowing; prone horizontal abduction (±external rotation)
Advanced	Neuromuscular control drills: rhythmic stabilization, circles, diagonal patterns	Progression of isotonic strengthening exercises

Physiologic Basis of Closed-kinetic–chain Activities

CKC exercises are often chosen over OKC exercises because the clinician wants to stress the joint in a weight-bearing position.[5] Weight-bearing exercises result in joint approximation, which produces stimulation of the articular receptors, whereas length tension changes excite tenomuscular receptors.[6] These mechanoreceptors provide the joint proprioceptive information, which is critical to the dynamic stability of the joint.

Re-establishment of proprioception is an important part of neuromuscular control of the joint. Proprioception arises from activation of afferent neurons located in the joint capsule, ligaments, and surrounding muscles. Muscle spindles and Golgi tendon organs (GTOs) detect changes in length and tension of the muscle, respectively. In addition, ligaments and joint capsules contain pacinian corpuscles, Ruffini endings, and GTO-like mechanoreceptors. These mechanoreceptors respond to changes in joint position, velocity, and direction.[4,7]

The joint compression seen with weight bearing facilitates muscular cocontractions of force couples, which provide a dynamic reflex stabilization.[8] Also, CKC exercises rely on the joint musculature to contract concentrically and eccentrically to generate joint mobility and stability farther along the kinetic chain.

Proprioceptive and muscular cocontraction training plays a complementary role in neuromuscular re-education. Adequate intensity and timing of muscular force–couple interaction allows for maximum joint congruency and inherent joint stability. Mechanoreceptors within the static and dynamic structures are cooperatively responsible for the neuromuscular control of the joint when the joint is in a weight-bearing position.

In addition, CKC exercises may be extremely beneficial in the neuromodulation of pain via the activation of type I and II mechanoreceptors. Therefore, when the client is experiencing significant pain and inflammation, the early initiation of low-level CKC exercises in the acute phase of rehabilitation may be warranted.

CLINICAL GUIDELINES

CKC exercises are often initiated in early phases of rehabilitation to facilitate cocontraction of joint force couples. Often used as precursors to the more advanced demands of plyometric training (Chapter 9), CKC exercises prepare the joint's ability to establish adequate muscular cocontraction and neuromuscular control to prevent potential overuse injuries.

Many clinicians base their rationale of choosing CKC exercises on the assumptions of increased safety and function. Obvious correlations exist between CKC squatting exercises and functional stopping and CKC step-up and step-down exercises and stair ambulation. Although some exceptions do occur in sports, such as a baseball pitcher's need for OKC proprioceptive exercises, most injured athletes often require the benefits of proprioceptive and neuromuscular rehabilitation observed with CKC exercises.

Weight-bearing during CKC exercises provides joint compression through the summation of ground-reaction forces, long believed to result in increased neuromuscular control and subsequently increased joint stability. Dynamic joint stabilization is achieved by cocontraction of the muscles surrounding a joint; lack of this stability often leads to injuries. During sport-specific movements such as running, cutting, and landing from a jump, the athlete relies on muscular cocontraction and eccentric control to dissipate ground-reaction forces. Consequently, athletes with reduced cocontraction and strength imbalances have been shown to have an increase risk of knee ligament injuries.[9] The athlete becomes susceptible to injury when he or she cannot dynamically control the ground-reaction forces muscularly, which places excessive stress on other static tissues, such as ligaments.

For preparing a patient for competition when dynamic stability is vital to the prevention of injuries, CKC exercises may very well be the best option. But a limitation of CKC exercises is that if specific muscle weakness is present, other agonistic muscles within the kinetic chain can generate forces to help compensate. In comparison, OKC exercise calls for a more isolated contraction of a muscle or muscle group and therefore may best be used for specific muscle strengthening. However, isolated open-chain exercise should be employed in combination with weight-bearing exercises.[10]

An integrated approach using both OKC and CKC exercise is recommended, although weight-bearing functional exercises are used in rehabilitation programs more often than isolated joint movements. Weight-bearing exercises are emphasized because such movements produce a greater stabilizing effect on the joint and may diminish ligament strain. Weight-bearing exercise also elicits muscular cocontractions and muscular recruitment in a manner that simulates functional activities. In turn, these activities stimulate mechanoreceptors throughout the kinetic chain. The importance of proprioception training in the rehabilitation program has been well established and cannot be overemphasized (see Chapters 10 and 11).

TECHNIQUES

This section provides the physical therapist assistant (PTA) with specific CKC and plyometric drills, programs, and progressions for the upper[11] and lower[12] extremities.[13] We present examples of possible exercises that can be incorporated into the rehabilitation of an injured patient. The demands of each sport should be considered when choosing the most appropriate drills because the program should be as patient and sport specific as possible.

Upper-extremity Closed-kinetic–chain Exercise

The clinical use of weight-bearing or axial compression exercises for the upper extremity is based on patient selection and the ultimate goal. The use of weight-bearing exercises for the upper extremity without careful consideration of the biomechanical forces imparted onto the glenohumeral and scapulothoracic joints is not recommended. For example, using push-ups against a wall or on the floor may increase instability in patients with multidirectional instability or posterior instability because the humeral head translates posteriorly during these exercises, stressing the posterior capsule of the glenohumeral joint. A list of commonly used CKC exercises for the glenohumeral and scapulothoracic joints is presented in Tables 8-1 and 8-2. General guidelines for the progression of CKC exercises for the upper extremity can be found in Table 8-3.

TABLE 8-3	General Guidelines for Progression of Closed-kinetic–chain Exercises
Static stabilization	→ Dynamic stabilization
Stable surfaces	→ Unstable surfaces
Single plane movements	→ Multiplane movements
Straight planes	→ Diagonal planes
Wide base of support	→ Small base of support
No resistance	→ Resistance
Rhythmic stabilization	→ Resistance throughout range of motion
Fundamental movements	→ Dynamic challenging movements
Bilateral support	→ Unilateral support
Consistent movements	→ Perturbation training

Acute Phase

Glenohumeral Joint

In the acute rehabilitation phase of most glenohumeral joint pathologies (including postglenohumeral-joint dislocations, subluxations, and rotator-cuff pathologies), the primary goal is to re-establish motion. However, equally as important is the re-establishment of dynamic glenohumeral joint stability and prevention of rotator-cuff shutdown. Weight-bearing exercises can be used to promote and enhance dynamic joint stability via the application of various techniques.[14] Often these weight-bearing techniques are employed with the hand fixed and no motion occurring; the resistance is applied either axially or rotationally. These exercises can be used early in the rehabilitation program because motion is not occurring with heavy resistance, which may irritate the joint.

Therefore, immediately after glenohumeral joint subluxation or dislocation, the injured patient may perform exercises such as isometric press-ups, isometric weight-bearing and weight shifts, and axial compression against a table or wall (Figs. 8-1 to 8-3). These movements produce both joint compression and joint approximation, which should enhance muscular cocontraction about the joint, producing dynamic stability.[14–16] In addition, these exercises may be extremely beneficial in the neuromodulation of pain if the patient is experiencing significant pain and inflammation. These activities are performed with the patient standing or kneeling, placing a proportionate amount of body weight through the hands as tolerated. The patient is instructed to shift his or her weight from side to side, forward to backward, and diagonally on and off of the affected side. These exercises may be progressed to using manual resistance rhythmic stabilization techniques that enhance the recruitment of the musculature involved in the force couples about the glenohumeral joint. These types of weight-bearing and shift exercises can be progressed by the patient placing his

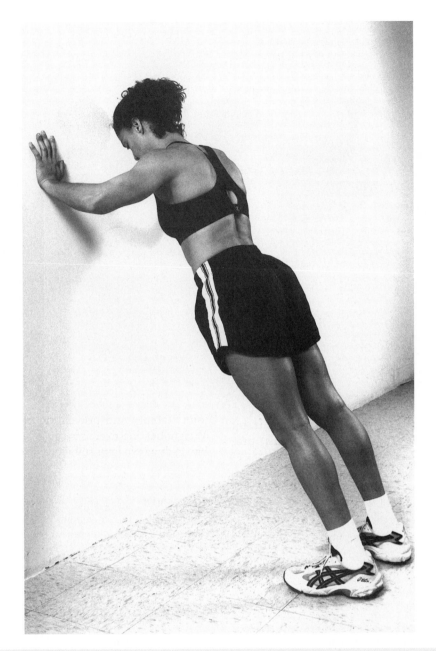

Figure 8-1   Axial compression against table or wall—beginning phase.

PURPOSE: Closed-kinetic–chain exercise to strengthen the muscles of the glenohumeral joint.

POSITION: Client standing with feet away from wall and arms extended against wall.

PROCEDURE: Using arms, client lowers chest half the distance to wall, keeping hips in (do not allow hips to protrude). Client maintains position for 3 to 5 seconds.

or her feet on a large therapeutic ball (Fig. 8-4) and then on a smaller ball; finally the patient places one hand on top of the other to increase the difficulty.

Hence, the PTA may manually resist the anterior and then posterior musculature via proprioceptive neuromuscular fa-cilitation (PNF) rhythmic stabilization exercises to enhance stabilization of the joint, thereby increasing the efficiency of the musculature involved in the compression of the humeral head within the glenoid (Fig. 7-23). The muscles on both sides of the joint are referred to as muscular force couples.

Figure 8-2   Isometric push-up—beginning phase.

PURPOSE: Closed-kinetic–chain exercise to strengthen muscles of the glenohumeral joint.

POSITION: Client in push-up position; arms extended.

PROCEDURE: Using arms, client lowers chest half the distance to ground, keeping hips in (do not allow hips to protrude). Client maintains position for 3 to 5 seconds.

Scapulothoracic Joint

Specific exercises can be used for the scapular musculature in much the same fashion as those described for the glenohumeral joint. In the early phases of rehabilitation for an upper-extremity injury, scapular musculature–strengthening movements must be integrated into the program. In the acute phase, various movements are used to promote specific musculature activity. Exercises such as isometric protractions or punching motions with resistance applied to the hand and lateral border of the scapula are excellent for promoting serratus anterior recruitment (Fig. 8-5). Isometric retractions of the scapular muscles may also be integrated into the program to recruit middle trapezius and rhomboid activity. Isometric press-ups can be employed to recruit cocontractions of the glenohumeral joint and to elicit activity of the latissimus dorsi and teres major (Fig. 8-3).

Subacute Phase

Glenohumeral Joint

In the subacute phase, resistance is applied to the distal segment, but some motion is allowed. Examples of these exercises include resisted arm circles against the wall, resisted axial load side-to-side motions either against a wall or on a slide board (Fig. 14-24), and push-ups. In addition, a multitude of resisted quadruped exercises can be employed during the subacute rehabilitative phase, including manual proximal resistance to the shoulder and pelvis. Resistance can be applied in different amounts to multiple positions in a rhythmic stabilization fashion. This form of exercise can also be progressed to a tripod of the involved extremity or even to a therapeutic ball (Figs. 14-15, 14-16, and 14-31).

Figure 8-3 Isometric press-up—beginning phase.

PURPOSE: Closed-kinetic–chain exercise to strengthen pectoralis major and latissimus dorsi muscles.

POSITION: Client sitting on edge of support surface; hands at sides on support surface.

PROCEDURE: Client presses down with arms, lifting hips off support surface. Client maintains position for 3 to 5 seconds.

By using weight-bearing exercises, the PTA attempts to enhance dynamic stability while the patient produces a superimposed movement pattern. This activity is a higher level of function than that performed in the acute phase and requires dynamic stabilization and controlled mobility.

Scapulothoracic Joint

In the subacute phase, several CKC exercises, such as push-ups with a plus, military press, and press-ups, are recommended. These exercises are performed to recruit significant muscular activity of the muscles that stabilize the scapula.

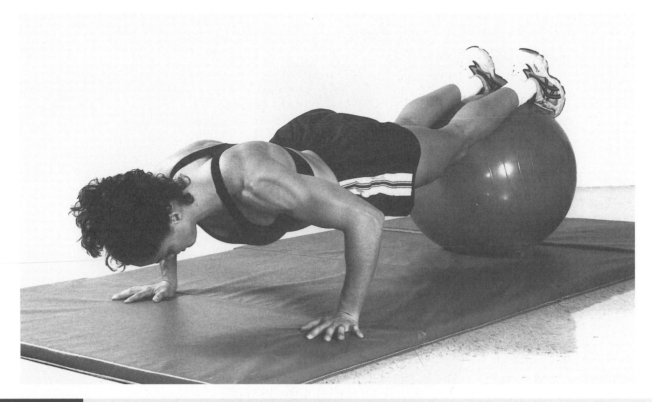

| **Figure 8-4** | Axial compression using therapeutic ball—beginning phase. |

PURPOSE: Closed-kinetic–chain exercise to strengthen muscles of the glenohumeral joint.

POSITION: Client in push-up position with feet on large therapeutic ball.

PROCEDURE: Using arms, client lowers chest half the distance to ground, keeping hips in (do not allow hips to protrude). Client maintains position for 3 to 5 seconds.

Advanced Phase

Glenohumeral Joint

In the advanced phase, the weight-bearing exercises employed are usually high-demand movements that require a tremendous degree of dynamic stability. One example is a push-up with the hands placed on a ball, which produces axial load on the joint but keeps the distal segment somewhat free to move (Fig. 8-6). This push-up may be performed on a balance board, balance system, or movable platform with feet elevated on a therapeutic ball. Other exercises include lateral step-ups using the hands and retrograde or lateral walking on the hands on a treadmill or stair stepper. In this last rehabilitative phase, the exercises are tremendously dynamic and require adequate strength to be carried out properly.

Scapulothoracic Joint

The exercises that may be included in the last, advanced phase of rehabilitation for the scapular musculature were already presented. In addition, a neuromuscular control exercise for the scapular muscles may be used (Fig. 8-7). In this exercise, the involved hand is placed on a table to fix the distal segment, which produces a greater magnitude of scapular activity. The individual is asked to slowly protract and retract and then elevate and depress the scapula to produce a circle or square movement. When these combined movement patterns are performed, tactile stimulus in the form of manual resistance is imparted onto the scapula and then is removed once the athlete produces the motion. The goal of this exercise is to enhance neuromuscular control and isolate dynamic control of the scapular muscles.

Lower-extremity Closed-kinetic–chain Exercise

The rationale for the use of OKC and CKC exercises for lower-extremity rehabilitation is similar to that for upper-extremity rehabilitation. Just as not all OKC exercises produce an isolated muscle contraction, not all CKC exercises produce muscular cocontraction of the surrounding musculature. With this in mind, lower-extremity kinetic-chain

Figure 8-5   Scapular protraction (punches)—beginning phase.

PURPOSE: Closed-kinetic–chain exercise to strengthen serratus anterior muscle.

POSITION: Client lying supine with shoulder flexed 90 degrees; elbow extended; hand in fist.

PROCEDURE: Physical therapist assistant (PTA) places one hand at fist and one hand at lateral border of scapula or on upper arm. PTA isometrically resists client's attempt to punch (keeping elbow extended).

exercises can be organized into three groups by the muscular activity produced: muscular cocontractions, isolated quadriceps contractions, and isolated hamstring contractions (Table 8-4). Using these categories, the physical therapist (PT) can prescribe exercises based on the desired muscle recruitment pattern.

CKC exercise can also be used to develop muscular endurance in the lower extremity. The stair stepper and bicycle are two beneficial and common machines used for developing increased muscular endurance capacity (Chapter 12) in a CKC, whereas aquatic therapy (Chapter 16) is extremely valuable for total body muscular conditioning.

Figure 8-6   Push-up with hands placed on ball—advanced phase.

PURPOSE: Closed-kinetic–chain exercise to strengthen muscles of the scapulothoracic joint.

POSITION: Client in push-up position with hands on ball; arms extended.

PROCEDURE: Using arms, client lowers chest half the distance to ball, keeping hips in (do not allow hips to protrude). Client maintains position for 3 to 5 seconds.

Figure 8-7   Neuromuscular control exercises—advanced phase.

PURPOSE: Closed-kinetic–chain exercise to enhance neuromuscular control and isolate dynamic control of scapular muscles.

POSITION: Client lying on side, with hand on support surface to fix distal segment.

PROCEDURE: Client slowly protracts/retracts and elevates/depresses scapula (proximal segment) to produce circular motion. Physical therapist assistant alternates between manual resistance and no resistance.

TABLE 8-4 Muscle Recruitment Patterns of Lower-Extremity Closed-kinetic-chain Activities

Class	Exercises
Muscular cocontractions	Vertical squats (0–30 degrees)
	Lateral lunges with knee flexed to 30 degrees
	Sliding board (including Fitter)
	Balance drills with knee flexed to 30 degrees
Quadriceps contractions	Wall squats
	Leg press (45–90 degrees)
	Lateral step-ups
Hamstring contractions	Retrograde stair machines
	Squats >45 degrees
	Front lunges onto box

Numerous exercises involve CKC and weight bearing for the lower extremity. The PT must choose the exercises that are most functional and sport specific and must decide if cocontraction or isolated muscle action is indicated for each client. Finally, when particular structures are healing, exercises must be altered based on clinical and biomechanical evidence to avoid stressing those tissues. The clinical guidelines suggested for the progression of the lower extremity are, in fact, the same as the clinical guidelines for upper-extremity progression and are presented in Table 8-3.

Acute Phase

CKC rehabilitation programs can begin in the acute phase. Early goals include re-establishment of motion, dynamic joint stability, and retardation of muscular atrophy (in particular, the vastus medialis oblique). The acute phase begins with weight bearing and shifting to provide axial compression and joint approximation, leading to the facilitation of muscular cocontraction and dynamic joint stabilization. Weight-shifting exercises are performed by the patient standing with bilateral support and shifting from side to side and forward to backward, independently controlling the amount of weight bearing on the involved extremity. Standing mini-squats from 0 to 30 degrees also begin in this stage (Fig. 8-8). As the tissues heal and the patient is able to perform the weight shifting and mini-squats without symptoms, lateral step-ups are initiated onto a step of low intensity; the height of the step controls the intensity of the exercise (Fig. 8-9). Also in the sagittal plane, forward lunges can be initiated if the PTA pays attention to the length and depth of the lunge (Fig. 8-10). Mini-squats are progressed near the end of the acute phase; the client may perform wall slides, if an isolated quadriceps contraction is indicated.

Subacute Phase

The subacute phase progresses the exercises performed in the acute phase. The squat is progressed to a range of 0 to 60 degrees or 75 degrees. The step-up and lunge are progressed to include lateral movements, and exercise-tubing resistance is used. The tubing can be applied from forward, backward, or either side to force the athlete to dynamically stabilize while the tubing produces a weight-shifting movement in the direction of application (Chapter 11).

The initiation of cone drills can begin during the subacute phase. They can be performed forward and laterally and involve the athlete stepping over the cones with a high knee raise and landing with a slightly flexed knee to develop balance and control of joint movements of the hip, knee, and ankle (Fig. 8-11).

Uneven surfaces can also be integrated into the rehabilitation program at this point to increase the demands on the mechanoreceptors. Patients can begin by balancing on foam, then a gym mat, and eventually a rocker board (Fig. 10-18). As the patient progresses, dumbbells of different weights can be placed in each hand to offset the patient's center of gravity. The patient is then instructed to maintain balance while randomly extending and abducting the arms, which alters the center of gravity.

Advanced Phase

As the athlete progresses to the advanced phase of rehabilitation, increased dynamic stability and an adequate base of strength are necessary to perform the high-demand exercises. Squats and lunges can be performed on an uneven surface with and without manual perturbations to begin training the athlete to respond to quick, unexpected outside forces.

Cone drills can be progressed in intensity (increased speed without deterioration of technique) and duration. Medicine balls can be incorporated into the cone drills and the uneven surface drills. During these drills the patient must perform the exercise as earlier described but must also catch and throw a ball without deterioration of technique (Fig. 8-12). Progressing to a medicine ball trains the patient to stabilize while loading and unloading external forces.

| Figure 8-8 | Standing mini-squats—beginning phase. |

PURPOSE: Closed-kinetic–chain exercise to strengthen muscles of lower extremity.

POSITION: Client standing; hands on support surface for balance control.

PROCEDURE: Client performs small (mini) squat from 0 to 30 degrees of knee flexion.

| Figure 8-9 | Lateral step-ups—beginning phase. |

PURPOSE: Closed-kinetic–chain exercise to strengthen muscles of lower extremity.

POSITION: Client standing with one foot on top of stool.

PROCEDURE: Client slowly extends hip and knee of extremity on stool to lift body up on stool. Client then slowly lowers body to floor.

Figure 8-10 Lunges—beginning phase.

PURPOSE: Closed-kinetic–chain to strengthen muscles of the lower extremity.

POSITION: Client standing with feet together.

PROCEDURE: Client takes step forward, lowering body until forward knee flexes to 90 degrees. Client maintains position for 1 to 2 seconds and then returns to starting position.

Functional equipment can be used to further progress the patient. Standing on a sliding board develops lateral strength and stability and simulates motions that occur frequently in sports such as hockey (Fig. 10-19). Increase the challenge on the sliding board by asking the patient to perform upper-extremity exercises while incorporating dynamic lower-extremity side-to-side activities to facilitate the development of balance and agility. The sliding board can be used to train quadriceps, hamstring, and gastrocnemius muscular cocontraction.

SUMMARY

- CKC exercises take place when the terminal segment (hand or foot) of an extremity is fixed or is weight bearing with the ground or surface, such as performing a squat, leg press, or push-up exercise.

- CKC exercises are often chosen instead of OKC exercises because of the stress that is desired in the weight-bearing portion of the extremity. Weight-bearing allows increases in joint stability and cocontraction of muscles surrounding the joint. CKC exercises are more functional than open-chain exercises and frequently are what the patient needs during the performance of sport-specific movements.

- When designing a rehabilitaiton program for a patient, the PT should formulate an integrated program that uses both OKC and CKC exercises. Unique advantages exist to each form of exercises, and the PT should carefully consider these advantages when developing the program.

Figure 8-11	Cone drills—intermediate phase.

PURPOSE: Closed-kinetic–chain exercise to develop balance and control the joint movements of hip, knee, and ankle.

POSITION: Client standing; two to three cones lined up 6 to 8 inches apart.

PROCEDURE: Using exaggerated high knees (hip flexion), client steps over cones.

Figure 8-12	Cone drills with medicine ball throws—advanced phase.

PURPOSE: Closed-kinetic–chain exercise to develop balance and control the joint movement of hip, knee, and ankle and to train client to stabilize lower extremity while loading and unloading external forces.

POSITION: Client standing; two to three cones lined up 6 to 8 inches apart.

PROCEDURE: Using exaggerated high knees (hip flexion), client steps over cones while catching and throwing a ball.

CASE STUDY 1

PATIENT INFORMATION

The patient was a 13-year-old male soccer player who had been practicing and playing for 5 weeks during the fall season. He had "left foot/heel" pain for 1 week without having experienced a specific injury. The parent recalled the child sliding feet first into the goal upright several weeks earlier but could not recall if the patient hit with his left or right foot. The patient did not complain of foot problems after that incident and had been playing up until the previous week, when he stopped playing because of pain. The child was referred for examination and treatment and for advice concerning return to play.

The patient arrived for examination with a report of pain in the left heel when running during soccer games and in gym class at school; he reported minimal to no pain when walking. His goals were to return to playing soccer as soon as possible. The patient had been seen by the physician and was told to use heat and to wear an over-the-counter lace-up–type ankle brace. Radiographs were negative for the left foot and ankle.

During the examination by the PT the patient reported pain in the heel with bilateral toe raises and had decreased push off on the left foot with jogging. Attempts to run faster or to perform cutting activities were difficult because of heel pain. Palpation indicated tenderness at the superior third of the posterior calcaneus and no pain in the Achilles tendon and bursa. Range of motion and strength were normal except for pain when rising up on the toes. All ligament tests to the ankle were negative.

The patient was diagnosed with calcaneal apophysitis (Sever's disease). This condition is relatively common in active, growing children.

ⓛ LINK TO
GUIDE TO PHYSICAL THERAPIST PRACTICE

According to the *Guide*,[17] calcaneal apophysitis is classified as musculoskeletal pattern 4E. This pattern is described as "impaired joint mobility, motor function, muscle performance, and range of motion associated with localized inflammation." Goals included coordinating care with the patient, parents, and volunteer soccer coach; reducing the disability associated with chronic irritation; enhancing physical function and sport participation; and improving sport-specific motor function and self-management of symptoms.

INTERVENTION

Apophysitis is caused by musculotendinous traction forces on the immature epiphysis. Initial goals were to decrease inflammation, increase strength, and maintain muscle length. The child was instructed to discontinue use of the ankle brace and to stop all activities (running) that caused pain. The PT discussed the goals and plan of care with the PTA, as well as with the parents. The PTA was instructed to perform the following initial intervention consisting of the following program with return feedback to the supervising PT on patient tolerance and understanding of treatment plan.

1. Mild stretching to maintain length and motion of the gastrocnemius and soleus muscles (Figs. 4-17 and 4-18).
2. Bicycle to maintain cardiovascular conditioning and lower-extremity endurance (Fig. 12-5).
3. Ice for discomfort and irritation.

PROGRESSION

One Week After Initial Examination

One week after examination the PT noted the patient's ability to raise up on his toes without pain. Goals at this point were updated to increase strength with more advanced, CKC activities. The PT discussed the updated goals with the PTA and instructed the PTA to progress the intervention as follows:

1. Elastic tubing strengthening to the calf muscles.
2. Toe raises and partial squats (Fig. 8-8).

3. Continue lower-extremity bicycling.

4. Lateral step-ups on 4-inch box (Fig. 8-9)

5. Pain-free lunges (Fig. 8-10).

Three Weeks After Initial Examination

At the 3-week follow-up the PT noted that the patient had no complaints of pain when rising up on his toes, walking, or jogging. Goals were to advance the program to include functional progression activities to prepare the patient for return to sport. Again after discussion with the PTA regarding the treatment plan, the patient was instructed on the following exercise progression by the PTA.

1. Lateral cone drills (Fig. 8-11)

2. Slide training for lateral movements (Fig. 10-19).

3. Low-velocity, low-vertical force plyometrics on 2-inch box (Fig. 9-15).

Four Weeks After Initial Examination

At the 4-week follow-up the patient had no complaints of pain at any time during the day and no pain with any of the exercises. The PT's goals were to continue to advance the program to include functional progression activities to prepare the patient for ultimate return to sport. The PTA, under the direction of the PT, instructed the progression of functional activities as follows:

1. Progress vertical force plyometrics to 4-inch box.

2. Low-level agility jumping (Fig. 9-14).

3. Lower-extremity functional progression, including running, cutting, changing directions.

OUTCOME

The patient returned to soccer without difficulty after 5 weeks. Clinicians should remember that the epiphyses and apophyses in young athletes are at risk for overuse and injury. The patient's injury may have been sparked by the collision into the goal post, but it really was the result of microtraumatic or repetitive use. Immobilization is not necessary for healing; instead, the athlete should decrease participation in activities that aggravate the symptoms.

SUMMARY—AN EFFECTIVE PT-PTA TEAM

This case study demonstrates an effective collaborative effort and good communication between the PT and the PTA. The PTA is able to follow the instruction of the PT after their re-examination of the patient and advance the exercise program with the PTA returning feedback to the supervising PT on patient tolerance and understanding. It is important in this scenario that the PT receives the feedback from the PTA due to the patient's young age. A clear understanding must exist on the patient's and parent's part of the treatment plan since increased activity that causes pain may aggravate symptoms. The PT expects that the PTA fully understands the interventions and is able to progress the patient under his or her direction. The PT also expects that the PTA can instruct the patient independently, reporting any adverse effects of the session. This type of working relationship allows the PT to be aware of the patient's status but at the same time allows him or her to perform examinations on other patients in the clinic, demonstrating effective and efficient teamwork while still providing quality care.

GERIATRIC PERSPECTIVES

■ Functional assessment of older adults should include examination of specific CKC task performances requiring integration of dynamic multijoint motion and incorporating concentric, eccentric, and isometric muscle activities.[1] Examination of task performance in dynamic movements involves the whole individual and his or her interaction with the environmental aspects of the tasks (e.g., the height of steps or other surfaces). Functional tests to examine CKC control may include bilateral stance with knee flexion, unilateral stance with knee flexion, and bilateral and unilateral balance reactions and equilibrium responses when standing with eyes open and closed.[1]

■ Older adults need to perform exercises directed toward gains in function and independence. Independent performance of activities of daily living (ADLs) require that the lower extremities function in closed-chain tasks.[1] Examples of such ADLs are dressing oneself and toileting.

■ Strengthening programs should include both CKC and OKC (Chapter 6) exercises to maximize physical performance.[2] Closed-chain exercises emphasize control while the distal end is fixed, whereas open-chain exercises improve control when the distal end is free moving. A good example of such interaction between closed- and open-chain exercise is walking, in which the cyclic movement requires that the distal point of contact alternate between fixed and free.

■ Because older adults are more prone to falls in challenging postural tasks, special attention should be given to the placement of the center of mass (Chapter 10) and the placement of the foot during CKC exercise. In addition, the exercise should be performed slowly with control and with external support, as needed for safety.

1. Scott KF. Closed kinetic chain assessment: rehabilitation of improved function in the older patient. *Top Geriatr Rehabil.* 1995;11:1–5.
2. Judge JO. Resistance training. *Top Geriatr Rehabil.* 1993;8: 38–50.

PEDIATRIC PERSPECTIVES

■ In children, as in adults, the muscles of postural support must be strong enough to withstand the stresses of high levels of activity among children. When CKC exercises are used, the training level and muscular conditioning base of the participant must be taken into account. For children who are essentially "untrained" and who lack basic muscular strength, endurance, and neuromuscular coordination, low-intensity CKC activities are a good place to begin to develop the muscles of postural support required for more strenuous exercise.[1,2]

■ Concentric strengthening may be preferable as children develop mature muscles ("Pediatric Perspectives" in Chapter 5) and bones. Therefore, good judgment must be used when prescribing CKC exercises to children as the intervention may have signifi-

cant eccentric muscle actions, even at low levels, which can lead to muscle soreness and possible injury.

■ For highly trained child athletes, CKC exercises may be a requisite for complete return to function. For example, a young female gymnast must be able to perform many complex CKC movements of both the upper and lower extremities. To complete a well-designed functional progression, sport-specific movements should be incorporated into the rehabilitation program via CKC exercises.[2]

1. Davies GJ, Heiderscheit BC, Manske R, et al. The scientific and clinical rationale for the integrated approach to open and closed kinetic chain rehabilitation. *Orthop Phys Ther Clin North Am.* 2000;9:247–267.
2. Straker JS, Stuhr PJ. Clinical application of closed kinetic chain exercises in the lower extremities. *Orthop Phys Ther Clin North Am.* 2000;9:185–207.

References

1. Steindler A. *Kinesiology of the human body under normal and pathological conditions.* Springfield, IL: Thomas; 1955.

2. Panariello RA. The closed kinetic chain in strength training. *Natl Strength Condition Assoc J.* 1991;13:29–33.

3. Dillman CJ, Murray TA, Hindermeister RA. Biomechanical differences of open and closed chain exercises with respect to the shoulder. *J Sport Rehabil.* 1994;3:228–238.

4. Lephart SM, Henry TJ. The physiological basis for open and closed kinetic chain rehabilitation for the upper extremity. *J Sport Rehabil.* 1996;5:71–87.

5. Heiderscheit BC, Rucinski TJ. Biomechanical and physiologic basis of closed kinetic chain exercises in the upper extremities. *Orthop Phys Ther Clin North Am.* 2000;9:209–229.

6. Clark FJ, Burgess PR. Slowly adapting receptors in cat knee joint. Can they signal joint angle? *J Neurophysiol.* 1975;38: 1448–1463.

7. Lephart SM, Pincivero JR, Giraldo JL, et al. The role of proprioception in the management and rehabilitation of athletic injuries. *Am J Sports Med.* 1997;25:130–137.

8. Voight M, Draovitch P. Plyometrics. In: Albert M, ed. *Eccentric muscle training in sports and orthopedics.* New York: Churchill Livingston; 1991:45–73.

9. Barratta R, Solomonow M, Zhou B. Muscular coactivation: the role of the antagonist musculature in maintaining knee stability. *Am J Sports Med.* 1998;16:113–122.

10. Davies GJ, Heiderscheit BC, Manske R, et al. The scientific and clinical rationale for the integrated approach to open and closed kinetic chain rehabilitation. *Orthop Phys Ther Clin North Am.* 2000;9:247–267.

11. Ellenbecker TS, Cappel K. Clinical application of closed kinetic chain exercises in the upper extremities. *Orthop Phys Ther Clin North Am.* 2000;9:231–245.

12. Straker JS, Stuhr PJ. Clinical application of closed kinetic chain exercises in the lower extremities. *Orthop Phys Ther Clin North Am.* 2000;9:185–207.

13. Hall CM, Brody LT. Impaired joint mobility and range of motion. In: *Therapeutic exercise: moving toward function.* 2nd ed. Philadelphia: Lippincott Williams & Wilkins; 2005: 291–306.

14. Wilk K, Arrigo C. Current concepts in the rehabilitation of the athletic shoulder. *J Orthop Sports Phys Ther.* 1993;18:364–378.

15. Davies G, Dickoff-Hoffman S. Neuromuscular testing and rehabilitation of the shoulder complex. *J Orthop Sports Phys Ther.* 1993;18:449–458.

16. Wilk KE, Arrigo CA, Andrews JR. The stabilizing structures of the glenohumeral joint. *J Orthop Sports Phys Ther.* 1997;15: 364–379.

17. American Physical Therapy Association. *Guide to physical therapist practice.* 2nd ed. Alexandria, VA; 2003.

Plyometrics

Kevin E. Wilk, PT, DPT and Michael M. Reinold, PT, DPT, ATC

OBJECTIVES

Upon completion of this chapter, the reader will be able to:

- Define plyometrics and identify the role of plyometrics in specificity training of athletes.
- Identify the neurophysiologic principles that are used for maximum force production in plyometrics.
- Identify three phases of plyometric exercise and the duration of each.
- Identify specific contraindications to performing upper- and lower-extremity plyometric exercise.
- Apply techniques appropriate for upper-extremity, trunk, and lower-extremity plyometric exercise programs within the established plan of care.

The concept of specificity of training is an important parameter in determining the proper exercise program. The imposed demands during training must mirror those incurred during competition, especially during the advanced phases of the rehabilitation process. In most advanced phases of rehabilitation, the essential element to enhance performance is the capacity of the muscle to exert maximal force output in a minimal amount of time. Most advanced skills depend on the ability of the muscle to generate force rapidly. To simulate the explosive strength needed in athletics, Verkhoshanski[1] advocated the shock method of training when he introduced the concept of plyometrics in Russia. During many athletic activities—such as playing tennis, throwing a ball, or jumping—the athlete performs a plyometric type of muscular contraction.

It should be noted that before initiation of a plyometric program, closed-kinetic–chain (CKC) drills are required. For example, generally CKC squats or CKC leg press exercises are performed before initiating plyometric jumping drills. Therefore, an integration of CKC (Chapter 8) and plyometric drills is imperative.

SCIENTIFIC BASIS

Terminology

Although the term *plyometric* is relatively new, its basic concepts are well established. The roots of plyometric training can be traced to eastern Europe, where it was simply known as jump training or shock training.[1,2] The word *plyometrics* originates from the Greek words *plythein* and *metric*. *Plyo* originates from the Greek word for "more," and *metric* literally means "to measure."[3] The term was first introduced in 1975 by American track coach Fred Wilt.[3]

The practical definition of plyometrics is a quick powerful movement involving a prestretching of the muscle, thereby activating the stretch–shortening cycle of the muscle. Therefore, one purpose of plyometric training is to increase the excitability of the neurologic receptors for improved reactivity of the neuromuscular system. Wilk and Voight[4] referred to this type of muscle training as muscular stretch–shortening exercise drills.

The literature demonstrates that since 1979 many authors have used variations of the Verkhoshanski methodology in an attempt to establish the best stretch–shortening or plyometric training techniques.[2,4–7] There appears to be agreement on the benefits of basic stretch–shortening principles, but controversy exists regarding an optimal training routine.[8,9] Historically the chief proponents of the plyometrics training approach were in the area of track and field,[10]

but authors have also discussed programs for baseball,[4,11] football,[12] and basketball.[13] Thus, it appears that plyometric training has become an accepted form of training and rehabilitation in many sports medicine areas.

Adaptation of plyometric stretch–shortening principles can be used to enhance the specificity of training for sports that require a maximum amount of muscular force in a minimum amount of time. All movements in competitive athletics involve a repeated series of stretch–shortening cycles.[7,8,10] For example, during the overhead throwing motion, an athlete externally rotates his arm during the cocking phase to produce a stretch on the powerful internal rotator/adductor muscle group. Once the stretch stimulus is completed (full external rotation is achieved), the athlete forcefully accelerates the arm forward into adduction and internal rotation during the acceleration and ball release phases of the throw. Thus, the stretch (cocking phase) precedes the shortening (acceleration, ball release) phases. When an athlete performs a vertical jump, such as to jump to catch a ball or shoot a basketball, he/she exhibits a stretch–shortening cycle. The athlete first squats or slightly lowers him/herself before jumping. When the squatting movement is performed first, a stretch is generated on the plantarflexors, quadriceps, and gluteal muscles. This is the stretch phase of the jump. After the stretch phase is the shortening phase: an explosive push-off that allows the athlete to elevate. Therefore, whether throwing a ball, jumping rope, or swinging a golf club, all the movements involve a stretch–shortening cycle of the muscle.

Consequently, specific exercise drills should be developed to prepare athletes for activities specific to their sports. Plyometric exercise provides a translation from traditional strength training to the explosive movements of various sports. In this chapter, specific examples of plyometric exercise drills are presented for the upper and lower extremities.

Physiologic Basis of Plyometrics

Stretch–shortening exercises use the elastic and reactive properties of a muscle to generate maximum force production. In normal muscle function, the muscle is stretched before it contracts concentrically. This eccentric–concentric coupling (i.e., the stretch–shortening cycle) employs the stimulation of the body's proprioceptors to facilitate an increase in muscle recruitment over a minimum amount of time.

The proprioceptors of the body include the muscle spindle, the Golgi tendon organ (GTO), and the joint capsule/ligamentous mechanoreceptors.[14] Stimulation of these receptors can cause facilitation, inhibition, and modulation of agonist and antagonist muscles.[14,15] Both the

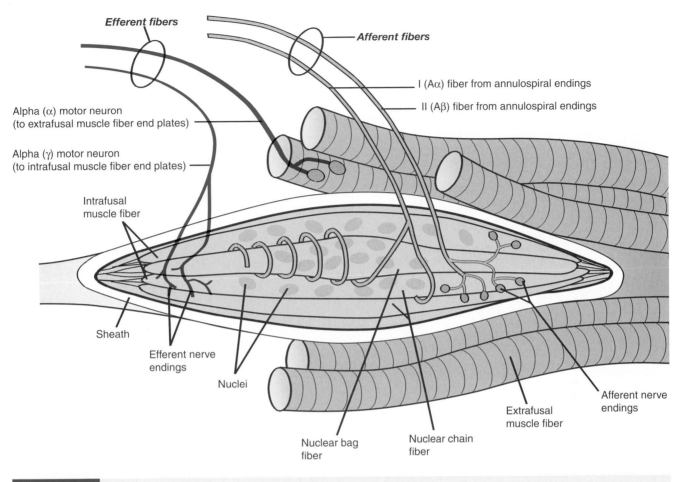

Efferent fibers

Afferent fibers

I (Aα) fiber from annulospiral endings

II (Aβ) fiber from annulospiral endings

Alpha (α) motor neuron
(to extrafusal muscle fiber end plates)

Alpha (γ) motor neuron
(to intrafusal muscle fiber end plates)

Intrafusal
muscle fiber

Sheath

Efferent nerve
endings

Nuclei

Afferent nerve
endings

Extrafusal
muscle fiber

Nuclear bag
fiber

Nuclear chain
fiber

Figure 9-1 The muscle spindle.

muscle spindle and GTO provide the proprioceptive basis for plyometric training.

The muscle spindle functions mainly as a stretch receptor (Fig. 9-1). The muscle spindle components that are primarily sensitive to changes in velocity are the nuclear bag intrafusal muscle fibers, which are innervated by type Ia phasic nerve fiber. The muscle spindle is provoked by a quick stretch, which reflexively produces a quick contraction of the agonistic and synergistic extrafusal muscle fibers (Fig. 9-2). The firing of the type Ia phasic nerve fibers is influenced by the rate of stretch; the faster and greater the stimulus, the greater the effect of the associated extrafusal fibers. This cycle occurs in 0.3 to 0.5 milliseconds and is mediated at the spinal cord level in the form of a monosynaptic reflex.[14]

The GTO, which is sensitive to tension, is located at the junction between the tendon and muscle at both the proximal and distal attachments. The unit is arranged in series with the extrafusal muscle fibers and therefore becomes activated with stretch. Unlike the muscle spindle, the GTO

has an inhibitory effect on the muscle. Upon activation, impulses are sent to the spinal cord, causing an inhibition of the α motor neurons of the contracting muscle and its synergists and thus limiting the force produced. It has been postulated that the GTO is a protective mechanism against overcontraction or stretch of the muscle. Because the GTO uses at least one interneuron in its synaptic cycle, inhibition requires more time than monosynaptic excitation by type Ia nerve fibers (Fig. 9-2).[14]

During concentric muscle contraction, the muscle spindle output is reduced because the muscle fibers are either shortening or attempting to shorten. During eccentric contraction the muscle stretch reflex serves to generate more tension in the lengthening muscle.[16] When the muscle tension increases to a high or potentially harmful level, the GTO fires, generating a neural pattern that reduces the excitation of the muscle. Consequently, the GTO receptors may act as a protective mechanism; however, in a correctly carried out plyometric exercise, the reflex arc pathway

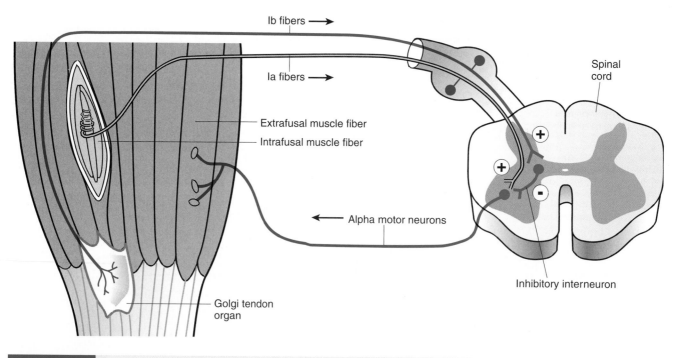

| Figure 9-2 | Passive stretch reflex. |

incorporated with excitation of type Ia nerve fibers overshadows the influence of the GTO.

In addition to the neurophysiologic stimulus, the positive results of the stretch–shortening exercise can also be attributed to the recoil action of elastic tissues.[7,8,17] Several authors have reported that an eccentric contraction will significantly increase the force generated concentrically as a result of storage of elastic energy.[5,6,17,18] The mechanism for this increased concentric force is the ability of the muscle to use the force produced by the elastic component. During the loading of the muscle that occurs when stretching, the load is transferred to the elastic component and stored as elastic energy. The elastic elements can then deliver increased energy, which is recovered and used for the concentric contraction.[5,17]

The ability of the muscle to use the stored elastic energy is affected by the duration, magnitude, and velocity of stretch. Increased force generated during the concentric contraction is most effective when the preceding eccentric contraction is of short range and performed quickly, without delay.[5,18] The improved or increased muscle performance that occurs by prestretching the muscle is the result of the combined effects of both the storage of elastic energy and the myotatic reflex activation of the muscle.[5,18] The percentage of contribution from each component is not yet known. In addition, the degree of enhanced muscular performance depends on the time between the eccentric and concentric contractions.[8]

Phases of Stretch–shortening Exercise

Three phases of the plyometric exercise have been described: the setting (stretch) or eccentric phase, amortization phase, and concentric (shortening) response phase (Table 9-1). The eccentric, or setting, phase begins when the athlete mentally prepares for the activity and ends when the stretch stimulus is initiated. The advantages of a correct setting phase include increasing the muscle spindle activity by stretching the muscle before activation and mentally biasing the α motor neuron for optimal extrafusal muscle contraction.[19] The duration of the setting phase is determined by the degree of impulse desired for facilitation of the contraction. With too much or prolonged loading, the elapsed time from eccentric to concentric contraction will prevent optimal exploitation of the stretch–shortening myotatic reflex.[1,20]

TABLE 9-1 Phases of Plyometric Exercises

Phase	Description
I	Eccentric: stretch or setting period
II	Amortization: time between eccentric and concentric phases
III	Concentric response: facilitated shortening contraction

The next phase of the stretch–shortening response is amortization. This phase begins as the eccentric contraction starts to wane and ends with the initiation of a concentric force. By definition, amortization is the electromechanical delay between the eccentric and concentric contractions, during which the muscle must switch from overcoming work to imparting the necessary amount of acceleration in the required direction.[2] Successful training using the stretch–shortening technique relies heavily on the rate of stretch rather than the length of the stretch. If the amortization phase is slow, elastic energy is wasted as heat and the stretch reflex is not activated. The more quickly the individual is able to switch from yielding work to overcoming work, the more powerful the response.

The final period of the stretch–shortening exercise is the concentric response phase. During this phase the athlete concentrates on the effect of the exercise and prepares for initiation of the second repetition. The response phase is the summation of the setting and amortization phases. This stage is often referred to as the resultant or payoff phase because of the enhanced concentric contraction.[2,9,21,22]

Theoretically, stretch–shortening exercise assists in the improvement of physiologic muscle performance in several ways. Although increasing the speed of the myotatic stretch-reflex response may increase performance, such information has not been documented in the literature. Research does exist to support the idea that the faster a muscle is loaded eccentrically, the greater the concentric force produced.[23] Eccentric loading places stress on the elastic components, thereby increasing the tension of the resultant rebound force.

A second possible mechanism for the increased force production involves the inhibitory effect of the GTO on force production. Because the GTO serves as a protective mechanism to limit the amount of force produced within a muscle, its stimulation threshold becomes the limiting factor. Desensitization of the GTO through a plyometric-training program may be possible, which will raise the level of inhibition and ultimately allow increased force production with greater loads applied to the musculoskeletal system.

The last mechanism by which plyometric training may increase muscular performance centers on neuromuscular coordination. The ultimate speed of movement may be limited by neuromuscular coordination. Explosive plyometric training may improve neural efficiency and increase neuromuscular performance. Using the prestretch response, the athlete may better coordinate the activities of the muscle groups. This enhanced neuromuscular coordination could lead to a greater net force production, even in the absence of morphologic change within the muscles themselves (referred to as neural adaptation).[2] In other words, the neurologic system may be enhanced, becoming more automatic.

The implementation of a stretch–shortening program begins with the development of an adequate strength and physical condition base. The development of a greater strength base leads to greater force generation owing to the increased cross-sectional area of both the muscle and the resultant elastic component. Therefore, to produce optimal strength gains and prevent overuse injuries, a structured strengthening program must be instituted before beginning plyometrics.

CLINICAL GUIDELINES

Plyometric exercise trains the neuromuscular system by teaching it to better accept and apply increased system loads. Using the stretch reflex helps improve the ability of the nervous system to react with maximum speed to the lengthening muscle. The improved stretch reflex allows muscle to contract concentrically with maximal force. Because the plyometric program attempts to modify and retrain the neuromuscular system, the program should be designed with sport specificity in mind.

Plyometric exercises are common for lower-extremity rehabilitation but can also be incorporated into upper-extremity rehabilitation.[24–26] Athletes often use the upper extremity in an open-kinetic–chain fashion, e.g., when throwing, golfing, shooting a basketball, and performing a tennis stroke. However, some athletes do bear weight on their distal upper extremities, either to protect themselves from a fall or to perform specific sports endeavors (e.g., gymnasts, boxers, football players, and wrestlers). In addition, athletic endeavors such as swimming, throwing, cross-country skiing, and wheelchair propulsion all use principles of rapid opening and closing of the kinetic chain to propel the body or an object through space. Athletes involved in these sports use the upper extremity in much the same way as athletes use the lower extremities when jumping or running. Thus, the theories of enhanced neuromuscular control from plyometric drills can be applied to the upper extremities.

Plyometric exercises have the capacity to condition the upper and lower extremities while being sport specific. Developing intervention protocols that incorporate sport-specific drills not only potentiates the effect of the overall rehabilitation program but may lead to prevention of further athletic injuries.

Precautions

Contraindications to performing upper- and lower-extremity plyometric exercises include acute inflammation or pain, immediate postoperative pathology, and gross instabilities.

The most significant contraindication to an intense stretch–shortening exercise program is for individuals who have not been involved in a weight-training program. Intense stretch–shortening exercise programs are intended to be advanced strengthening programs for the competitive athlete to enhance athletic performance and are not recommended for the recreational athlete. Athletes appear to exhibit the greatest gain from a well-designed plyometric program. The clinician should be aware of the adverse reactions secondary to this form of exercise, such as delayed-onset muscular soreness. In addition, it should be noted that this form of exercise should not be performed for an extended period of time because of the large stresses that occur during exercise. More appropriately, stretch–shortening exercise is used during the first and second preparation phases of training, using the concept of periodization (Chapter 5).

TECHNIQUES

This section provides the physical therapist assistant (PTA) with specific plyometric drills, programs, and progressions for the upper and lower extremities. We present examples of possible exercises that can be incorporated into the rehabilitation of an injured patient. The demands of each sport should be considered when choosing the most appropriate drills because the program should be as patient and sport specific as possible.

Upper-extremity Plyometric Drills

As noted, implementation of the stretch–shortening program begins with the development of an adequate strength and physical condition base. A sample upper-extremity stretch–shortening exercise program is presented to illustrate its clinical applications. The program is organized into four groups: warmup exercises, throwing movements, trunk exercises, and wall exercises (Table 9-2). General suggestions for progressing the program are presented in Table 9-3.

Warmup

Warmup exercises are designed to provide the body (especially the shoulder, arm, and trunk) an adequate physiologic preparation before beginning a plyometric program. An active warmup should facilitate muscular performance by increasing blood flow, muscle and core temperatures, speed of contraction, oxygen use, and nervous system transmission. The first three warmup exercises—trunk

TABLE 9-2 Upper-extremity Plyometric Program

Group	Exercises
Warmup	Trunk rotation with medicine ball
	Side bends
	Wood chops
	Push-ups
	Internal and external shoulder rotation with tubing (90-degree abduction)
Throwing movements	Two-hand chest pass
	Two-hand soccer throw
	Internal and external shoulder rotation with tubing (90-degree abduction; fast speed)
	One-hand baseball throw
Trunk exercises	Sit-ups with medicine ball
	Sit-ups with rotation
	Sit-ups with throws and rotation
Wall exercises	Two-hand overhead soccer throw
	Two-hand chest pass
	One-hand baseball throw (standing; kneeling)
	One-hand wall dribble
	Multiple jumps

rotations (Fig. 9-3), trunk side bends, and wood chops (Fig. 9-4)—use a 9-pound medicine ball. Some warmup exercises are performed with exercise tubing and include internal and external rotation movements of the shoulder with the arm in 90 degrees of shoulder abduction and 90 degrees of elbow flexion to simulate the throwing position. Finally, push-ups with both hands on the ground can enhance the warmup period. Patients should perform two to three sets of 10 repetitions each of these warmup exercises before beginning the exercise session.

TABLE 9-3 General Guidelines for Progression of Lower-extremity Plyometric Activities

Two-hand drills → One-hand drills
Bilateral drills → Unilateral drills
Light Plyoball → Heavy Plyoball
Movements close to body → Movements away from body
Single-joint movements → Multiple-joint movements
Straight planes → Diagonal planes
Single planes → Multiple planes
Specific drills → Sport-specific drills

| Figure 9-3 | Trunk rotation. |

PURPOSE: Warmup exercise for upper extremity before plyometric drills.

POSITION: Client standing, holding medicine ball in both hands in front with elbows extended.

PROCEDURE: Client rotates trunk to right and to left keeping ball in front of body with elbows extended. It is important to pause at each extreme of rotation before rotating in opposite direction.

A **B**

| Figure 9-4 | Wood chops. |

PURPOSE: Warm-up exercise for upper extremity before plyometric drills.

POSITION: Client standing, holding medicine ball in both hands in front with elbows extended.

PROCEDURE: Client bends forward, pauses at full trunk flexion (**A**) and then extends spine fully while raising ball overhead (**B**). It is important to pause at each extreme of flexion and extension.

Throwing Movement

Throwing-movement stretch–shortening exercises attempt to isolate the muscles and muscle groups necessary for throwing. These exercises are performed in combined movement patterns similar to the throwing motion. Beginning drills are throwing-movement plyometrics using a 4-pound Plyoball (Integrated Functional Products, Dublin, CA). The first drill is a two-hand overhead soccer throw (Fig. 9-5), followed by a two-hand chest pass (Fig. 9-6). These exercises can be performed with a partner or with the use of a spring-loaded bounce-back device called the Plyoback (Integrated Functional Products).

In addition, several of the stretch–shortening drills require exercise tubing. The first movement involves stretch–shortening movement for the external rotators in which the athlete brings the tubing back into external rotation and holds that position for 2 seconds (Fig. 9-7). The athlete then allows the external rotator musculature to release the isometric contraction, allowing the tubing to pull the arm into internal rotation. Thus, the external rotators eccentrically control the movement. Once the arm reaches full internal rotation (horizontal), the external rotators contract concentrically to bring the tubing back into external rotation. This constitutes one stretch–shortening repetition.

Similar movements are performed for the internal rotators and for proprioceptive neuromuscular facilitation diagonal patterns, including D2 flexion and D2 extension of the upper extremity (Figs. 7-7 and 7-8). The stretch–shortening technique can also be performed for the elbow flexors using exercise tubing.

Push-ups to enhance the strength of the serratus anterior, pectoralis major, deltoid, triceps, and biceps musculature can also be incorporated into the program. Push-ups can be advanced to a plyometric exercise by using the assistance of a PTA, performing push-ups against a wall (Fig. 9-8), and using a 6- to 8-inch box and the ground in a depth-jump–training manner (Fig. 9-9). Two to four sets of six to eight repetitions of all of these exercise drills are performed two to three times weekly.

Another group of exercises or drills uses a 2-pound medicine ball or Plyoball and a wall, which allows the patient the opportunity to perform plyometric medicine ball drills. Using a 2-pound medicine ball, the patient can perform a one-handed plyometric baseball throw (Fig. 9-10). To further challenge the patient, exercises can be performed in the kneeling position to eliminate the use of the lower extremities and increase the demands on the trunk and upper extremities. A commonly used exercise drill is called wall dribbling. The patient quickly dribbles a 2-pound ball against a wall, making a half circle. This drill is usually performed for a specific time period, e.g., 30 to 120 seconds.

The purpose of the stretch–shortening throwing exercises is to provide the patient with advanced strengthening exercises that are more aggressive and at a higher exercise level than a simple isotonic dumbbell exercise program. Stretch–shortening programs can be implemented only after the patient has undergone a strengthening program for an extended period of time and has a satisfactory clinical examination.

Trunk Exercises

Two groups of stretch–shortening drills for trunk-strengthening purposes emphasize the abdominal and trunk extensor muscles. Exercises in this group include medicine ball sit-ups, sit-ups with rotation, and sit-ups with throws (Fig. 9-11). Trunk exercise drills are performed two to three times a week for three to four sets of six to eight repetitions. Performing trunk exercises is extremely important for the overhead athlete.

Lower-extremity Plyometric Drills

Implementation criteria of plyometric exercises for the lower extremity follow the same guidelines as those for the upper extremity. Lower-extremity plyometric drills can be divided into four different categories: warmup, jump drills, box drills, and depth jumps (Table 9-4). Sport-specific drills should always be chosen to enhance the rehabilitation of the injured athlete. The PTA should observe the techniques of jumping and should stress correct posture, minimum side to side and forward to backward deviations, landing with toe-heel motion, landing with slightly flexed knees, and instant preparation for subsequent jumps. As the patient progresses and the plyometric drills become more advanced, drills should concentrate on the development of strength and power. As the patient masters proper technique, the focus shifts to quality, distance, height, or speed of jumping, depending on the goals of the athlete.

Chu[27] suggests counting the number of foot contacts as a measure of frequency when using plyometrics for the lower extremity. A range of 60 to 100 foot touches per training session is considered appropriate for the beginner; 100 to 150 for the intermediate exerciser; and 150 to 200 for the advanced exerciser.

Warmup

As with any plyometric-training program, an adequate warmup is essential to avoid overuse injuries. Warmup begins with stretching the lower extremities, followed by light running. Running can be progressed to include skipping, lateral side shuffles, backward running, and carioca drills.

| Figure 9-5 | Two-hand overhead soccer throw. |

PURPOSE: Plyometric drill to facilitate movement patterns similar to throwing motion.

POSITION: Client standing and holding medicine ball with both hands behind head.

PROCEDURE: Client takes one step forward and throws ball with both hands.

| Figure 9-6 | Two-hand chest pass. |

PURPOSE: Plyometric drill to facilitate movement patterns similar to throwing motion.

POSITION: Client standing and holding medicine ball in both hands against chest.

PROCEDURE: Client takes one step forward and extends elbows, throwing ball by pushing with both hands.

Figure 9-7	External rotation with elastic tubing—throwing movement.

PURPOSE: Plyometric drill to facilitate stretch–shortening activities for external rotator muscles.

POSITION: Client standing and facing elastic tubing, which is attached to the wall at eye level, shoulder in 90-degree abduction and neutral external and internal rotation. Client holding elastic tubing.

PROCEDURE: Client pulls tubing back into external rotation (concentric contraction), holds position for 2 seconds (isometric contraction), and then releases external rotator muscles to allow tubing to pull arm into internal rotation (eccentric contraction).

A   **B**

Figure 9-8	Plyometric push-ups on wall—advanced phase.

PURPOSE: Plyometric drill to strengthen muscles of the glenohumeral and scapulothoracic joints.

POSITION: Client standing with feet 8 to 10 inches from wall with hands in push-up position against wall. Physical therapist assistant (PTA) standing behind client.

PROCEDURE: Keeping feet in place, client pushes body from wall by extending arms (concentric contraction). PTA catches patient and pushes patient back toward wall **(A)**. Patient catches body against wall with hands (eccentric contraction) **(B)** and immediately pushes away again (concentric contraction).

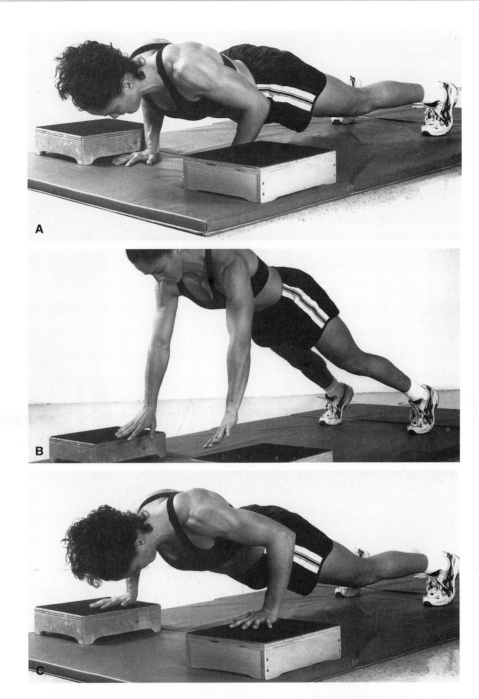

| Figure 9-9 | Plyometric push-ups with boxes—advanced phase. |

PURPOSE: Plyometric drills to strengthen muscles of the glenohumeral and scapulothoracic joints.

POSITION: Client in push-up position between two 6- to 8-inch boxes **(A)**.

PROCEDURE: From the support surface, client pushes with arms hard enough to lift body from ground (concentric contraction) **(B)**. When high enough off ground, client moves upper extremity slightly laterally and catches body with hands on boxes (eccentric contraction) **(C)**. Client then pushes off boxes to lift body from boxes (concentric contraction) and catches body on support surface (eccentric contraction).

| Figure 9-10 | One-handed plyometric baseball throw on wall—throwing movement. |

PURPOSE: Plyometric drills to facilitate stretch–shortening activities for external rotator muscles.

POSITION: Client standing directly in front of wall with shoulder in 90-degree abduction and full external rotation and elbow in 90-degree flexion. Client holding small medicine ball in one hand.

PROCEDURE: Client repeatedly internally rotates shoulder to throw (concentric exercise) ball against wall and catches ball as it returns from wall (eccentric contraction).

| Figure 9-11 | Sit-up with throw—trunk. |

PURPOSE: Strengthen abdominal muscles.

POSITION: Client lying supine with knees flexed, holding medicine ball in both hands overhead.

PROCEDURE: Client sits up and simultaneously throws ball with overhead soccer throw.

Jumps

Jump drills begin with basic hops in place on both extremities (double-ankle hop) using full ankle range of motion (ROM) for hopping momentum. This activity can be progressed to performing the exercise on one extremity (single-ankle hops). These exercises are of low intensity, and the client should focus on technique and amortization phase length. It is essential for the patient to develop the proper recoil from each jump to minimize the length of the amortization phase. Squat jumping involves dropping into a squat position before jumping with maximal extension of the lower extremities (Fig. 9-12). Tuck jumps begin with a slight squat; then the athlete brings both knees up to the chest and holds until extending to land in a vertical position (Fig. 9-13). The vertical and tuck jumps should focus on the production of power; they require a period of recovery between jumps.

The 180-degree jumps begin with a two-footed jump; the patient rotates 180 degrees in midair, holding the landing, and then reverses direction. Cones or tape on the floor can be used for multiple forward, lateral, diagonal, or zigzag jumps and hops on one or two limbs (called agility jumps) (Fig. 9-14). The patient is instructed to jump as quickly as possible to the cone or tape. One of the most important aspects of plyometric training is the landing after the jump. A soft landing is strongly encouraged, and the patient is told to land as light as a feather. The soft landing aids in controlling ground-reaction forces.

Box Jumps

Box jumps (aerobic benches can be used) begin with basic front and lateral box jumps (Fig. 9-15). The patient begins on level ground and jumps onto a box of prescribed height. To do box push-off drills, the patient faces a box and puts one foot on it. Then the patient extends the lower extremity that is on the box, achieving maximal height and landing on top of the box. The patient returns to the original position. The patient can alternate the lower extremities, working each one in turn. Lateral push-off drills can also be incorporated.

Multiple box jumps can be performed in the forward or lateral direction, with the athlete jumping up onto the box, down from the box, and then back up to another box (Fig. 9-16). In addition, turns can be added (Fig. 9-17). Box drills can be progressed from low intensity to high intensity by adjusting the height of the box. Furthermore, the individual can be progressed from performing the exercise on two legs to performing it on one extremity.

Depth Jumps

Box jumps are progressed to include depth jumps. Depth jumps from atop a box use the athlete's potential energy to vary the ground-reaction forces produced during landing. The simplest form of depth jumping involves the athlete stepping from the top of a box and landing flexed and holding the landing (Fig. 9-18). The patient should not jump from the box but rather step off the edge of the box so the exercise can be reliably reproduced at different prescribed heights.

Once the proper landing technique is learned and tolerated by the patient, depth jumps can be followed by a maximal vertical jump, the patient recoiling as rapidly as possible after absorbing the impact. The patient recoils after landing and jumps up from landing as rapidly as possible to decrease the amortization phase. A squat depth jump begins with the patient stepping off a box and landing in a squat position, followed by a quick explosion out of the squat and again landing in a squat position. For added difficulty, the athlete can land on a second box.

Progression

Plyometric exercises for the lower extremity can be progressed by adding weight (using medicine balls), altering the height of box drills and depth jumps, and jumping from and landing on uneven surfaces. Each progression stresses the patient's force production, eccentric control of landing, and modulation of proprioceptive input. In addition, all plyometric exercises can be progressed by advancing the activity from two legs to one leg for a very aggressive plyometric exercise program.

TABLE 9-4 Lower-extremity Plyometric Program

Group	Exercises
Warmup	Stretching of lower-extremity muscles
	Running
	Skipping
	Lateral side shuffles
	Backward running
	Carioca
Jump drills	Double-ankle hops
	Single-ankle hops
	Squat jumps
	Vertical jumps
	Tuck jumps
	180-degree jumps
	Agility jumps
Box drills	Front jumps
	Lateral jumps
	Multiple jumps
Depth jumps	Forward jumps
	Squat depth jumps

Figure 9-12   Squat jumps.

PURPOSE: Plyometric drill to strengthen lower-extremity muscles.

POSITION: Client in squat position.

PROCEDURE: From squat position **(A)**, client jumps vertically as high as possible (concentric contraction) **(B)**. Upon landing, client absorbs shock into squat (eccentric contraction). Repeat.

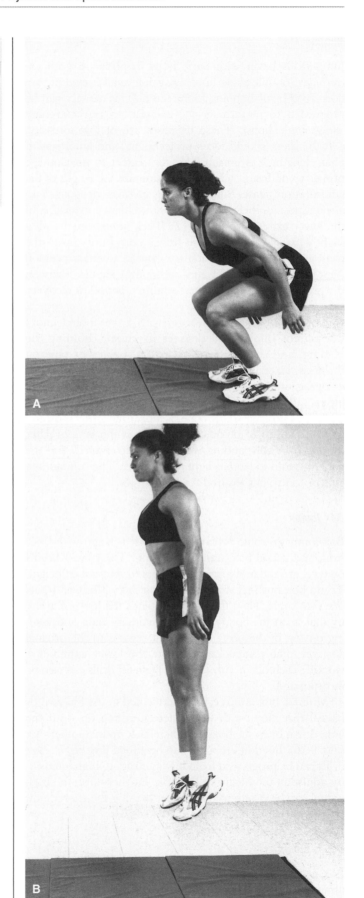

Figure 9-13	Tuck jumps.

PURPOSE: Plyometric drill to strengthen lower-extremity muscles.

POSITION: Client standing.

PROCEDURE: Client jumps vertically as high as possible (concentric contraction). During jump, client brings both knees up to chest and holds briefly (accentuation of concentric contraction). Client absorbs shock on landing (eccentric contraction). Repeat.

Figure 9-14	Agility jumps.

PURPOSE: Plyometric drill to enhance agility.

POSITION: Client standing; tape on floor marks four quadrants.

PROCEDURE: Client quickly jumps from one quadrant to next quadrant, jumping as quickly as possible and landing lightly.

| Figure 9-15 | Front box jumps. |

PURPOSE: Plyometric drills to facilitate stretch–shortening of lower-extremity muscles.

POSITION: Client standing and facing box.

PROCEDURE: Facing box, client jumps up to land on box (concentric contraction). After landing (eccentric contraction), client immediately jumps from box back to floor (concentric contraction). Repeat.

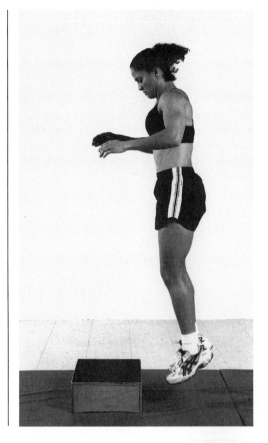

| Figure 9-16 | Multiple box jumps. |

PURPOSE: Plyometric drills to facilitate stretch–shortening of lower-extremity muscles.

POSITION: Client standing between two boxes but not facing either box.

PROCEDURE: Facing same direction during entire drill, client jumps laterally up to land on first box (concentric contraction). After landing (eccentric contraction), patient immediately jumps back to floor (concentric contraction). Patient lands on ground (eccentric contraction), immediately jumps laterally to land on second box (concentric contraction), and then immediately jumps back to original position (concentric contraction).

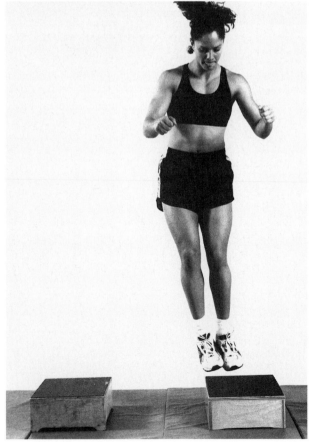

Figure 9-17   Multiple box jumps with turns.

PURPOSE: Plyometric drills to facilitate stretch–shortening for lower-extremity muscles.

POSITION: Client standing between two boxes but not facing either box.

PROCEDURE: Client jumps up and simultaneously turns to land on first box (concentric contraction). After landing (eccentric contraction), patient immediately jumps from box while turning in original direction (concentric contraction). Client lands on ground (eccentric contraction) and immediately jumps and simultaneously turns toward second box (concentric contraction). Client lands on second box (eccentric contraction) and then immediately jumps from box and turns back to original position (concentric contraction).

Figure 9-18   Depth jumps.

PURPOSE: Plyometric drills to facilitate stretch–shortening for lower-extremity muscles.

POSITION: Client standing on top of box.

PROCEDURE: Client steps off edge of box (should not jump) **(A)** and sticks the landing in a squat position (eccentric contraction) **(B)**.

NOTE: The exercise can end in squat position or client can jump up out of squat position (concentric contraction). For added difficulty, client can jump (concentric contraction) and land on second box (eccentric contraction).

CASE STUDY 1

PATIENT INFORMATION

The patient was an 18-year-old who played high school football and ran track. He injured his knee during football practice while he was trying to block a lineman. He reported that his left knee was planted when he felt the knee pop and shift out of place. He stated that pain was immediate and he was unable to walk without limping.

The patient presented to the clinic 1 day after injury. Examination by the physical therapist (PT) indicated an antalgic flexed knee gait and moderate joint effusion. He was able to perform a straight leg raise with 0-degree extension. Active ROM was 0 to 116 degrees and 0 to 146 degrees for the involved and noninjured knees, respectively. The Lachman's test was positive on the involved extremity.

Examination was consistent with a diagnosis of sprain to the anterior cruciate ligament (ACL). The patient was referred by the PT to an orthopedic surgeon, who recommended autogenous bone–patellar tendon–bone ACL reconstruction.

LINK TO
GUIDE TO PHYSICAL THERAPIST PRACTICE

According to the *Guide to Physical Therapist Practice,*[28] pattern 4D relates to the diagnosis of this patient. The pattern is described as "impaired joint mobility, motor function, muscle performance, and range of motion associated with other connective tissue dysfunction" and includes sprains of the knee and leg. Direct intervention includes "strengthening and power, including plyometric" exercises and "neuromuscular education and reeducation."

INTERVENTION

One Week After Surgery

One week after surgery the patient returned, demonstrating a slight antalgic gait without assistive devices. He reported using the continuous passive motion (CPM) machine on his ACL-reconstructed knee (Fig. 3-33). Examination by the PT noted that he presented with moderate joint effusion; pain was rated at 1/5; ROM was 0 to 100 degrees and 0 to 142 degrees for the involved and noninvolved knees, respectively.

Initial goals by the PT included decreasing swelling, obtaining full passive knee extension, and obtaining 110 degrees of flexion. The PT instructed the PTA to instruct the patient on the intervention consisting of the following home exercise program:

1. Discontinue use of CPM.
2. Heel props: 10 minutes every hour (while lying supine, patient props heel up on towel roll and places weight over the anterior knee to promote increased extension).
3. Prone hangs with weight: 10 minutes every hour.
4. Wall slides and heel slides (Fig. 3-6): three times a day.

Two Weeks After Surgery

At 2 weeks after surgery, upon re-examination by the PT, the patient reported that his knee had improved daily and he had worked on his home exercises daily. He presented with normal gait but still rated his pain at 1/5. A mild effusion was present. ROM was 0 to 126 degrees for the reconstructed knee.

The goals noted by the PT at this point were to maintain full extension, control swelling, increase flexion, and begin early strengthening. The PT discussed the goals and updated the home exercise program with the PTA and asked the PTA to instruct the patient on the following home exercise program:

1. Standing mini-squats from 0 to 30 degrees (Fig. 8-8).
2. Forward step-ups.
3. Stationary bicycle (Fig. 12-5).
4. Continue wall slides and prone hangs.

One Month After Surgery

One month after surgery, upon re-examination by the PT, the patient stated that his knee continued to improve and he rated his reconstructed knee at 60%. He presented with normal gait, mild effusion, and no reports of pain. ROM was 0 to 135 degrees.

Goals were updated to achieve full flexion ROM and to progress to more advanced strengthening activities. After receiving instruction from the PT, the PTA instructed the patient on the following program and was to report back to the PT about the patient's status and ability to perform the new exercise program.

1. Progress squats to a range of 0 to 60 degrees.
2. Progress step-ups to include forward and lateral movements (Fig. 8-9).
3. Forward lunges (Fig. 8-10).
4. Initiation of balance activities (Figs. 10-11 and 10-12).
5. Continue bicycle.

Two Months After Surgery

Examination by the PT at the 2-month follow-up indicated that ROM was equal bilaterally. The PT updated the home exercise program and instructed the PTA to instruct the patient on the following exercise program with a return status report after completion.

1. Continue bicycle
2. Continue closed-chain step-ups, mini-squats, and lunges.
3. Begin closed-chain cone drills (Fig. 8-11).
4. Begin calf raises.
5. Step machine (Fig. 12-7).
6. Open-chain hamstring curls with weight.

Three Months After Surgery

At 3 months the patient reported that he continued to improve and feel stronger. He also reported no problem with the home exercise program. Isokinetic examination indicated that the left quadriceps strength was 70% of the right. The exercise program was revised by the PT and instructed by the PTA. The program consisted of the following:

1. Jogging
2. Plyometric program: warmup exercises (jogging; hamstring, quadriceps, and gastrocnemius stretching; Figs. 4-7 to 4-10, 4-17), double-ankle jumps, and tuck jumps (Fig. 9-13).
3. Open-chain quadriceps strengthening (Fig. 6-33).
4. Continue closed-chain exercise program.

Four Months After Surgery

After 4 months the patient was progressing well. The exercise program was revised by the PT and instructed by the PTA. The program consisted of the following:

1. Continue open-chain strengthening.
2. Continue plyometric program.
3. Single-ankle jumps
4. Box jumps (Figs. 9-15 to 9-17).
5. Continue jogging program.

Five Months After Surgery

At the 5-month follow-up the patient reported no problems with any activities during the previous month. Functional testing performed by the PT, using a one-legged hop for distance and a one-legged vertical hop, indicated no deficit in the injured knee. The goal for the patient at this point was to prepare the athlete to return to full activities and competition. The home exercise program was progressed by the PT to include running and agility drills with his football coach. In addition, the athlete was instructed to perform depth jumps two times per week (Fig. 9-18).

OUTCOME

Examination by the PT at the end of 6 months indicated no deficits in the left knee. The athlete was cleared to participate in all activities. He completed an uneventful season in football and track the following year.

SUMMARY—AN EFFECTIVE PT-PTA TEAM

This case study demonstrates an effective collaborative effort between the PT and PTA that is conducive to a busy sport medicine clinic. The PTA is able to follow the instruction of the PT after their re-examination of the patient and is able to instruct the patient about the home exercise program. The PT is aware of the patient's status and ability to advance the home exercise program due to the good communication between the PT and PTA after the instruction. The PT expects that the PTA fully understands the interventions included in the home exercise program. The PT also expects that the PTA can instruct the patient independently and report any adverse effects of the session. This type of working relationship allows the PT to be aware of the athlete's status but at the same time allows him/her to perform examinations on other patients in the clinic, demonstrating effective and efficient teamwork while still providing quality care.

▼ ▼ ▼ GERIATRIC PERSPECTIVES ▼ ▼ ▼

■ With the exception of the older athlete, plyometrics may not be the optimal choice for rehabilitation of the aged. Movements requiring quick power and rapid muscle reactivity should be used with caution because of age-related changes in muscle tissue.

▲ ▲ ▲ PEDIATRIC PERSPECTIVES ▲ ▲ ▲

■ Plyometrics can be used to train children in fun, play-related movements such as hopscotch and bouncing activities.[1] Use of plyometrics during rehabilitation is determined by the needs of the patient for his or her chosen activity.[1] Children who are not competitive athletes may engage in many common activities that do not require aggressive plyometric training. Take into account the patient's age, experience, maturity, and attention span when considering use of plyometrics.[1] Lack of sufficient attention span may contraindicate the use of plyometrics in rehabilitation of children.

■ Examples of low-intensity exercises that may be used are single-leg squats and jump/play activities. Use discretion and close supervision when medium-intensity skills are required.[2] It is probably wise to avoid high-intensity and large vertical dimensions when using plyometrics with most children.

■ It is common for children to lack coordination, which suggests the need to pay attention to proper technique during training. Ongoing supervision during plyometric programs used with children is essential. Be certain that children's performances are routinely evaluated and that youngsters are able to demonstrate mastery of a skill before they are given clearance to move to the next level of difficulty in a program.

1. Chu D. *Jumping into plyometrics.* Champaign, IL: Leisure; 1992.
2. Albert M. *Eccentric muscle training in sports and orthopedics.* New York: Churchill Livingston; 1995.

SUMMARY

- Plyometric exercises are quick powerful movements involving a prestretching of the muscle, thereby activating the stretch–shortening cycle of the muscle.

- The purpose of plyometric training is to increase the excitability of the neurologic receptors (stretch reflex) for improved reactivity of the neuromuscular system.

- The physiologic rationale and clinical application for plyometrics for the upper and lower extremity are presented.

- Plyometrics are designed to provide a functional form of exercise just before the initiation of sport-specific training (Chapter 15). These exercises are an excellent form of training for the competitive athlete.

References

1. Verkhoshanski Y. Depth jumping in the training of jumpers. *Track Tech.* 1983;51:1618–1619.

2. Voight M, Draovitch P. Plyometrics. In: Albert M, ed. *Eccentric muscle training in sports and orthopedics.* New York: Churchill Livingston; 1991:45–73.

3. Wilt F. Plyometrics, what it is and how it works. *Athl J.* 1975; 55:76–90.

4. Wilk K, Voight M. Plyometrics for the shoulder complex. In: Andrews J, Wilk K, eds. *The athlete's shoulder.* New York: Churchill Livingston; 1993:543–566.

5. Bosco C, Komi P. Potentiation of the mechanical behavior of the human skeletal muscle through prestretching. *Acta Physiol Scand.* 1979;106:467–472.

6. Bosco C, Tarkka J, Komi P. Effects of elastic energy and myoelectric potentiation of triceps surca during stretch-shortening cycle exercise. *Int J Sports Med.* 1982;2:137–141.

7. Cavagna GA. Elastic bounce of the body. *J Appl Physiol.* 1970; 29:279–282.

8. Cavagna G, Disman B, Margarai R. Positive work done by previously stretched muscle. *J Appl Physiol.* 1968;24:21–32.

9. Chu D. Plyometric exercise. *Natl Strength Cond Assoc J.* 1984; 6:56–62.

10. Blattner S, Noble L. Relative effects of isokinetic and plyometric training on vertical jumping performance. *Res Q Exerc Sport.* 1979;50:583–588.

11. Gambetta V, Odgers S, Coleman A, et al. The science, philosophy, and objectives of training and conditioning for baseball. In: Andrews J, Zarins B, Wilk K, eds. *Injuries in baseball.* Philadelphia: Lippincott–Raven Publishers; 1998:533–536.

12. Arthur M, Bailey B. *Complete conditioning for football.* Champaign, IL: Human Kinetics; 1998:165–237.

13. Hewett T, Riccobene J, Lindenfeld T. The effect of neuromuscular training on the incidence of knee injury in female athletes: a prospective study. *Am J Sports Med.* 1999;27:699–706.

14. Pearson K, Gordon J. Spinal reflexes. In: Kandel E, Schwartz JH, Jessell TM, eds. *Principles of neural science.* 3rd ed. New York: Elsevier; 2000:713–734.

15. Knott M, Voss D. *Proprioceptive neuromuscular facilitation.* New York: Harper & Row; 1968.

16. Komi P, Buskirk E. Effects of eccentric and concentric muscle conditioning on tension and electrical activity of human muscle. *Ergonomics.* 1972;15:417–422.

17. Cavagna G, Saibene F, Margaria R. Effect of negative work on the amount of positive work performed by an isolated muscle. *J Appl Physiol.* 1965;20:157–160.

18. Assmussen E, Bonde-Peterson F. Storage of elastic energy in skeletal muscle in man. *Acta Physiol Scand.* 1974;91:385–392.

19. Eldred E. Functional implications of dynamic and static components of the spindle response to stretch. *Am J Phys Med.* 1967;46:129–140.

20. Komi P, Bosco C. Utilization of stored elastic energy in leg extensor muscles by men and women. *Med Sci Sports Exerc.* 1978;10:261–265.

21. Chu D. The language of plyometrics. *Natl Strength Cond Assoc J.* 1984;6:30–31.

22. Voight M. Stretch-strengthening: an introduction to plyometrics. *Orthop Phys Ther Clin North Am.* 1992;1:243–252.

23. Lundin P. A review of plyometric training. *Natl Strength Cond Assoc J.* 1985;7:65–70.

24. Davies GJ, Matheson JW. Shoulder plyometrics. *Sports Med Arthro Rev.* 2001;9:1–18.

25. Schulte-Edelmann JA, Davies GJ, Kernozek TW, et al. The effects of plyometric training of the posterior shoulder and elbow. *J Strength Cond Res.* 2005;19:129–134.

26. Swanik KA, Lephart SM, Swanik CB, et al. The effects of shoulder plyometric training on proprioception and selected muscle performance characteristics. *J Shoulder Elbow Surg.* 2002;11:579–586.

27. Chu D. *Jumping into plyometrics.* Champaign, IL: Human Kinetics; 1992.

28. American Physical Therapy Association. *Guide to physical therapist practice.* 2nd ed. Alexandria, VA; 2003.

Balance

Balance Training

Bridgett Wallace, PT

OBJECTIVES

Upon completion of this chapter, the reader will be able to:

■ Describe the roles of base of support, limits of stability, and center of gravity in static and dynamic balance.

■ Identify sensory systems vital to the maintenance of balance.

■ Discuss appropriate clinical examination tools used to measure each sensory system input.

■ Identify automatic postural reaction strategies.

■ Discuss how and when each postural reaction strategy is used by the muscular system to prevent falls and maintain balance during locomotion.

■ Apply proper techniques to improve ankle strategies, hip strategies, and stepping strategies within the established plan of care.

Balance is essential for individuals to move about their environments and successfully carry out daily activities. Although the definition of balance and its neural mechanisms have changed over the years, this chapter will focus on the systems theory.[1] The systems model focuses on a dynamic interplay among various systems by integrating both motor and sensory strategies to maintain static and dynamic balance. This integration is a complex process that depends on (a) sensory inputs, (b) sensorimotor integration by the central nervous system (CNS), and (c) postural responses.[2] Since about 1980 the literature has expanded on the systematic approach to postural stability for developing more clinical tests and a better understanding of balance. Specifically, this chapter focuses on much of the pioneering work by Nashner.[3,4] The information is presented from a systematic approach to balance that includes biomechanical factors, sensory organization, and coordination of postural movements (musculoskeletal components).

SCIENTIFIC BASIS

Biomechanical Components of Balance

Balance is the process of controlling the body's center of gravity over the support base or, more generally, within the limits of stability, whether stationary or moving. Balance can be divided into static and dynamic balance. Static balance refers to an individual's ability to maintain a stable antigravity position while at rest by maintaining the center of gravity within the available base of support. Dynamic balance involves automatic postural responses to the disruption of the center of gravity position.[1]

Base of Support

The base of support is defined as the area within the perimeter of the contact surface between the feet and the support surface.[4] In normal stance on a flat surface, the base of support is almost square. Although a tandem stance (standing with one foot in front of the other, heel touching toe) and walking extend the length of the person's support surface, the width is narrow. When the support base becomes smaller than the feet (tandem) or unstable, the base of support is decreased and the individual's stability is reduced.

Limits of Stability

To maintain balance in standing, the center of gravity must be kept upright within specific boundaries of space, referred to as limits of stability. Thus, limits of stability can be defined as the greatest distance a person can lean away from the base of support without changing that base.[5] Limits of stability allow individuals to overcome the destabilizing

effect of gravity by performing small corrective sways in the anterior–posterior (AP) dimension as well as laterally. The limits of stability for a normal adult who is standing upright is approximately 12 degrees AP and 16 degrees laterally.[3] These limits of stability are sometimes illustrated by a "cone of stability." If sway occurs outside the cone, a strategy must be used to restore balance. Figure 10-1 demonstrates the limits of stability boundaries during standing, walking, and sitting.[3]

Center of Gravity

The center of gravity is defined as the central point within the limits of stability area.[4] When a normal person stands upright, the center of gravity is centered over the base of support provided by the feet. A centralized center of gravity allows the individual's sway boundaries to be as large as the stability limits. On the other hand, a person with an abnormal center of gravity will not be as stable within the limits of stability. The relationships among the limits of stability, sway envelope, and center of gravity are shown in Figure 10-2.[3]

From a biomechanical standpoint, postural stability is the angular distance between the center of gravity and the limits of stability.[3] Therefore, a person's static postural alignment and the dynamic sway affect his or her stability.

Sensory Components of Balance

Balance requires accurate information from sensory input, effective processing by the CNS, and appropriate responses of motor control.[2] Therefore, imbalance can occur from neuropathy, involvement of the CNS, and decreased muscle strength. Proper examination of each component is critical for determining a client's underlying problem and the appropriate treatment plan.

Sensory Organization

The CNS relies on information from three sensory systems: proprioception, visual, and vestibular. No single system provides all the information. Each system contributes a different yet important role in maintaining balance. The ability of the CNS to select, suppress, and combine appropriate inputs under changing environmental conditions is called "sensory organization."[6]

Proprioception inputs provide information about the orientation of the body and body parts relative to each other and the support surface. Information is received from joint and skin receptors, deep pressure, and muscle proprioception.[6,7] Proprioception cues are the dominant inputs for maintaining balance when the support surface is firm and fixed.[6,8] Visual inputs provide information to an individual about the physical surroundings relative to the position and

Figure 10-1 Boundaries of the limits of support during standing, walking, and sitting.

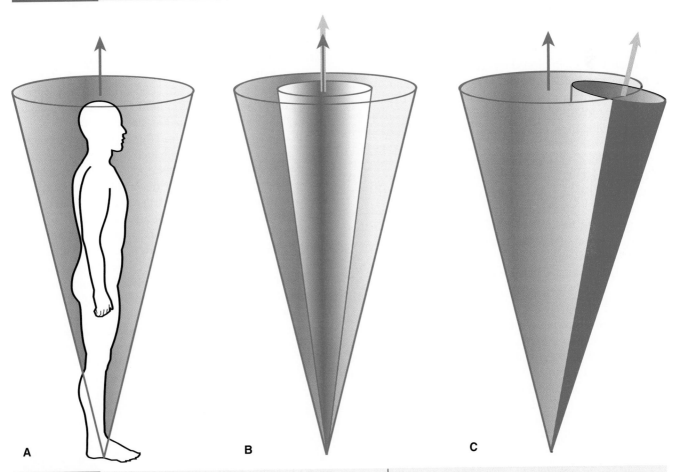

A B C

Figure 10-2 **A.** Relationship among the limit of support, sway envelope, and center of gravity alignment. **B.** The center of gravity alignment centered within the limit of support.

C. An offset center of gravity (leaning forward) requires the individual to make an adjustment to maintain balance.

movement of the head. Visual cues are particularly important when proprioceptive inputs are unreliable.[6,9]

Vestibular inputs provide both sensory and motor functions to the individual. The sensory component of the vestibular system measures the angular velocity and linear acceleration of the head and detects the position of the head relative to gravity.[6] The motor component, however, uses motor pathways for postural control and coordinated movement. One mechanism within the vestibular motor system is the vestibulospinal reflex. The vestibulospinal reflex initiates a person's appropriate body movements to maintain an upright posture and to stabilize the head and trunk.[10,11] The vestibulo-ocular reflex, on the other hand, stabilizes vision during head and body movements, thus allowing for accurate dynamic vision.[6,10] Because the system has sensory and motor components, the vestibular system plays an important role in balance. This system is dominant when a conflict exists between proprioceptive and visual cues and for postural stability during ambulation.[6,7]

Examination of Sensory Organization

These three sensory inputs (proprioceptive, visual, and vestibular) provide the individual with redundant information regarding orientation. This redundancy allows normal individuals to select, suppress, or combine the appropriate inputs to maintain balance under changing environmental conditions.[3] Nashner[3,4] pioneered technologic advances for examining appropriate sensory integration. One such advancement is known as computerized dynamic posturography, which examines sensory and motor components of the postural control system. The two protocols of this system are the sensory organization test (SOT), which isolates and compares the three sensory inputs, and the movement coordination test (MCT), discussed later in this chapter. A less sophisticated test for examining the sensory and motor components of balance is the clinical test of sensory interaction on balance (CTSIB).

Sensory Organization Test

The SOT protocol is used to examine the relative contributions of vision, vestibular, and proprioceptive inputs to the control of postural stability when conflicting sensory input occurs (Fig. 10-3). Postural sway can be examined under six increasingly challenging conditions (Fig. 10-4). Baseline sway is recorded with an individual quiet and standing with the eyes open. The reliance on vision is then examined by asking the patient to close the eyes. A significant increase in sway or loss of balance suggests an overreliance on visual input.[3,12]

Sensory integration is also examined when the surrounding visual field moves in concert with sway (sway-referenced vision), creating inaccurate visual input. The patient is then retested on a support surface that moves with sway (sway-referenced support), thereby reducing the quality and

availability of proprioceptive input for sensory integration. With the eyes open, vision and vestibular input contribute to the postural responses. With the eyes closed, vestibular input is the primary source of information because proprioceptive input is altered. The most challenging condition includes sway-referenced vision and sway-referenced support surface.[3,12]

Clinical Test for Sensory Interaction and Balance

A less sophisticated tool for examining sensory organization is the CTSIB, also known as the "foam and dome."[10,12] The CTSIB requires the patient to maintain standing balance under six different conditions (Fig. 10-5). During the first three conditions the individual stands on a firm surface for 30 seconds with eyes open, eyes closed, and while wearing a "dome" to produce inaccurate visual cues. The individual repeats these tasks while standing on a foam surface. The tester uses the first condition as a baseline for comparing sway under the other conditions.[10,12]

Less Sophisticated Balance Assessment Tools

There are additional less sophisticated tests for use as quick screen tools or preliminary clinical assessments. These are listed in Table 10-1.

The Romberg Test is a simple standing test. The client is instructed to stand with his or her feet parallel and together about shoulder width apart. The client is observed to see if balance is maintained for at least 30 seconds with eyes open; if not possible, the test is terminated. If completed, then the client is asked to close his or her eyes to see if balance can be maintained for 15 seconds or longer. Increased sway with eyes closed is normal; loss of balance is not. This quickly tests for balance when visual cues are removed.[12]

The one-limb stance test tests balance on each leg by asking the client to cross the arms across the chest. While being timed, the client stands on one leg for as long as possible, switches legs, and again stands as long as possible while being timed. There is little functional validity, but this test may be helpful to determine if there is a symmetric issue with balance since 20% to 40% of gait time is spent on one leg.

The functional reach test was described by Duncan et al.[13] It is an easily used test since the only equipment necessary is a wall with a yardstick attached. So quick and easy, this test is one of the tests included in the Funfitness Program, Special Olympics. Once the yardstick is set up, the client is asked to stand parallel with the wall and extend the hand and arm with the shoulder at 90 degrees of flexion. The client is instructed to reach as far forward as possible without losing his or her balance. This distance is recorded; after three trials the distance is averaged, and the opposite limb is measured using the same protocol.

The Berg Scale is a performance-based assessment of function. The test needs minimal equipment: an armchair, an armless chair, a stop watch, and a step. The patient is

Figure 10-3

The sensory organization test performed on a SMART Balance Master, a type of computerized posturography. Postural sway is examined under six increasingly challenging conditions illustrated in Figure 10-4. (Courtesy of Neurocom International, Inc., Clackamas, OR)

assessed in both static and dynamic balance activities while completing 14 functional tasks such as getting in and out of a chair, reaching forward, and picking up an object from the floor. The tasks are graded on a five-point scale with points awarded based on time or distance. The Berg Scale looks at many different aspects, has both reliability and validity, and takes only 15 minutes to implement.[14-16]

The Tinetti Balance and Gait Tests are also easy to complete and correlate well with the Berg Scale ($r = 0.91$). This assessment tool has nine balance items and seven gait items. It also requires minimal equipment.[17]

The Timed Up and Go Test (TUG) is another easy tool to evaluate balance during mobility. The client is asked to stand and walk 3 meters, then turn around, return, and sit. The timed performance has good interrater and intrarater reliability ($r = 0.99$). It requires no equipment and is easy to administer. Standards exist that indicate if it takes less than 10 seconds, there are no mobility issues. More than 30 seconds indicates that there is limited mobility and assistance may be required.[18]

Musculoskeletal Components of Balance

Many muscles are involved in the coordination of postural stability. This section focuses on key muscle groups and joint actions involved in balance and automatic postural reactions.

Key Muscle Groups

Figure 10-6 shows the major muscle groups that control the body's center of gravity during standing.[4] Postural stability primarily depends on coordinated actions between the trunk and lower extremities. The motions around the hip, knee, and ankle include joint-specific muscle actions and indirect, inertial forces of neighboring joints.[2-4] Therefore, the anatomic classification of a muscle may differ from the functional classification. For example, the anatomic classification of the tibialis anterior muscle is dorsiflexion. In walking, however, the functional classification of the tibialis anterior is knee flexion, even though no insertion of this muscle occurs at the knee. As the ankle dorsiflexes, the lower leg begins to move forward during gait and inertia causes the thigh to lag behind, resulting in knee flexion.

By the same inertial interactions, the gastrocnemius muscle is defined as an ankle extensor (plantarflexion) and a knee flexor anatomically, but it functionally acts as a knee extensor in standing. The anatomic actions of the quadriceps muscle are hip flexion and knee extension, but it indirectly acts as ankle plantarflexion (extensors). The direct actions of the hamstring muscles are hip extension and knee flexion, but they have an indirect effect on ankle dorsiflexion (flexors).[3,4] These actions are summarized in Table 10-2.[3]

Figure 10-4 Six balance testing conditions.

(Courtesy of Neurocom International, Inc., Clackamas, OR)

Figure 10-5 The clinical test of sensory interaction on balance.

(Courtesy of Neurocom International, Inc., Clackamas, OR)

TABLE 10-1   Balance Assessment Tools

Quiet Standing Tests	Equipment Needed	Time	Construct Measured
Nudge test (sitting, standing)		<5 minutes	Automatic/anticipatory postural responses; ankle, hip, stepping strategies (standing)
Romberg	Stop watch	<5 minutes	Somatosensation, vestibular, motor strategies (ankle, hip, stepping)
Sharpened Romberg	Stop watch	<5 minutes	Somatosensation, vestibular, motor strategies
One-limb stance test	Stop watch	<5 minutes	Somatosensation, vestibular, motor strategies

Active Standing Tests	Equipment Needed	Time	Construct Measured
Functional reach	Yard stick	10 minutes	Screener tool; anticipatory postural response; limits of stability (forward)
Limits of stability (LOS)	Computerized forceplate	10 minutes	Movement strategies; actual vs perceived LOS

Sensory Manipulation Tests	Equipment Needed	Time	Construct Measured
Clinical test of sensory interaction on balance (CTSIB)	Stop watch, T-foam, dome	30 minutes	Sensory strategies; ability to select appropriate input with sensory conflict
Modified CTSIB	Computerized forceplate OR modify above—eliminate conditions 3 and 6 (dome)	15–20 minutes	Sensory strategies

Functional Tests	Equipment Needed	Time	Construct Measured
Berg scale	Armchair, armless chair, stopwatch, yardstick, shoe, step	30 minutes	Static and dynamic balance abilities during functional tasks
Tinetti balance and gait tests (perform oriented mobility assess)	Armless chair	15 minutes	Screener for balance and mobility skills
Timed up & go	Armchair, stop watch	10 minutes	Screener tool for balance during mobility tasks
Functional reach	Yardstick	10 minutes	Screener for active standing balance
Dynamic gait index	Stop watch, 2 cones, shoebox, 3–4 steps with handrail	30 minutes	Ability to modify gait in response to changing task demands
Three-minute walk	Stop watch	5 minutes	Endurance

Figure 10-6 Key muscle groups that control the center of gravity when an individual is standing.

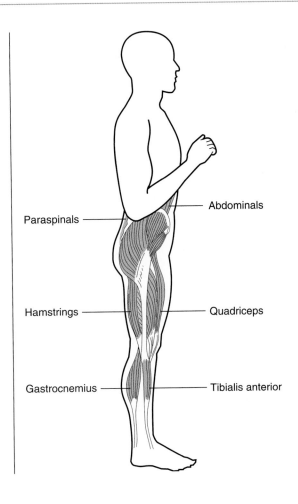

Paraspinals

Abdominals

Hamstrings

Quadriceps

Gastrocnemius

Tibialis anterior

Automatic Postural Reactions

To maintain balance, the body must make continual adjustments. Most of what is currently known about postural control is based on stereotypical postural strategies activated in response to AP perturbation or displacement.[3,10] Horak and Nashner[19] described three primary strategies used for controlling AP sway: ankle, hip, and stepping (Figs. 10-7 to 10-9). These strategies adjust the body's center of gravity so that the body is maintained within the base of support, preventing the loss of balance or falling. Several factors determine which strategy is the most effective response to a postural challenge: speed and intensity of the displacing forces, characteristics of the support surface, and magnitude of the displacement of the center of mass.

The responses an individual makes during sudden perturbations are called automatic postural reactions.[4,19] These responses occur before voluntary movement and after reflexes yet are similar to both. Automatic postural movements are like reflexes because they respond quickly and are relatively similar among individuals. However, like voluntary movements, they primarily depend on coordination responses between the lower trunk and the leg muscles.[4,20]

TABLE 10-2 Anatomic and Functional Classifications of Muscles Involved in Balance Movements

	Extension		Flexion	
Joint	Anatomic	Functional	Anatomic	Functional
Hip	Paraspinals	Paraspinals	Abdominal	Abdominal
	Hamstrings	Quadriceps	Quadriceps	Hamstrings
Knee	Quadriceps	Gastrocnemius	Hamstrings, gastrocnemius	Tibialis anterior
Ankle	Gastrocnemius	Quadriceps	Tibialis anterior	Hamstrings

Figure 10-7	Ankle strategy.

STRATEGY USED: Center of mass is repositioned after small, slow-speed pertubation.

EXAMPLE: Posterior sway of the body is counteracted by tibialis anterior muscles pulling the body anteriorly.

Figure 10-8	Hip strategy.

STRATEGY USED: Center of mass is repositioned using rapid, compensatory hip flexion or extension to redistribute body weight.

EXAMPLE: Hip flexion and extension in response to standing on a bus that is rapidly accelerating.

Figure 10-9	Stepping strategy.

STRATEGY USED: Center of mass can only be repositioned by taking a step to enlarge the base of support. New postural control is then established.

EXAMPLE: Stumbling on an unexpectedly uneven sidewalk.

These responses can be thought of as a class of functionally organized responses that activate muscles to bring the body's center of mass into a state of equilibrium.[3] Each of the strategies has reflex, automatic, and volitional components that interact to match the response to the challenge. Table 10-3 compares reflexes, automatic postural responses, and voluntary movements.[4] To prevent a fall after a sudden perturbation or to maintain balance during locomotion, the healthy individual responds with appropriate muscular actions, called postural strategies.

Ankle Strategy

Small disturbances in the center of gravity can be compensated by motion at the ankle (Fig. 10-7). The ankle strategy repositions the center of mass after small displacements caused by slow-speed perturbations, which usually occur on a large, firm, supporting surface. The oscillations around the ankle joint with normal postural sway are an example of the ankle strategy. Anterior sway of the body is counteracted by gastrocnemius muscle activity, which pulls the body posteriorly. Conversely, posterior sway of the body is

TABLE 10-3 Properties of the Three Movement Systems

Property	Reflex	Automatic	Voluntary
Mediating pathway	Spinal cord	Brainstem, subcortical	Brainstem, subcortical
Mode of activation	External stimulus	External stimulus	Self-stimulus
Response properties	Localized to point of stimulus; highly stereotypical	Coordinated among leg and trunk muscles; stereotypical but adaptable	Unlimited variety
Role in posture	Regulate muscle forces	Coordinate movements across joints	Generate purposeful behaviors
Onset time	Fixed at 35–40 msec	Fixed at 85–95 msec	Varies 150+ msec

counteracted by contraction of the anterior tibialis muscles, which pulls the body anteriorly.

Hip Strategy

If the disturbance in the center of gravity is too great to be counteracted by motion at the ankle, the patient will use a hip or stepping strategy to maintain the center of gravity within the base of support. The hip strategy uses a rapid compensatory hip flexion or extension to redistribute the body weight within the available base of support when the center of mass is near the edge of the sway envelope (Fig. 10-8). The hip strategy is usually employed in response to a moderate or large postural disturbance, especially on an uneven, narrow, or moving surface. For example, the hip strategy is often used while standing on a bus that is rapidly accelerating.

Stepping Strategy

When sudden, large-amplitude forces displace the center of mass beyond the limits of control, a step is used to enlarge the base of support and redefine a new sway envelope (Fig. 10-9). New postural control can then be re-established. An example of the stepping strategy is the uncoordinated step that often follows a stumble on an unexpectedly uneven sidewalk.

Examination of Automatic Postural Movements

Automatic postural movements can be analyzed at a range of velocities and directions using the MCT (Fig. 10-10). As noted, the MCT is the second protocol of computerized dynamic posturography. This test requires the patient to maintain standing balance as the support surface repeats various unexpected displacements. Testing includes changing magnitudes of forward and backward displacements as well as tilts of toes up and toes down.[2,3] Diener et al.[20] noted that automatic postural reactions in normal individuals were proportional to the size of the perturbation; hence, the forward and backward translations of the MCT vary in magnitude (small, medium, and large).

CLINICAL GUIDELINES

Biomechanical Deficits

When inputs are impaired, such as with inadequate range of motion (ROM) or weakness in the lower extremities, the postural control system receives distorted information.

| Figure 10-10 | The movement coordination test, a type of computerized posturography. Test requires patient to maintain standing balance as support surface tilts the toes up and down and displaces patient forward and backward. |

This inaccurate information can result in a malaligned center of gravity within the stability limits, which causes altered movement and increases the risk of falling. For example, if the center of gravity is offset to the left, just a small amount of sway in that direction (left) will cause the individual to exceed the limits of stability. Once this happens, the individual must step or use external support to prevent a fall.

Pain can decrease the patient's normal stability limits. If a patient has knee pain with full weight bearing, he or she compensates by leaning away from the affected side. Thus, the patient develops an offset center of gravity, and movement patterns are compromised.

Sensory Deficits

Lack of balance is usually multifactorial; however, examination for sensory organization provides valuable information. Once the deficit or deficits have been appropriately identified, the physical therapist (PT) can design a specific treatment plan to improve the impaired sensory system or can teach the patient compensatory strategies. For example, a patient with neuropathy has impaired proprioceptive cues but could compensate by using an assistive device and depending more on visual and vestibular cues.[1] Increasing the use of the remaining sensory systems is crucial for this patient. In contrast, a person who suffers from an inner-ear disorder may have impaired use of vestibular cues for balance.[1] Treatment should focus on decreasing the intact sensory systems (visual and proprioception), allowing the vestibular system to adapt.

Balance impairment with neurologic involvement can be much more complex. For example, the client may have impaired use of individual sensory systems (e.g., decreased proprioception and visual deficits) along with impaired central processing of the sensory organization mechanisms.[1,21] Treatment should focus on improving the use of individual sensory systems and teaching the client strategies to optimize sensory selection.

Musculoskeletal Deficits

Ankle strategies require adequate ROM and strength in the ankles and intact proprioception for the individual to adequately sense the support base. Muscle weakness and decreased ROM also limit the use of hip strategies, but proprioception input is not as critical.[7] However, more recent studies have shown that individuals who suffer from vestibular loss are unable to use hip strategies, although their ability to use ankle strategies is unaffected.[7,22]

Postural stability not only requires adequate strength and ROM from the musculoskeletal system but also the ability of the CNS to adequately generate these forces. For instance, abnormal muscle tone (hypertonicity and hypotonicity) may limit the individual's ability to recruit muscles required for balance. Impaired coordination of postural strategies can also be a problem. Deficits in these areas are seen with neurologic involvement such as stroke, head injury, and Parkinson's disease.[1,23]

Treatment of musculoskeletal problems includes strengthening and ROM exercises, techniques to correct abnormal tone (facilitation or inhibition), and various coordination activities to improve timing of postural reactions. The following section focuses on major points of clinical application for biomechanical, sensory, and musculoskeletal deficits.

TECHNIQUES

Biomechanical Factors

A malaligned center of gravity decreases one's limits of stability, compromising normal movement patterns. As noted, these biomechanical deficits can be a result of inadequate ROM, decreased strength, pain, swelling, and joint instability. Treatment includes appropriate modalities such as ice, heat, massage, ROM (Chapter 3), stretching (Chapter 4), and strengthening (Chapters 5 to 9) exercises are also used.

Sensory Organization Training

The postural control system depends on the demands of the individual's activity and the surroundings; therefore, treatment needs to be task and environmental specific. Sensory systems respond to environmental changes so exercises should focus on isolating, suppressing, and combining the different inputs under different conditions. To isolate a patient's proprioceptive inputs, visual cues must be removed (eyes closed) or destabilized. Visual inputs are destabilized when the patient moves his or her eyes and head together in a variety of planes (horizontal, vertical, diagonal), decreasing gaze stability. Prism glasses and moving visual fields are also used to produce inaccurate cues for orientation.[1] During all of these exercises the patient is asked to stand on a firm, stable surface to optimize proprioceptive inputs. This technique is particularly important for visually dependent patients.

To stimulate vestibular inputs, the patient's reliance on visual and somatosensory cues needs to be reduced simultaneously. The patient's level of function determines the difficulty of the task. For example, patient A may be able to decrease surface cues only by changing from her normal stance (feet apart and eyes open on a firm surface) to a stance with feet together and eyes closed on a firm surface. Patient B's exercises, on the other hand, may require him to stand on a foam surface with feet together and eyes closed. Regardless of the sensory deficit, activities should require the patient to maintain balance under progressively more difficult static and dynamic activities.[1,24]

Musculoskeletal Exercises

As discussed, sensory systems respond to environmental changes, whereas the musculoskeletal system responds more to task constraints. The goal of treatment is to optimize the patient's use of movement strategies for improving postural stability under changing conditions.

Static balance skills can be initiated once the individual is able to bear weight on the lower extremity. The general progression of static balance activities is to progress from bilateral to unilateral and from eyes open to eyes closed. The logical progression of balance training to destabilizing proprioception is from a stable surface to an unstable surface, such as a mini-trampoline or balance board. As joint position changes, dynamic stabilization must occur for the patient to maintain control on the unstable surface.

The patients should initially perform the static balance activities while concentrating on the specific task (position sense and neuromuscular control) to facilitate and maximize sensory output. As the task becomes easier, activities to distract the patient's concentration (catching a ball or performing mental exercises) should be incorporated into the training program. These distraction activities help facilitate the conversion of conscious to unconscious motor programming.

Techniques to Improve Ankle Strategies

To improve ankle strategies, the patient should perform the exercises on a broad stable surface, concentrating on AP sway. The patient maintains slow, small sways while standing on a firm surface to minimize the use of hip strategies. Examples of activities that can be used to facilitate and improve ankle strategies are presented in Figures 10-11 to 10-14.

Figure 10-11   One-foot standing balance.

PURPOSE: Facilitate and improve ankle strategies.

POSITION: Client standing with feet shoulder width apart on firm surface.

PROCEDURE: Client lifts right leg off ground and establishes balance on left leg.

| **Figure 10-12** | One-foot standing balance with hip flexion. |

PURPOSE: Facilitate and improve ankle strategies.

POSITION: Client standing with feet shoulder width apart on firm surface.

PROCEDURE: Client lifts right leg off ground and establishes balance on left leg. The client flexes right hip and knee.

| **Figure 10-13** | One-foot standing balance using weights. |

PURPOSE: Facilitate and improve ankle strategies.

POSITION: Client standing with feet shoulder width apart on firm surface.

PROCEDURE: Client lifts right leg off ground and establishes balance on left leg. Then client lifts lightweight dumbbell to horizontal position.

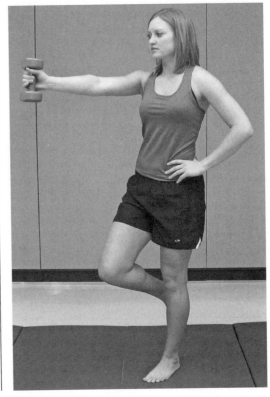

Figure 10-14	One-foot standing balance while playing catch—beginning.

PURPOSE: Facilitate and improve ankle strategies.

POSITION: Client standing with feet shoulder width apart on firm surface.

PROCEDURE: Client lifts right leg off ground and establishes balance on left leg. Physical therapist assistant gently tosses ball to client, who catches it.

NOTE: Initially ball should be thrown near client's body.

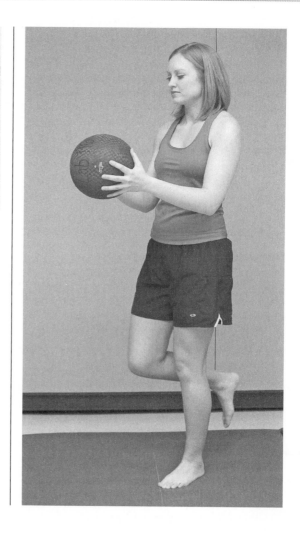

Techniques to Improve Hip Strategies

Exercises to improve the use of hip strategies should be performed on unstable surfaces and at high-sway frequencies. These exercises exceed the capabilities of ankle strategies and usually result in movement and adjustments of the trunk. Figures 10-15 to 10-21 demonstrate exercises that can be used to improve hip strategies.

Techniques to Improve Stepping Strategies

Stepping strategies are used once the stability limits have been exceeded. Although stepping strategies are normal reactions for preventing falls, many patients avoid this pattern and prefer to reach for external support. Reaching for support is especially common in elderly patients, who are proprioceptive and hip dependent. Patients should practice step-ups (Fig. 10-22), step-downs (forward and lateral), and step-overs (also called carioca and braiding) (Fig. 10-23) to help with stepping strategies. To make the training more difficult, the patient can increase the speed at which the step-overs are performed.

A particularly helpful technique is the push and nudge. For example, the patient stands with feet together. The physical therapist assistant's (PTA's) hands are placed on the patient's shoulders, offering support. The patient maintains an upright posture and leans forward into the PTA's hands until the limit of stability is reached. The PTA—without warning—removes the support, forcing the patient to step to prevent a fall (Fig. 10-24). This exercise can be performed in all directions (anterior, posterior, and lateral).

Figure 10-15	One-foot standing balance with forward bending.

PURPOSE: Facilitate and improve hip strategies.

POSITION: Client standing with feet shoulder width apart on firm surface.

PROCEDURE: Client lifts right foot off ground and establishes balance on left leg. Then client bends forward as far as possible while maintaining balance.

NOTE: Modifications include bending backward and to each side.

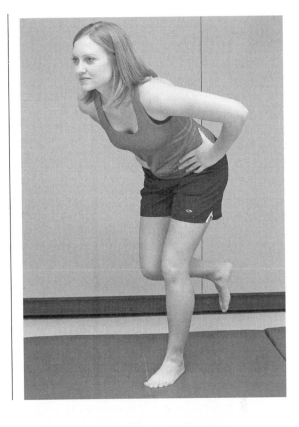

Figure 10-16	One-foot standing balance while playing catch—advanced.

PURPOSE: Facilitate and improve hip strategies.

POSITION: Client standing with feet shoulder width apart on firm surface.

PROCEDURE: Client lifts right foot off ground and establishes balance on left leg. Physical therapist assistant (PTA) throws ball to client, who catches it and throws it back to PTA. PTA gradually shifts direction and angle of ball toss so that client must reach away from body.

NOTE: Ball should be thrown so that patient must reach away from body.

Figure 10-17 One-foot standing balance on mini-trampoline.

PURPOSE: Facilitate and improve hip strategies.

POSITION: Client standing with feet shoulder width apart on mini-trampoline.

PROCEDURE: Client lifts right foot off ground and establishes balance on left leg **(A)**.

NOTE: Activity can be progressed to a more difficult level by asking patient to catch and throw a ball while standing on one leg on mini-trampoline **(B)**.

A

B

| Figure 10-18 | Two-foot standing balance on rocker (balance) board. |

PURPOSE: Facilitate and improve hip strategies.

POSITION: Client standing with feet shoulder width apart on rocker board.

PROCEDURE: Client establishes balance with both feet remaining on rocker board while attempting to keep all surfaces of board off ground.

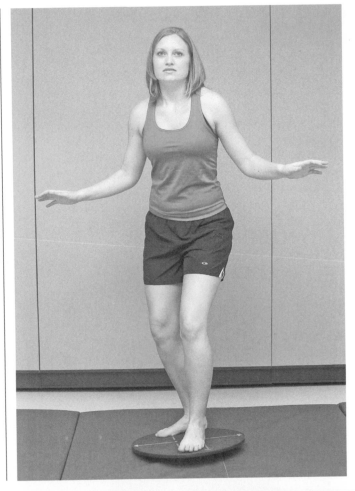

| Figure 10-19 | Two-foot standing balance on sliding board. |

PURPOSE: Facilitate and improve hip strategies.

POSITION: Client standing with feet shoulder width apart on sliding board.

PROCEDURE: Client establishes balance with both feet remaining on sliding board while attempting to shift weight at hips to move sliding piece laterally back and forth on base.

| Figure 10-20 | Two-foot standing balance in surfer position on foam roller. |

PURPOSE: Facilitate and improve hip strategies.

POSITION: Client standing with feet shoulder width apart on foam roller.

PROCEDURE: Client establishes and maintains balance with one foot in front of the other, assuming a surfer position.

A

B

| Figure 10-21 | One-foot hop from stool. |

PURPOSE: Facilitate and improve hip strategies.

POSITION: Client standing on one foot on top of foot stool **(A)**.

PROCEDURE: Client establishes balance, hops down from stool, and maintains balance **(B)**.

Figure 10-22 Forward step-up on stool.

PURPOSE: Facilitate and improve stepping strategies.

POSITION: Client standing with feet shoulder width apart facing step stool.

PROCEDURE: Client maintains balance while stepping up onto stool with lead foot and then brings up trailing foot. Client reverses process, stepping down.

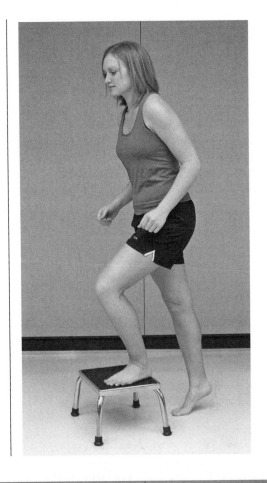

Figure 10-23 Slow and controlled step-overs.

PURPOSE: Facilitate and improve stepping strategies.

POSITION: Client standing with feet shoulder width apart on firm surface.

PROCEDURE: Client crosses one leg over in front of the other and slowly steps in a controlled movement.

NOTE: This technique can be progressed to faster controlled movements

Figure 10-24 Push and nudge in anterior direction.

PURPOSE: Facilitate and improve stepping strategies.

POSITION: Client standing with feet shoulder width apart on firm surface. Physical therapist assistant (PTA) places hands on client's shoulders.

PROCEDURE: Client leans forward into PTA's support as far as balance allows **(A)**. PTA quickly removes support, forcing client to compensate by taking a step **(B)**.

NOTE: PTA may change direction of support to posterior or lateral.

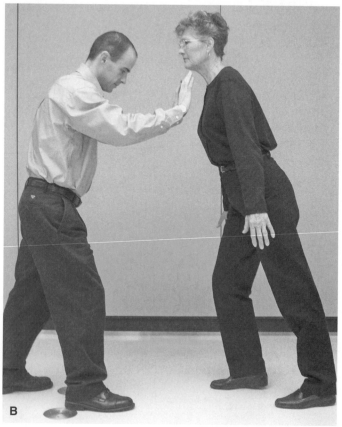

CASE STUDY 1

PATIENT INFORMATION

The patient was a 43-year-old man who had left ankle pain and edema. The patient reported that he "twisted" his left ankle 2 days before the appointment while stepping off a ladder onto uneven ground. He complained of moderate lateral ankle pain and had been unable to walk without limping since his injury.

The PT evaluation revealed that the patient presented with localized swelling and pain over the lateral aspect of the ankle. The patient's strength with eversion and plantarflexion was 4/5, secondary to pain with resistance. He was particularly tender to palpation of the anterior talofibular ligament. All ankle laxity tests were negative. Based on these findings, the patient was diagnosed with a first-degree inversion ankle sprain.

LINKS TO
GUIDE TO PHYSICAL THERAPIST PRACTICE

According to the *Guide to Physical Therapist Practice*,[25] pattern 4D relates to the diagnosis of this patient and the pattern is described as "impaired joint mobility, muscle performance, and range of motion associated with connective tissue dysfunction" and includes ligamentous sprain. Tests and measures of this diagnosis include quantification of static and dynamic balance. Anticipated goals are improving balance through direct intervention using "balance and coordination training" and "posture awareness training."

INTERVENTION

The PT instructed the patient to use ice, wear a compression wrap, elevate the leg, and rest for the first 48 hours. The PT then asked the PTA to instruct the patient in the following home exercise program (in the morning and evening, as per instructions provided to the patient by the PTA).

1. Stretch the calf muscles, using a towel for assistance: three repetitions, each held for 20 seconds.
2. Ankle plantarflexion and dorsiflexion ROM and circumduction of the ankle: 20 repetitions (Fig. 3-8).
3. Pick up objects (e.g., marbles) one at time and place them in a container: 20 repetitions.

PROGRESSION

Two Weeks After Initial Examination

The patient reported that he was able to complete the home exercise program without pain and with minimal swelling. The patient's chief complaints were a mild limp when walking that worsened when he was fatigued and instability when walking on uneven surfaces. Further examination by the PT using computer-assisted technology showed decreased limits of stability (75% of normal to the left, including AP planes) and decreased weight bearing on the left in 60-degree to 90-degree squats.

The PTA continued treatment consisting of stretching, riding a bicycle (Fig. 12-5), walking on the treadmill (Fig. 12-8) in all directions (forward, backward, sidestepping), and using a rocker (balance) board (Fig. 10-18). The patient's home program was advanced according to the plan of care as follows:

1. Resistive ankle exercise with tubing in all directions (Fig. 6-31).
2. Continue stretching.
3. Step-ups and step-downs (Fig. 8-9).
4. Squats (Fig. 8-8).
5. Toe raises while standing.
6. Balance activities on balance and sliding boards (Figs. 10-18 and 10-19).

OUTCOMES

Four weeks after the initial examination the patient had no complaints of pain. His primary goal was to return to playing basketball on the weekends. Re-examination by the PT noted no significant swelling and strength of 5/5 (using manual muscle test). Computerized testing revealed a normal center of gravity and normal limits of stability. The patient was discharged from intervention. He was told to continue with his home exercise program, except the tubing exercises were discontinued and jogging and jump roping were added.

SUMMARY—AN EFFECTIVE PT–PTA TEAM

This case study demonstrates an effective PT/PTA team for patient care. The PT utilized the PTA to perform the home exercise program and then continued treatment with the patient in the clinic. The PT intervened at the appropriate times to re-examine the patient. The PT also determined the timing on discharge and follow-up care. The PTA in this case study could have assisted the PT in predetermined screenings such as the computerized-assisted technology that was used to assess limits of stability and weight bearing. The PT chose not to use the PTA for this procedure after considering the specific knowledge, education, and skills of this PTA with this procedure. The PT must consider many factors when determining what should be delegated to the PTA.

▼ ▼ ▼ GERIATRIC PERSPECTIVES

- Under circumstances of low-task demand, age-related changes in postural control (control of balance and coordination) are minimal through age 70. With advancing age, anatomic and physiologic changes occur in biomechanical capabilities that affect static and dynamic balance, such as decline in proprioceptive, vestibular, and visual responses; decrease in muscle mass; increase in postural sway; slowing of motor reaction time; and alterations in central control of balance.

- In addition, the sensing threshold for postural stimuli is affected by age, resulting in increased muscle onset latencies. Compared with younger adults, older adults require 10 to 30 milliseconds longer to volitionally develop the same levels of ankle torque or to begin to take a step to recover balance after a disturbance.[1]

- The visual system is a major contributor to balance, giving the older individual information on location in space and the environment. However, vision is affected by aging and may provide distorted or inaccurate information.[2] In addition, corrective lenses (e.g., bifocals) tend to blur images on the ground or in the distance.

- The number of vestibular neurons and the size of the nerve fibers decrease with aging.[3] With increasing age over 40, a slow reduction in the number of myelinated nerve fibers is evident. By age 70+, a loss of 40% to 50% may be noted compared with younger adults.[4]

- Synergist motor responses responsible for restoration of balance after a disturbance are also affected by aging, resulting in altered muscle activation sequences, agonist–antagonist stiffness (cocontraction), slowed postural responses, and use of disordered postural strategies.[5] In response to a small disturbance, older adults will generally use a hip strategy rather than an ankle strategy typically observed in young adults.

- Research has determined that restoration of balance is not a fixed reflexive response to disturbance but rather

is a multifactorial event involving interaction of the body (musculoskeletal and neuromuscular), the magnitude of the disturbance, and the attentional demands placed on the older individual by the environment.[6-8]

- Older adults are at greater risk of experiencing an injurious fall requiring hospitalization. Therefore, all examinations of adults over age 60 should include a balance screening (functional reach test[9]) and falls risk assessment (Elderly Fall Screening Test[10]).

1. Stelmach GE, Populin L, Muller F. Postural muscle onset and voluntary movement in the elderly. *Neurosci Lett.* 1990;117:188–193.
2. Simoneau M, Teasdale N, Bourdin C, et al. Aging and postural control: postural perturbations caused by changing visual anchor. *J Am Geriatr Soc.* 1999;47:235–241.
3. Spirduso WW. Balance, posture, and locomotion. In: Spirduso WW, ed. *Physical dimensions of aging.* Champaign, IL: Human Kinetics; 1995:155–184.
4. Rees TS, Duckert LG, Carey JP. Auditory and vestibular dysfunction. In: Hazard WR, Blass JP, Ettinger WH, et al, eds. *Principles of geriatric medicine and gerontology.* 4th ed. New York: McGraw-Hill; 1998:617–632.
5. Woollacott MH. Changes in posture and voluntary control in the elderly: research findings and rehabilitation. *Top Geriatr Rehabil.* 1990;5:1–11.
6. Maylor EA, Wing AM. Age differences in postural stability are increased by additional cognitive demands. *J Gerontol Psychol Sci.* 1996;51B:P143–P154.
7. Shumway-Cook A, Woollacott MH. Attentional demands and postural control: the effect of sensory context. *J Gerontol Med Sci.* 2000;55A:M10–M16.
8. Brown L, Shumway-Cook A, Woollacott MH. Attentional demands and postural recovery: the effects of aging. *J Gerontol Med Sci* 1999;54A:M165–M171.
9. Duncan PW, Weiner DK, Chandler J, et al. Functional reach: a new clinical measure of balance. *J Gerontol Med Sci.* 1990;45:M192–M197.
10. Cwikel JG, Fried AV, Biderman A, et al. Validation of a fall-risk screening test, the Elderly Fall Screening Test (EFST), for community-dwelling elderly. *Disabil Rehabil.* 1998;20: 161–167.

SUMMARY

- Balance is a complex process of controlling the body's center of gravity over the base of support, whether the individual is stationary or moving. Balance requires accurate information from sensory input, effective processing by the CNS, and appropriate responses of motor control.

- The CNS relies on information from three sensory systems: proprioceptive, visual, and vestibular. Each system contributes a unique role in maintaining balance. The ability of the CNS to select, suppress, and combine these inputs is called sensory organization. Proprioceptive inputs are dominant when the surface is firm and fixed. Visual cues are particularly important when somatosensory inputs are unreliable (changing surfaces). The vestibular system, on the other hand, is dominant when a conflict exists between somatosensory and visual cues; the vestibular system plays a major role in ambulation.

- Technologic advances in the examination of appropriate sensory organization provide valuable information of both sensory organization and motor control.

- The major muscle groups that control the center of gravity over the base of support include the paraspinals, abdominals, hamstrings, quadriceps, gastrocnemius, and tibialis anterior. Coordinated actions among muscles result in joint-specific movements and indirect, inertial forces on the neighboring joints. Therefore, the anatomic classification of a muscle may differ from its functional classification.

- The primary movement patterns for controlling balance include ankle, hip, and stepping strategies. The strategies vary in muscle recruitment, body movements, and joint axes. Inadequate ROM, decreased strength, pain, swelling, and joint instability can decrease the normal limits of stability. Dysfunction in any of these factors creates an offset center of gravity, compromising movement patterns.

- Treatment of musculoskeletal problems include strengthening and ROM, techniques to effect abnormal tone, and several coordination activities to improve the timing of postural reactions.

▲ ▲ ▲ PEDIATRIC PERSPECTIVES ▲ ▲ ▲

- Control of balance and coordination progresses throughout childhood. The concepts of balance, coordination, and postural control are closely interrelated. Much continued research is needed to understand the development and refinement of postural control in children as they acquire adult postural and movement skills.[1]

- Children begin to learn anticipatory postural strategies to coordinate posture and locomotion with the onset of voluntary sitting and crawling.[2] During perturbations of stance, 4- to 6-year-old children have greater and more variable responses than do younger children. It has been suggested that the difference may be the result of a period of transition, as visual sensory input becomes less important and other somatosensory information becomes more important in postural control and balance.[3] Children do not demonstrate adult values for muscle onset latencies for postural responses and control of movement until 10 to 15 years.[2]

- Childhood deficits in balance and postural stability may be related to deficits in the proprioceptive system, owing to incomplete development or injury. Balance and coordination in sports may be adversely affected by attention deficit hyperactivity disorder.[4] Chronic otitis media and effusion in the inner ear significantly affect balance and coordination skills in 4- to 6-year-old children. These skills improve after tympanostomy tube insertion.[5]

- Children with neurologic and musculoskeletal diagnoses may have impaired balance and coordination, which may be related to multiple factors such as sensory system deficits, impaired ROM and strength, and abnormal muscle tone. Patients must be treated at developmentally correct stages of balance and control. For example, children with cerebral palsy show deficits in sensorimotor organization and muscular coordination. These deficits affect their anticipatory activities.[6]

1. Horak FB. Assumptions underlying motor control for neurologic rehabilitation. In: Lister MJ, ed. *Contemporary management of motor control problems: proceedings of the II step conference.* Alexandria, VA: Foundation for Physical Therapy; 1991:11–28.

2. Haas G, Diener HC, Rupp H, et al. Development of feedback and feedforward control of upright stance. *Dev Med Child Neurol.* 1989;31:481–488.

3. Shumway-Cook A, Woollacott M. The growth of stability: postural control from a developmental perspective. *J Motor Behav.* 1985;17:131–147.

4. Hickey G, Frider P. ADHD: CNS function and sports. *Sports Med.* 1999;27:11–21.

5. Hart MC, Nichols DS, Butler EM, et al. Childhood imbalance and chronic otitis media with effusion: effect of tympanostomy tube insertion on standardized tests of balance and locomotion. *Laryngoscope.* 1998;108:665–670.

6. Nashner LM, Shumway-Cook A, Marin O. Stance posture control in select groups of children with cerebral palsy: deficits in sensory organization and muscular coordination. *Exp Brain Res.* 1983;49:393–409.

References

1. Shumway-Cook A, McCollum G. Assessment and treatment of balance disorders. In: Montgomery PC, Connolly BH, eds. *Motor control and physical therapy*. Hixson, TN: Chattanooga Group, Inc; 1993:123–138.

2. Kauffman TL, Nashner LM, Allison LK. Balance is a critical parameter in orthopedic rehabilitation. *New Technol Phys Ther*. 1997;6:43–78.

3. Nashner LM. Sensory, neuromuscular, and biomechanical contributions to human balance. In: Duncan PW, ed. *Balance: proceedings of APTA forum*. Alexandria, VA: American Physical Therapy Association; 1990:33–38.

4. Nashner LM. Evaluation of postural stability, movement and control. In: Hasson S, ed. *Clinical exercise physiology*. St. Louis: Mosby; 1994:199–234.

5. McCollum G, Leen T. Form and exploration of mechanical stability limits in erect stance. *J Motor Behav*. 1989;21:225–238.

6. Hobeika CP. Equilibrium and balance in the elderly. *Ear Nose Throat J*. 1999;78:558–566.

7. Horak FB, Shupert CL. Role of the vestibular system in postural control. In: Herdman SJ, ed. *Vestibular rehabilitation*. Philadelphia: FA Davis Co; 1994:22–46.

8. Dietz V, Horstmann GA, Berger W. Significance of proprioceptive mechanisms in the regulation of stance. *Prog Brain Res*. 1989;80:419–423.

9. Dorman J, Fernie GR, Holliday PJ. Visual input: its importance in the control of postural sway. *Arch Phys Med Rehabil*. 1978;59:586–591.

10. Horak FB. Clinical measurement of postural control in adults. *Phys Ther*. 1987;67:1881–1885.

11. Hain TC, Hillman MA. Anatomy and physiology of the normal vestibular system. In: Herdma SJ, ed. *Vestibulare rehabilitation*. Philadelphia: FA Davis Co. 1994:3–21.

12. Shumway-Cook A, Horak FB. Assessing the influence of sensory interaction on balance. *Phys Ther*. 1986;66: 1548–1550.

13. Duncan PW, Weiner DK, Chandler J, et al. Functional reach: a new clinical measure of balance. *J Gerontol Med Sci*. 1990;45:M192–M197.

14. Berg K, Wood-Dauphinee S, Williams J, et al. Measuring balance in the elderly: preliminary development of an instrument. *Physiother Can*. 1989;41:304–311.

15. Berg K, Maki B, Williams J, et al. Clinical and laboratory measures of postural balance in an elderly population. *Arch Phys Med Rehabil*. 1992;73:1073–1080.

16. O'Sullivan S. Assessment of motor function. In: O'Sullivan S, Schmitz TJ, ed. *Physical rehabilitation, assessment and treatment*. Philadelphia, PA: FA Davis Co; 2001:208–209.

17. Tinetti M, Williams T, Mayewski R. A fall risk index for elderly patients based on number of chronic disabilities. *Am J Med*. 1986;80:429–434.

18. Podsiadlo D, Richardson S. The timed "Up & Go": a test of basic functional mobility for frail elderly persons. *J Am Geriatr Soc*. 1991;39:142–148.

19. Horak FB, Nashner LM. Central programming of posture control: adaptation to altered support surface configurations. *J Neurophysiol*. 1986;55:1369–1381.

20. Diener HC, Horak FB, Nashner LM. Influence of stimulus parameters on human postural responses. *J Neurophysiol*. 1988;59:1888–1905.

21. DiFabio RP, Badke MB. Relationships of sensory organization to balance function in patients with hemiplegia. *Phys Ther*. 1990;70:543–548.

22. Horak FB, Diener HC, Nashner LM. Postural strategies associated with somatosensory and vestibular limits of stability. *Exp Brain Res*. 1992;82:167–171.

23. Badke MB, DiFabio RP. Balance deficits in patients with hemiplegia: considerations for assessment and treatment. In: Duncan PW, ed. *Balance: proceedings of the APTA forum*. Alexandria, VA: American Physical Therapy Association; 1990:130–137.

24. Shumway-Cook A, Horak FB. Rehabilitation strategies for patients with peripheral vestibular disorders. *Neurol Clin*. 1990;8:441–457.

25. American Physical Therapy Association. *Guide to physical therapist practice*. 2nd ed. Alexandria, VA; 2003.

Reactive Neuromuscular Training

Michael L. Voight, PT, DHSC, OCS, SCS, ATC, and William D. Bandy PT, PhD, SCS, ATC

OBJECTIVES

Upon completion of this chapter, the reader will be able to:

- Define neuromuscular control.

- Identify four crucial elements involved in neuromuscular control programs.

- Apply proper clinical techniques to a reactive neuromuscular-training program focusing on single-leg stance, uniplanar, and isometric activities within the established plan of care.

- Apply proper clinical techniques to a reactive neuromuscular-training program focusing on exercises that use controlled eccentric and concentric contractions through a full range of motion (ROM) within the established plan of care.

- Apply proper clinical techniques to a reactive neuromuscular-training program focusing on ballistic and impact activities within the established plan of care.

SCIENTIFIC BASIS

Observing the coordinated and integrated movements of the triple jump, a dismount from the parallel bars, or dribbling a basketball around a screen for a jump shot, it is obvious that there must be something more to functional progression than breaking down skills step by step and hoping for skill integration. Some activities are complex movements requiring a variety of movements and positions and a smooth transition from one position or movement to another. In the competitive environment, the client does not routinely think about each of the basic movement patterns required to perform complex skills. As the client becomes more proficient in a given activity, the basic skills become second nature. In other words, the client is able to perform these activities at a subconscious level. Therefore, primitive skills in the exercise program are integrated from the conscious to the subconscious level.

A patient's ability to function at the subconscious level involves integration of incoming information from the environment, which involves neuromuscular control. To re-establish neuromuscular control after injury, the program must incorporate activities that entail balance, proprioception, coordination, power, and agility.[1-5] Neuromuscular control is the motor response to sensory information from the environment and is under the influence of four crucial elements: proprioception and kinesthetic awareness, functional motor patterns, dynamic joint stability, and reactive neuromuscular control.[6] Lower-extremity activities in the closed-kinetic chain facilitate proprioceptive and kinesthetic re-education of the weight-bearing joints. Functional motor patterns are the heart and soul of exercises, beginning at the conscious level and progressing to the subconscious.

Reactive neuromuscular training is a specialized training program designed to re-establish neuromuscular control after injury. The program entails the shifting of the patient's center of gravity by pulling the upper body in a given direction over the fixed lower extremity. The patient is required to generate lower-extremity isometric contractions to offset this weight shift and thereby maintain stability of the lower extremity. These oscillating techniques of isometric stabilization to offset the shift in the center of gravity aid in the integration of visual, mechanoreceptors, and equilibrium reaction.

Reactive neuromuscular training is an example of a program designed to restore dynamic stability and enhance cognitive appreciation of the joint's position and movement of the joint after it is injured. The design and implementation of this type of training program are critical for restoring the synergy and synchrony of muscle-firing patterns required for dynamic stability and fine motor control, thereby restoring both functional stability about the joint and enhanced motor-control skills.[7,8]

The reactive neuromuscular-training program can be progressed from slow- to fast-speed activities, from low- to high-force activities, and from controlled to uncontrolled activities. Initially, these exercises should evoke a balance reaction or weight shift in the lower extremities and ultimately progress to a movement pattern.[7-9] Examples of specific reactive neuromuscular-training techniques are presented in this chapter.

CLINICAL GUIDELINES

Reactive neuromuscular training can be as simple as static control with little or no visible movement or as complex as a dynamic plyometric response (Chapter 9) requiring explosive acceleration, deceleration, or change in direction. Early activities include single-leg stance, uniplanar activities in which the patient pulls on exercise tubing while maintaining balance, and isometric activities that include minimal joint motion. The patient can be progressed from isometric activities to exercises that used controlled concentric and eccentric contractions through a full ROM, such as the squat and lunge. Finally, ballistic and impact activities, such as resisted walking, running, and bounding, can be introduced in the advanced stages of rehabilitation.[7] (Note: the rest of this section provides examples of reactive neuromuscular training and are not inclusive of all exercises available.)

Single-leg Stance

The client should stand bearing full weight with equal distribution on the affected and unaffected lower extremity. Placing a 6- to 8-inch step stool under the unaffected lower extremity will cause a weight shift to the affected lower extremity, placing greater emphasis on the affected side. At the same time, the unaffected extremity can still assist with balance reactions (Fig. 11-1).

The exercise can be made more difficult by using an unstable surface, which will also increase the demands on the mechanoreceptor system. Single or multidirectional rocker devices or bolsters assist the progression to the next phase (Fig. 11-2).

Uniplanar Exercise

Exercise tubing can be used for uniplanar exercise by the pulling of two pieces of tubing toward the body and returning the tubing to the start position in a smooth, rhythmic fashion with increasing speed. Changes in direction (anterior, posterior, medial, or lateral weight shifting) create specific planar demands. Each technique is given a name that is related to the weight shift produced by the applied tension. The body reacts to the weight shift with an

Figure 11-1 Single-leg stance on step stool.

PURPOSE: Reflex stabilization using static compression of articular surfaces to facilitate isometric contraction of muscles of the lower extremity.

POSITION: Standing, feet shoulder width apart (assume left side is involved extremity).

PROCEDURE: Place uninvolved extremity on step stool, forcing greater weight shift to involved side.

Figure 11-2 Single-leg stance on unstable surface.

PURPOSE: Reflex stabilization using static compression of articular surfaces to facilitate isometric contraction of muscles of the lower extremity.

POSITION: Standing on involved extremity (left) on bolster.

PROCEDURE: Patient maintains balance while standing on bolster.

equal and opposite stabilization response. *Therefore, the exercise is named for the cause and not the effect.*

During performance of these exercises, the patient should make little or no movement of the lower extremity. If movement is noted, resistance should be decreased to achieve the desired stability. Uniplanar activities are described in Figures 11-3 to 11-6.

Multiplanar Exercises

The basic exercise program can be progressed to multiplanar activity by combining the proprioceptive neuromuscular facilitation (PNF) diagonal patterns and chop and lift patterns of the upper extremities (Fig. 11-7). The patterns from the unaffected and affected sides cause a multiplanar stress

Figure 11-3   Uniplanar anterior weight shift.

PURPOSE: Static stabilization, demonstrating stability required to achieve motor learning and control in single plane of motion.

POSITION: Standing on involved extremity (left) facing tubing.

PROCEDURE: Patient holds tubing in both hands **(A)**. Maintaining balance on involved extremity, patient pulls tubing toward body in smooth motion **(B)**. This positioning causes a forward weight shift, which is stabilized with isometric counterforce consisting of hip extension, knee extension, and ankle plantarflexion.

| Figure 11-4 | Uniplanar posterior weight shift. |

PURPOSE: Static stabilization, demonstrating stability required to achieve motor learning and control in single plane of motion.

POSITION: Standing on involved extremity (left) with back to tubing.

PROCEDURE: Maintaining balance on involved extremity, patient moves tubing away from body in smooth motion. This positioning causes posterior weight shift, which is stabilized by isometric counterforce consisting of hip flexion, knee flexion, and ankle dorsiflexion.

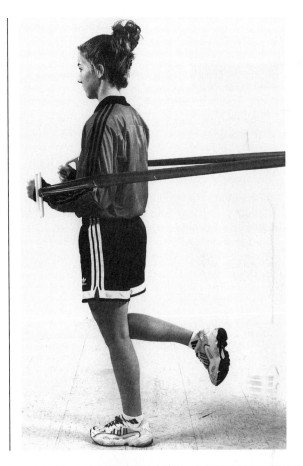

| Figure 11-5 | Uniplanar medial weight shift. |

PURPOSE: Static stabilization, demonstrating stability required to achieve motor learning and control in single plane of motion.

POSITION: Standing on involved extremity (left) with uninvolved extremity closest to tubing.

PROCEDURE: Maintaining balance on involved extremity, patient pulls tubing with one hand in front of body and other hand behind body in smooth motion. This positioning causes medial weight shift, which is stabilized with isometric counterforce consisting of hip adduction, knee cocontraction, and ankle inversion.

Figure 11-6   Uniplanar lateral weight shift.

PURPOSE: Static stabilization, demonstrating stability required to achieve motor learning and control in single plane of motion.

POSITION: Standing on involved extremity (left) with involved extremity closest to tubing.

PROCEDURE: Maintaining balance on involved extremity, patient pulls tubing with one hand in front of body and other hand behind body in smooth motion. The lateral shift is stabilized with isometric counterforce consisting of hip abduction, knee cocontraction, and ankle eversion.

Figure 11-7   Multiplanar proprioceptive neuromuscular facilitation (PNF) lift technique.

PURPOSE: Static stabilization, demonstrating stability required to achieve motor learning and control in multiple planes of motion.

POSITION: Standing on involved extremity (left).

PROCEDURE: Maintaining balance on involved extremity, patient performs PNF lift technique.

that requires isometric stabilization. The client is forced to automatically integrate the isometric responses that were developed in the previous uniplanar exercises.

Squat

The squat is used because it employs symmetric movement of the lower extremities, which allows the affected lower extremity to benefit from the proprioceptive feedback from the unaffected lower extremity. A chair or bench can be used as a ROM block (range-limiting device) if necessary. The block may minimize fear and increase safety (Figs. 11-8 to 11-10).

Lunge

The lunge is more specific than the squat in that it simulates sports and normal activity. The exercise decreases the base of support while producing the need for independent disassociation. The ROM can be stressed to a slightly higher degree. If the client is asked to alternate the lunge from the right to the left leg, the clinician can easily compare the quality of the movement between the limbs (Fig. 11-11 to 11-13).

Resisted Walking

Resisted walking uses the same primary components used in gait training. The applied resistance of the tubing, however, allows a reactive response unavailable in nonresisted activities. The addition of resistance permits increased loading and brings about the need for improved balance and weight shift.

Resisted Running

Resisted running simply involves jogging or running in place with tubing attached to a belt around the waist. The physical therapist (PT) and physical therapist assistant (PTA) can analyze the jogging or running activity because this is a stationary drill. The tubing resistance is applied in four different directions, which provides simulation of the different forces that the client will experience on return to full activity (Figs. 11-14 to 11-16).

Resisted Bounding

Bounding is an exercise in which the client jumps off one foot and lands on the opposite foot, essentially jumping from one

---

Figure 11-8 Squat: anterior weight shift (assisted).

PURPOSE: Stimulation of dynamic postural response, facilitating concentric and eccentric contractions.

POSITION: Standing, facing tubing, with belt around waist and feet shoulder width apart (assume involved side is left lower extremity).

PROCEDURE: Patient squats to height of chair in smooth, controlled motion and then returns to standing. The anterior weight shift facilitates the descent phase of the squat; the hip flexors, knee flexors, and ankle dorsiflexors are loaded dynamically with eccentric contractions during the return to standing. This activity is great for retraining shock absorption activities that occur during landing.

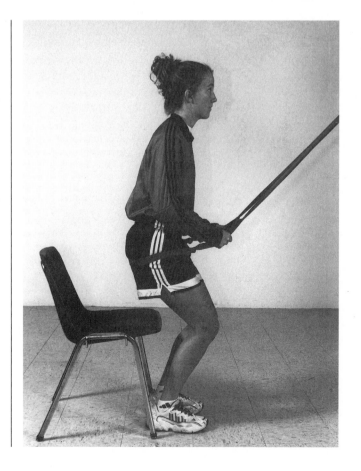

Figure 11-9   Squat: posterior weight shift.

PURPOSE: Stimulation of dynamic postural response, facilitating concentric and eccentric contractions.

POSITION: Standing on involved extremity (left), facing away from tubing, with belt around waist and feet shoulder width apart.

PROCEDURE: Patient squats to height of chair in smooth, cortrolled motion and then returns to standing. This technique facilitates the ascent phase of the squat; the hip extensors, knee extensors, and ankle plantarflexors are loaded dynamically with eccentric contractions during the return to sitting. The posterior weight shift is a great activity for learning the take-off position for sprinting and jumping.

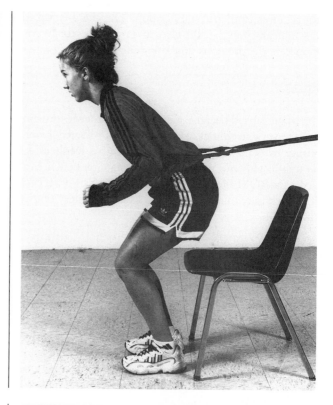

Figure 11-10   Squat: medial weight shift.

PURPOSE: Stimulation of dynamic postural response, facilitating concentric and eccentric contractions.

POSITION: Standing with uninvolved extremity closest to tubing, belt around waist, with feet shoulder width apart (assume involved extremity is left lower extremity).

PROCEDURE: Patient squats to height of chair in smooth, controlled motion and then returns to standing. This technique places less stress on the affected lower extremity and allows patient to lean onto the unaffected lower extremity without incurring excessive stress or loading.

NOTE: The lateral weight-shift technique is not illustrated, but it is the same as shown in Figure 11-10 except with tubing pulling laterally (to patient's left) instead of medially (to patient's right as is shown in Fig. 11-10). This lateral weight-shift exercise will place greater stress on the affected lower extremity, thereby demanding increased balance and control. The exercise simulates a single-leg squat but adds balance and safety by allowing the unaffected extremity to remain on the ground.

Figure 11-11 Lunge: anterior weight shift.

PURPOSE: Stimulation of dynamic postural response, facilitating concentric and eccentric contractions.

POSITION: Standing, facing tubing, with feet shoulder width apart (assume involved side is left lower extremity).

PROCEDURE: Leading with involved extremity, patient lowers into lunge position in smooth, controlled motion and then returns to standing. This positioning will increase the eccentric loading on the quadriceps with deceleration on the downward movement. For upward movement, patient is asked to focus on hip extension not knee extension.

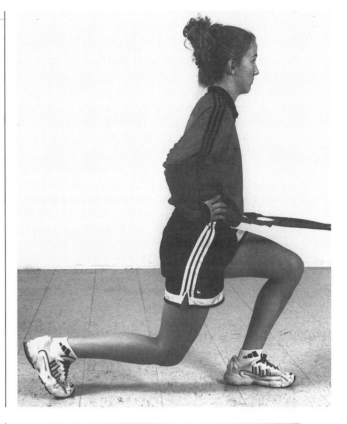

Figure 11-12 Lunge: posterior weight shift.

PURPOSE: Stimulation of dynamic postural response, facilitating concentric and eccentric contractions.

POSITION: Standing, facing away from tubing, with feet shoulder width apart (assume involved extremity is left lower extremity).

PROCEDURE: Leading with involved extremity, patient lowers into lunge position in smooth, controlled motion and then returns to standing. When lowering self into lunge, patient must work against resistance because tubing is stretched; when at the low point of lunge position, patient is assisted back up by tubing.

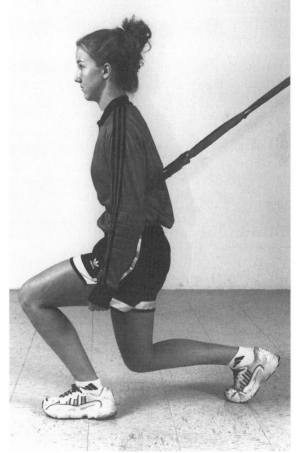

Figure 11-13 Lunge: medial weight shift.

PURPOSE: Stimulation of dynamic postural response, facilitating concentric and eccentric contractions.

POSITION: Standing with uninvolved extremity closest to tubing, with feet shoulder width apart (assume involved extremity is left lower extremity).

PROCEDURE: Leading with involved extremity, patient lowers into lunge position in smooth, controlled motion and then returns to standing. Medial weight shift causes ankle inverters to fire to maintain position, which may facilitate ankle stability.

NOTE: The lateral weight shift is not illustrated but is the same as shown in Figure 11-13 except with tubing pulling laterally (to patient's left) instead of medially (to patient's right as is shown in Fig. 11-13). The lunge with lateral weight shift is performed by positioning patient with the affected lower extremity closest to the resistance. This lateral weight shift causes firing of ankle everters, which may facilitate ankle stability.

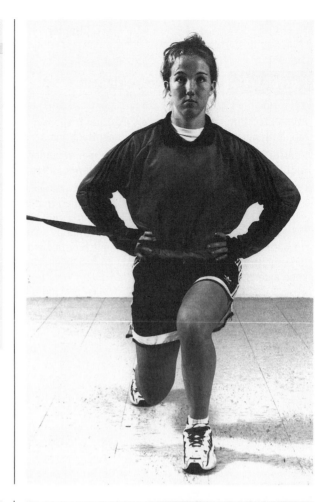

Figure 11-14 Stationary run: anterior weight shift.

PURPOSE: Stimulation of dynamic postural response, introducing impact and ballistic exercise and improving balance and weight shift.

POSITION: Standing, facing tubing, with feet shoulder width apart (assume involved side is left lower extremity).

PROCEDURE: Patient starts with light jogging in place and can progress to "butt kicks"; same distance from origin of tubing should be maintained. The anterior weight shift run is probably the most difficult technique to perform correctly and is therefore taught last. This technique simulates deceleration and eccentric loading of knee extensors

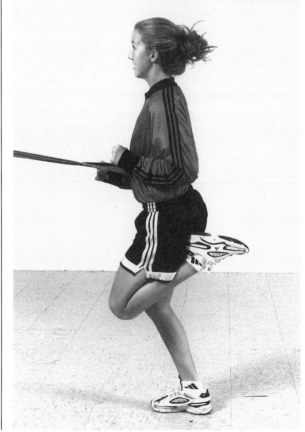

Figure 11-15   Stationary run: posterior weight shift.

PURPOSE: Stimulation of dynamic postural response, introducing impact and ballistic exercise and improving balance and weight shift.

POSITION: Standing, facing away from tubing, with feet shoulder width apart (assume involved extremity is left lower extremity).

PROCEDURE: Patient starts with light jogging in place and can progress to running in place; same distance from origin of tubing should be maintained. The most advanced form of the posterior weight-shift run involves exaggeration of hip flexion called "high knees." This technique simulates the acceleration phase of jogging or running.

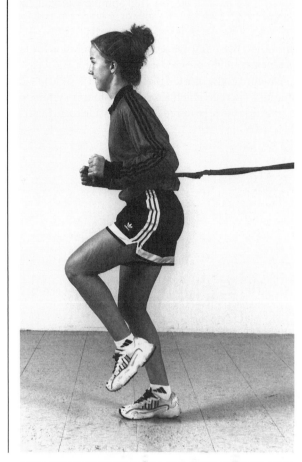

Figure 11-16   Stationary run: medial weight shift.

PURPOSE: Stimulation of dynamic postural response, introducing impact and ballistic exercise and improving balance and weight shift.

POSITION: Standing with uninvolved extremity closest to tubing, with feet shoulder width apart (assume involved extremity is left lower extremity).

PROCEDURE: Patient starts with light jogging in place and can progress to running in place; same distance from origin of tubing should be maintained. This technique simulates the forces that patient will experience when cutting or turning quickly away from affected side. (For example, the exercise will facilitate cutting left in a patient with a left lower extremity problem.)

NOTE: The lateral weight-shift technique is not illustrated, but it is the same as shown in Figure 11-10 except with tubing pulling laterally (to patient's left) instead of medially (to patient's right as is shown in Fig. 11-16). This technique simulates the forces that patient will experience when cutting or turning quickly towards affected side. (For example, this exercise will facilitate cutting right in a patient with a left lower extremity problem.)

foot to the other. Bounding places greater emphasis on the lateral movements, and its progression follows the same weight-shifting sequence as the resisted running exercise. Side-to-side bounding in a lateral-resisted exercise promotes symmetric balance and endurance required for progression to higher levels of strength and power applications. Before using the tubing, the client should learn the bounding activity by jumping over cones or other obstacles. The tubing can then be added to provide the secondary forces that cause anterior, posterior, medial, or lateral weight shifting (Figs. 11-17 to 11-19).

Figure 11-17   Bounding: anterior weight shift.

PURPOSE: Stimulation of dynamic postural response, promoting balance and endurance in preparation for progression to higher-level lower-extremity exercise.

POSITION: Standing, facing tubing, with feet shoulder width apart (assume involved extremity is left lower extremity).

PROCEDURE: Patient takes off of one foot, jumps over cones that are set at prescribed distance, and lands on opposite foot. The technique is then repeated in opposite direction. This exercise will assist in teaching deceleration and lateral cutting movements.

A

B

A

B

Figure 11-18 Bounding: posterior weight shift.

PURPOSE: Stimulation of dynamic postural response, promoting balance and endurance in preparation for progression to higher-level lower-extremity exercise.

POSITION: Standing, facing away from tubing, with feet shoulder width apart (assume involved extremity is left lower extremity).

PROCEDURE: Patient takes off of one foot, jumps over cones that are set at prescribed distance, and lands on opposite foot. The technique is then repeated in opposite direction. This exercise will assist in teaching acceleration and lateral cutting movements.

Figure 11-19 Bounding: medial weight shift.

PURPOSE: Stimulation of dynamic postural response, promoting balance and endurance in preparation for progression to higher-level lower-extremity exercise.

POSITION: Standing, with uninvolved extremity closest to tubing, with feet shoulder width apart (assume involved side is left lower extremity).

PROCEDURE: Patient takes off of one foot, jumps over cones that are set at prescribed distance, and lands on opposite foot. The technique is then repeated in opposite direction. The medial weight-shift bound is used as an assisted plyometric exercise because the impact on the involved extremity (left) is greatly lowered owing to the pull of the tubing.

NOTE: The lateral weight-shift technique is not illustrated but is the same as shown in Figure 11-19 except with tubing pulling laterally (to patient's left) instead of pulling medially (to patient's right as is shown in Fig. 11-19). This exercise is the most strenuous of the bounding activities since it actually accelerates the body weight onto the affected lower extremity. This shift to the affected extremity is, however, necessary so that the clinician can observe the ability of the affected limb to perform quick direction change and controlled acceleration/deceleration.

CASE STUDY 1

PATIENT INFORMATION

This case involved a 15-year-old female high school soccer player injured during an intrasquad game 2 days prior to the examination. The athlete sustained contact just after completing a crossing pass and sustained a valgus stress to the knee. She felt immediate medial knee pain and was unable to continue participation. The athlete was able to bear minimal weight on the leg following the injury. No immediate swelling was noted, no pop was felt or heard, and no episodes of the knee locking or catching was experienced. She was seen in the emergency department the same date of the injury and was placed in a 30-degree immobilizer and issued crutches.

The athlete presented to the initial visit able to bear partial weight with the assistance of axillary crutches. Examination by the PT indicated that active ROM of the knee was 20 to 100 degrees of knee flexion that was limited by medial knee pain. Passive knee ROM was 5 to 105 degrees of flexion and was limited by hamstring spasm and medial knee pain. Volitional quadriceps recruitment with an isometric contraction was decreased via palpation, as compared with the opposite side.

Tenderness to palpation was noted at the mid one third of the medial joint line. In the skeletally immature athlete, the distal femoral epiphysis can be injured in this same mechanism of injury in soccer players.[25] Palpation of the distal femoral epiphysis, however, did not reveal any tenderness. Ligamentous exam for lateral, anterior, and posterior straight-plane instability revealed no asymmetric instability. Examination of anteriomedial, anterolateral, and posterolateral instability likewise did not reveal asymmetric instability. Approximately 5 millimeters of instability was noted with valgus stress at 30 degrees of flexion, an end point was present which was accompanied by pain (six on a 0–10 scale). The minimal instability was present at the joint line and not at the distal femoral epiphysis. Based on the examination and evaluation, the PT diagnosed the patient with a second-degree medial collateral ligament sprain.

LINKS TO
GUIDE TO PHYSICAL THERAPIST PRACTICE

Using the *Guide to Physical Therapist Practice*,[10] this patient fell in musculoskeletal practice pattern 4E: "impaired joint mobility, muscle performance, and range of motion associated with ligament or other connective tissue disorders." Anticipated goals for this patient as they relate to functional progression include: increasing motor function; improved joint mobility; improved weight-bearing status; improved strength, power, and endurance; as well as protecting the injured body part and minimizing the risk of recurrent injury.

INTERVENTION

Goals for the early stage of intervention were initiated by the PT and focused on minimizing the inflammatory process that accompanies healing. The patient was instructed to utilize crutches with toe touch weight bearing. She was also instructed in ice application to the medial knee after exercise and for 10 to 15 minutes every 4 hours when awake. The athlete was instructed in quadriceps isometrics (10-second contractions, 10 repetitions, ten times per day) (Fig. 6-9) and bent-knee leg raising (Fig. 6-26) (three sets of 20 repetitions twice daily) while in the immobilizer. The immobilizer was to be removed four to five times a day and the athlete was to perform 90- to 40-degree open-chain, gravity-resisted knee extensions (three sets of 20 repetitions). The patient belonged to a health club with access to an upper-extremity ergometer, and she was instructed in monitoring her pulse, given a maximum heart rate (205 beats/minute), and instructed to perform 20- to 30-minute workouts at 80% of her target heart rate (164 beats/minute). (For more detail on exercise prescription, the reader is referred to Chapter 12). The PT asked the PTA to continue the plan of care that had been established and focus on decreasing flare-ups of inflammation.

PROGRESSION

One Week After Initial Examination

The PTA worked with the patient on exercises to promote full ROM. The PTA asked the PT if prone active-assisted flexion exercises through the full ROM (three sets of 15 repetitions twice a day) could be added (Fig. 3-5). Obtaining approval, the PTA initiated the full ROM exercises. Also, isotonic strengthening of the hip musculature in all planes was initiated (Figs. 6-26 to 6-28). The athlete was allowed to begin full weight-bearing ambulation in the immobilizer.

Bilateral support activities consisting of reactive neuromuscular training using oscillating techniques for isometric stabilization were instituted in three sets of 1 minute in straight-plane anterior, medial, and lateral weight shifts (Figs. 11-3, 11-5, and 11-6).

Conditioning efforts on the upper-extremity ergometer continued but were modified to also address anaerobic needs. Efforts on the upper-extremity ergometer were expanded to encompass two 20-minute workouts with a 10-minute rest between sessions. During each 20-minute session on the ergometer the athlete was instructed to perform 15- to 30-second "all out" sprints every 2 minutes per the PT-directed plan of care. The patient was determined to be a candidate for a functional knee brace, a prescription was secured, and she was measured for a brace at this time.

Two Weeks After Initial Examination

At this point prone active knee flexion was symmetric and the athlete lacked less than five degrees of seated knee extension per goniometer measurements. Functional progression activities were progressed to straight-plane bilateral nonsupport activities, which consisted of front to back line jumps (Fig. 9-14). Following the closed-chain activities, the athlete performed three sets of 15 repetitions of open-chain knee extension through the full ROM (Fig. 6-30).

Three Weeks After Initial Examination

The PTA consulted with the PT about progression of activities and sought clarification on expectations. The PTA continued with intervention after clarification from the PT. At this point active and passive ROM of the knee was full and symmetric. Functional progression activities in the brace were advanced to include elastic cord–resisted lateral stepping drills and stationary lateral bounding (Fig. 11-19). The lateral stepping drills were performed in the functional brace and were gradually increased to a distance of 8 feet after initial resistance of the cord was encountered. In-place stationary bounding began at a distance slightly greater than shoulder width apart and was progressed to a distance of 3 feet. Both of these activities were performed for three sets of 1 minute and were increased to three sets of 2 minutes. Straight-plane, unilateral, nonsupport activities and multiplane bilateral nonsupport drills were also added per the PT-directed plan of care. Straight-plane, unilateral, nonsupport activities (excluding valgus loading) consisted of front to back lines hops for three sets of 15 seconds and were progressed to 1 minute.

The PTA spoke with the PT and discussed discharge. At this point the athlete returned to the soccer field for early sport-related activities per the PT. Ball-handling skills and outside touch passing and kicking were allowed in the brace. She was also allowed to begin a straight-plane jogging program on level surfaces to address aerobic and anaerobic conditioning (Table 15-3). Open-chain knee extension through the full ROM continued to be performed three times a week following closed-chain functional progression drills per the home exercise program established by the PT and PTA.

OUTCOMES

As part of the formal exercise program that the PT and PTA established, the athlete was now ready for more strenuous unilateral support and nonsupport activities to stress valgus loading. Multiplane unilateral nonsupport drills consisted of diagonal hopping (Table 15-7). Inside kicking, passing, and shooting were instituted at this point. Agility drills consisting of the figure eight and cutting progression were instituted (Table 15-8). As she completed the lateral power hop sequence, the athlete was allowed to return to competition 30 days following injury per the PT.

SUMMARY—AN EFFECTIVE PT–PTA TEAM

This case study demonstrates components of an effective working relationship of the PT and PTA. The communication was effective and created efficient treatment of the patient. The PTA communicated needs of clarification of treatment expectations. Also, the PTA communicated possible discharge of the patient, and then the PT made the decision on discharge based on the information provided by the PTA. The PT and PTA collaborated on developing the home exercise program. Collaboration of the home exercise program demonstrates the mutual respect of the PT and the PTA.

SUMMARY

- Reactive neuromuscular training is a program designed to restore balance, proprioception, and dynamic stability and enhance cognitive appreciation of the joint's position and movement of the joint after injury.

- Reactive neuromuscular training entails the shifting of the patient's center of gravity by pulling the upper body in a given direction over the fixed lower extremity. The patient is required to generate lower-extremity isometric contractions to offset this weight shift and thereby maintain stability of the lower extremity. These oscillating techniques of isometric stabilization to offset the shift in the center of gravity aid in the integration of visual, mechanoreceptors, and equilibrium reactions.

- The reactive neuromuscular-training program can be progressed from slow to fast activities, from low-force to high-force activities, and from controlled to uncontrolled activities. In addition, the shift on the center of gravity can occur in a single plane or in multiple planes.

References

1. Anderson MA, Foreman TL. Return to competition: functional progression. In: Zachezewski JE, Magee DJ, Quillen WS, eds. *Athletic injuries and rehabilitation*. Philadelphia: WB Saunders. 1996:229–261.

2. Sandler-Goldstein T. *Functional rehabilitation in orthopaedics*. Gaithersburg, MD: Aspen; 1988.

3. Tippett SR. Closed chain exercise. *Orthop Phys Ther Clin North Am*. 1992;1:253–268.

4. Bandy WD. Functional rehabilitation of the athlete. *Orthop Phys Ther Clin North Am*. 1992;1:269–282.

5. Rivera JE. Open versus closed chain rehabilitation of the lower extremity: a functional and biomechanical analysis. *J Sport Rehabil*. 1994;3:154–167.

6. Swanik CB, Lephart SM, Giannantonio FP, et al. Reestablishing proprioception and neuromuscular control in the ACL-injured athlete. *J Sport Rehabil*. 1997;6:182–206.

7. Voight ML, Cook G. Clinical application of closed kinetic chain exercise. *J Sport Rehabil*. 1996;5:25–44.

8. Voight ML, Cook G. Lower extremity closed chain progression using reactive neuromuscular training. *J Orthop Sports Phys Ther*. 1997;25:69.

9. Hewett TE, Paterno MV, Myer GD. Strategies for enhancing proprioception and neuromuscular control of the knee. *Clin Orthop Rel Res*. 2002;402:76–94.

10. American Physical Therapy Association. *Guide to physical therapist practice*. 2nd ed. Alexandria, VA; 2003.

PART

V

Cardiopulmonary
Applications

Principles of Aerobic Conditioning and Cardiac Rehabilitation

Dennis O'Connell, PT, PhD, FACSM, and Janet Bezner, PT, PhD

OBJECTIVES

Upon completion of this chapter, the reader will be able to:

- Discuss the role of aerobic exercise and conditioning.

- Describe basic physiology of aerobic exercise.

- Discuss the evaluation procedures for exercise tolerance.

- Describe the components of exercise prescription.

- Discuss the breadth, scope, and purpose of cardiac rehabilitation.

- Describe the continuum of cardiac rehabilitation, including exercise programming and patient progression through cardiac rehabilitation.

PRINCIPLES OF
Aerobic Conditioning

The positive influence of exercise on general health and well-being has been hypothesized and studied with great interest by most of the world. Throughout Western history, dating back to and probably starting with Hippocrates (the father of preventative medicine), exercise has been recommended to improve health and physical function and to increase longevity.[1,2] Conversely, the notion that sedentary individuals tend to contract illness more readily than those who are active has been observed and documented since at least the 16th century.[2] In the 19th and 20th centuries these ideas led to the creation of physical education curricula; the study of exercise physiology as a science; and maturation of the literature regarding exercise, including clarification of the many terms used to describe movement of the body.[2]

Caspersen et al[3] defined physical activity as any bodily movement produced by skeletal muscles that results in energy expenditure. Exercise is a type of physical activity that is planned, structured, repetitive, and purposely aimed at improving physical fitness. Physical fitness is a set of attributes that people have or achieve and includes components of health-related (cardiorespiratory endurance, body composition, muscular endurance, muscular strength, flexibility) and athletic-related skills.[3] Being physically fit, therefore, enables an individual to perform daily tasks without undue fatigue and with sufficient energy to enjoy leisure-time activities and to respond in an emergency situation, if one arises. A primary activity used to achieve physical fitness is cardiorespiratory endurance training, whereby one performs repetitive movements of large muscle groups fueled by an adequate response from the circulatory and respiratory systems to sustain physical activity and eliminate fatigue.[2] Cardiorespiratory endurance training is the ability of the whole body to sustain prolonged exercise.[4]

Another term for cardiorespiratory endurance training is aerobic training, indicating the role of oxygen in the performance of these types of activities. The highest rate of oxygen that the body can consume during maximal exercise is termed aerobic capacity.[4] Maximal oxygen uptake ($\dot{V}O_{2max}$) is considered the best measurement of aerobic capacity and therefore cardiorespiratory endurance and fitness.[4] Maximal or submaximal oxygen uptake when divided by 3.5 is expressed as a metabolic equivalent (MET). This shorthand version of exercise intensity is easy to use and explain to clients or patients.

The literature contains convincing evidence that the regular performance of cardiorespiratory endurance activities reduces the risk of coronary heart disease and is associated with lower mortality rates in both older and younger adults.[2,5,6] Despite this evidence, recent surveys of exercise trends in the United States illustrate that approximately 15% of U.S. adults perform vigorous physical activity (three times per week for at least 20 minutes) during leisure time, 22% partake in sustained physical activity (five times per week for at least 30 minutes) of any intensity during leisure time, and 25% of adults perform no physical activity in leisure time.[2] Adolescents and young adults (ages 12 to 21) are similarly inactive and approximately 50% regularly participate in vigorous physical activity.[2]

Owing to the widespread prevalence of physical inactivity among the U.S. population, the U.S. Public Health Service created goals for exercise participation in the *Healthy People 2000*[7] and *Healthy People 2010*[8] documents, aimed at improving the quality of and increasing the years of healthy life. In addition, the U.S. Department of Health and Human Services, Centers for Disease Control and Prevention, National Council on Physical Fitness and Sports, and American College of Sports Medicine (ACSM) recommend that all adults should accumulate 30 minutes or more of moderate-intensity physical activity on most, and preferably all, days of the week.[2,9] Toward that end, clinicians have an opportunity to contribute to the overall well-being of the patients and clients served by prescribing meaningful exercise programs based on the most contemporary scientific evidence. The physical therapist assistant (PTA) can be instrumental in encouraging increased activity for their patients. It is also important to understand the role of cardiovascular fitness in overall health and well-being for the best outcomes of therapeutic exercise programs. The scientific basis of aerobic training is presented in this chapter, along with guidelines for prescribing and supervising aerobic exercise.

SCIENTIFIC BASIS

Energy Sources Used During Aerobic Exercise

The performance of aerobic exercise requires readily available energy sources at the cellular level. Ingested food (composed of carbohydrate, fat, and protein) is converted to and stored in the cell as adenosine triphosphate (ATP), the body's basic energy source for cellular metabolism and the performance of muscular activity. Each energy source has a unique route, whereby ingested food is converted to ATP. ATP is produced by three methods, or metabolic pathways.[4] To base an exercise prescription on sound scientific principles, understanding and differentiation of the fuel sources and metabolic pathways are paramount.

Fuel Sources

Carbohydrates (including sugars, starches, and fibers) are the preferred energy source for the body and are the only fuel capable of being used by the central nervous system

(CNS). In addition, carbohydrate is the only fuel that can be used during anaerobic metabolism. Carbohydrates are converted to glucose and stored in muscle cells and the liver as glycogen; 1,200 to 2,000 kcal of energy can be stored in the body. Each gram of carbohydrate ingested produces approximately 4 kcal of energy.[4]

Fat can also be used as an energy source and forms the body's largest store of potential energy; the reserve is about 70,000 kcal in a lean adult.[4] Fat is generally stored as triglycerides. Before triglycerides can be used for energy, they must be broken down into free fatty acids (FFAs) and glycerol; FFAs are used to form ATP by aerobic oxidation. The process of triglyceride reduction (lipolysis) requires significant amounts of oxygen; thus, carbohydrate fuel sources are more efficient than fat fuel sources[12] and are preferred during high-intensity exercise. Each gram of fat produces 9 kcal of energy.

Protein is used as an energy source in cases of starvation or extreme energy depletion and provides 5% to 12% of the total energy needed to perform endurance exercise. It is not a preferred energy source under normal conditions.[4] Each gram of protein produces approximately 4 kcal of energy.

Metabolic Pathways

ATP–phosphocreatine System

The first pathway for production of ATP is anaerobic, meaning that it does not require oxygen to function (although the pathway can occur in the presence of oxygen). This pathway is called the ATP–phosphocreatine (PCr, or creatine phosphate) system.[4] Phosphocreatine is a high-energy compound, like ATP, that replenishes ATP in a working muscle, extending the time to fatigue by 12 to 20 seconds.[12] Thus, energy released as a result of the breakdown of PCr is not used for cellular metabolism but to prevent the ATP level from falling. One molecule of ATP is produced per molecule of PCr. This simple energy system can produce 3 to 15 seconds of maximal muscular work[4] and requires an adequate recovery time, generally three times longer than the duration of the activity.

Glycolytic System

The production of ATP during longer bouts of activity requires the breakdown of food energy sources. In the glycolytic system, or during anaerobic glycolysis, ATP is produced through the breakdown of glucose obtained from the ingestion of carbohydrates or from the breakdown of glycogen stored in the liver. Anaerobic glycolysis, which also occurs without the presence of oxygen, is much more complex than the ATP–PCr pathway, requiring numerous enzymatic reactions to break down glucose and produce energy. The end product of glycolysis is pyruvic acid, which is converted to lactic acid in the absence of oxygen. The net energy production from each molecule of glucose used is two molecules of ATP, and each molecule of glycogen yields three molecules of ATP.

Although the energy yield from the glycolytic system is small, the combined energy production of the ATP–PCr and glycolytic pathways enables muscles to contract without a continuous oxygen supply, thus providing an energy source for the first part of high-intensity exercise until the respiratory and circulatory systems catch up to the sudden increased demands placed on them. Furthermore, the glycolytic system can provide energy for only a limited time because the end product of the pathway, lactic acid, accumulates in the muscles and inhibits further glycogen breakdown, eventually impeding muscle contraction.[4]

Oxidative System

The production of ATP from the breakdown of fuel sources in the presence of oxygen is termed aerobic oxidation, or cellular respiration. This process occurs in the mitochondria, which are the cellular organelles conveniently located next to myofibrils, the contractile elements of individual muscle fibers. The oxidative production of ATP involves several complex processes, including aerobic glycolysis, the Krebs cycle, and the electron transport chain.[4]

Carbohydrate, or glycogen, is broken down in aerobic glycolysis in a similar manner as the breakdown of carbohydrate in anaerobic glycolysis. But in the presence of oxygen, pyruvic acid is converted to acetyl coenzyme A, which can then enter the Krebs cycle, producing two molecules of ATP. The end result of the Krebs cycle is the production of carbon dioxide and hydrogen ions, which enter the electron transport chain, undergo a series of reactions, and produce ATP and water. The net ATP production from aerobic oxidation is 39 molecules of ATP from 1 molecule of glycogen, or 38 molecules of ATP from 1 molecule of glucose.[4]

Therefore, the presence of oxygen enables significantly more energy to be produced and results in the ability to perform longer periods of work without muscle contraction being impeded from the buildup of lactic acid. Figure 12-1 summarizes and compares the energy-production capabilities of the three metabolic pathways.[11]

Selection of Metabolic Pathway and Fuel Source During Exercise

High-intensity, brief-duration exercise (efforts of less than 15 seconds) generally relies on stored ATP in the muscle for energy and employs the ATP–PCr pathway. High-intensity, short-duration exercise (efforts of 1 to 2 minutes) relies on the anaerobic pathways, including the ATP–PCr and glycolysis systems for the provision of ATP. Both of these types of exercise use carbohydrate or glucose as a fuel source.[4]

Submaximal exercise efforts use carbohydrate, fat, and protein for energy. Low-intensity exercise (less than 50%

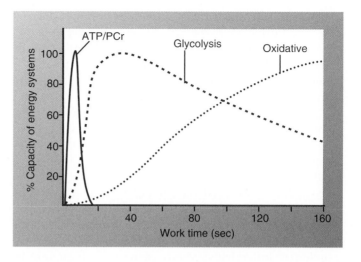

Figure 12-1

Energy production capabilities of the three metabolic pathways. This figure depicts the actions and interactions of the adenosine triphosphate (ATP)–phosphocreatine, glycolytic, and oxidative metabolic pathways. High-intensity, brief-duration exercise is fueled by the ATP–phosphocreatine pathway, whereas high-intensity, short duration exercise relies on the glycolytic pathway, both of which are anaerobic. The aerobic oxidative pathway provides energy for muscular contraction during prolonged exercise of low to moderate intensity.

of maximal oxygen consumption) performed for long durations uses both FFA and carbohydrate fuel sources within the aerobic oxidative pathway to produce ATP.[12] In the presence of an abundant supply of oxygen, as exercise duration increases or intensity decreases, the body uses more FFAs than carbohydrates for ATP production. During work loads of moderate to heavy intensity (more than 50% of maximal oxygen consumption), carbohydrates are used more than FFAs for ATP production. As the workload approaches maximal exercise capacity, the proportion of FFA oxidation decreases and that of carbohydrate oxidation increases. Above maximal levels, exercise is anaerobic and can be performed for only a short time.[12] As noted, protein participates as an energy source only in extremely deficient situations (starvation) and minimally during endurance exercise.[4]

To summarize, carbohydrate is the preferred fuel source for supplying the body with energy in the form of ATP during exercise. Exercise can occur anaerobically, via the ATP–PCr or anaerobic glycolysis pathways, or aerobically via the aerobic oxidative pathway. The oxidative pathway has the greatest ATP yield and enables exercise to continue for prolonged periods without the fatigue caused by lactic acid buildup. To support the aerobic needs of prolonged exercise, numerous changes occur in the cardiovascular and respiratory systems, which are discussed next.

Normal Responses to Acute Aerobic Exercise

Numerous cardiovascular and respiratory mechanisms aimed at delivering oxygen to the tissues contribute to the ability to sustain exercise aerobically. To examine an individual's response to exercise, it is important to understand the normal physiologic changes that occur as a result of physical activity. The following sections outline the changes expected during aerobic exercise and are considered normal responses.[4,11]

Heart Rate

Heart rate (HR) is measured in beats per minute (bpm). A linear relationship exists between HR and the intensity of exercise, indicating that as workload or intensity increases, HR increases proportionally. The magnitude of increase in HR is influenced by many factors, including age, fitness level, type of activity being performed, presence of disease, medications, blood volume, and environmental factors (e.g., temperature and humidity).[4]

Stroke Volume

The volume, or amount, of blood (measured in milliliters) ejected from the left ventricle per heart beat is termed the stroke volume (SV). As workload increases, SV increases linearly up to approximately 50% of aerobic capacity, after which it increases only slightly. Factors that influence the magnitude of change in SV include ventricular function, body position, and exercise intensity.[4]

Cardiac Output

The product of HR and SV is cardiac output ($\dot{Q}$), or the amount of blood (measured in liters) ejected from the left ventricle per minute. Cardiac output increases linearly with workload owing to the increases in HR and SV in response to increasing exercise intensity. Changes in $\dot{Q}$ depend on age, posture, body size, presence of disease, and level of physical conditioning.[4]

Arterial–venous Oxygen Difference

The amount of oxygen extracted by the tissues from the blood represents the difference between arterial blood oxygen content and venous blood oxygen content and is referred to as the arterial–venous oxygen difference ($\Delta a\text{–}\bar{v}O_2$; measured in milliliters per deciliter). As exercise intensity increases, $\Delta a\text{–}\bar{v}O_2$ increases linearly, indicating that the tissues are extracting more oxygen from the blood, creating a decreasing venous oxygen content as exercise progresses.[4]

Blood Flow

The distribution of blood flow (measured in milliliters) to the body changes dramatically during acute exercise. When at rest, 15% to 20% of the cardiac output goes to muscle, but during exercise 80% to 85% is distributed to working muscle and shunted away from the viscera. During heavy exercise, or when the body starts to overheat, increased blood flow is delivered to the skin to conduct heat away from the body's core, leaving less blood for working muscles.[4]

Blood Pressure

The two components of blood pressure (BP)—systolic (SBP) and diastolic (DBP) (measured in millimeters of mercury)—respond differently during acute bouts of exercise. To facilitate blood and oxygen delivery to the tissues, SBP increases linearly with workload. Because DBP represents the pressure in the arteries when the heart is at rest, it changes little during aerobic exercise, regardless of intensity. A change in DBP from a resting value of <15 mm Hg is considered a normal response. Both SBP and DBP are higher during upper-extremity aerobic activity than during lower-extremity aerobic activity.[4]

Pulmonary Ventilation

The respiratory system responds to exercise by increasing the rate and depth of breathing to increase the amount of air exchanged (measured in liters) per minute. An immediate increase in rate and depth occurs in response to exercise and is thought to be facilitated by the nervous system and initiated by movement of the body. A second, more gradual, increase occurs in response to temperature and blood chemical changes as a result of the increased oxygen use by the tissues. Thus, both tidal volume (the amount of air moved in and out of the lungs during regular breathing) and respiratory rate increase in proportion to the intensity of exercise.[4]

Abnormal Responses to Aerobic Exercise

Individuals with suspected cardiovascular disease (CVD), or any other type of disease that may produce an abnormal response to exercise, should be appropriately screened and tested by a physician before the initiation of an exercise program (discussed in greater detail later in this chapter). Abnormal responses may also occur in individuals without known or documented disease. Routine monitoring of exercise response is important and can be used to evaluate the appropriateness of the exercise prescription and as an

---

TABLE 12-1 Signs and Symptoms of Exercise Intolerance

Angina: chest, left arm, jaw, back, or lower neck pain or pressure
Unusual or severe shortness of breath
Abnormal diaphoresis
Pallor, cyanosis, cold and clammy skin
Central nervous system symptoms: vertigo, ataxia, gait problems, or confusion
Leg cramps or intermittent claudication
Physical or verbal manifestations of severe fatigue or shortness of breath

Reprinted with permission from American College of Sports Medicine. *Resource manual for guidelines for exercise testing and prescription.* 3rd ed. Baltimore: Williams & Wilkins; 1998.

---

indication that further diagnostic testing is indicated. In general, responses that are inconsistent with the normal responses described previously are considered abnormal. Of the parameters described, HR and BP are most commonly examined during exercise. Examples of abnormal responses to aerobic exercise are the failure of the HR to rise in proportion to exercise intensity, the failure of the SBP to rise during exercise, a decrease in the SBP of 20 mm Hg during exercise, and an increase in the DBP of 15 mm Hg during exercise.[11] The PTA should be able to recognize other signs and symptoms of exercise intolerance, which are presented in Table 12-1.

Knowledge of the normal and abnormal physiologic and symptom responses to exercise will enable the PTA to prescribe and monitor exercise safely and confidently and to minimize the occurrence of untoward events during exercise. Regular exposure to aerobic exercise results in changes to the cardiovascular and respiratory systems that can also be examined by monitoring basic physiologic variables during exercise.

Cardiovascular and Respiratory Adaptations to Aerobic Conditioning

The documented benefits of aerobic exercise are a result of the adaptations that occur in the oxygen-delivery system with the habitual performance of regular activity. These adaptations, considered chronic changes, enable more efficient performance of exercise and affect cardiorespiratory endurance and fitness level.

Cardiovascular Adaptations

Factors involving the heart that adapt in response to a regular exercise stimulus include heart size, HR, SV, and $\dot{Q}$. The weight and volume of the heart and the thickness and chamber size of the left ventricle increase with training. As a result, the heart pumps out more blood per beat (SV) and the force of each contraction is stronger. With training, the left ventricle is more completely filled during diastole, increasing SV (at rest as well as during submaximal and maximal exercise) and plasma blood volume.

Changes in the HR include a decreased resting rate and a decreased rate at submaximal exercise levels, indicating that the individual can perform the same amount of work with less effort after training. Maximal HR typically does not change as a result of training. The amount of time it takes for the HR to return to resting after exercise decreases as a result of training and is a useful indicator of progress toward better fitness. Since $\dot{Q}$ is the product of HR and SV ($\dot{Q}$ = HR × SV), no change occurs at rest or during submaximal exercise because HR decreases and SV increases. However, because of the increase in maximum SV, maximum $\dot{Q}$ increases considerably.[4,11]

Adaptations also occur to the vascular system, including blood volume, BP, and blood flow changes. Aerobic training increases overall blood volume, primarily because of an increase in plasma volume. The increase in blood plasma results from an increased release of hormones (antidiuretic and aldosterone) that promote water retention by the kidneys and an increase in the amount of plasma proteins (namely albumin). A small increase in the number of red blood cells may also contribute to the increase in blood volume. The net effect of greater blood volume is the delivery of more oxygen to the tissues.

Resting BP changes seen with training are most noteworthy in hypertensive or borderline hypertensive patients, in whom aerobic training can decrease both SBP and DBP by 12 mm Hg. During the performance of submaximal and maximal exercise, little change, if any, occurs in BP as a result of training. Several adaptations are responsible for the increase in blood flow to muscle in a trained individual, including greater capillarization in the trained muscles, greater opening of existing capillaries in trained muscles, and more efficient distribution of blood flow to active muscles.[4,11]

Respiratory Adaptations

The capacity of the respiratory system to deliver oxygen to the body typically surpasses the ability of the body to use oxygen; thus, the respiratory component of performance is not a limiting factor in the development of endurance. Nevertheless, adaptations in the respiratory system do occur in response to aerobic training. The amount of air in the lungs, represented by lung volume measures, is unchanged at rest and during submaximal exercise in trained individuals. However, tidal volume, the amount of air breathed in and out during normal respiration, increases during maximal exercise. Respiratory rate (RR) is lower at rest and during submaximal exercise and increases at maximal levels of exercise. The combined increase in tidal volume and RR during maximal exercise of trained individuals produces a

substantial increase in pulmonary ventilation, or the movement of air into and out of the lungs.

Pulmonary ventilation at rest is either unchanged or slightly reduced, and during submaximal exercise it is slightly reduced after training. The process of gas exchange in the alveoli, or pulmonary diffusion, is unchanged at rest and at submaximal exercise levels but increases during maximal exercise owing to the increased blood flow to the lungs and the increased ventilation, as noted. These two factors create a situation that enables more alveoli to participate in gas exchange and more oxygen perfuses into the arterial system during maximal exercise. Finally, $\Delta a\text{-}\bar{v}O_2$ increases at maximal exercise in response to training as a result of increased oxygen distraction by the tissues and greater blood flow to the tissues, owing to more effective blood distribution.[4,11]

Aerobic Capacity Adaptations

The net effect of these cardiovascular and respiratory adaptations on aerobic capacity is an increase in $\dot{V}O_{2max}$ as a result of endurance training. When $\dot{V}O_2$ is measured in leg mass, it is termed absolute $\dot{V}O_{2max}$; when it is in mL/kg/min, it is relative $\dot{V}O_{2max}$ because it is relative to body weight. A typical training program performed at 75% of $\dot{V}O_{2max}$ (described in a later section) three times per week at 30 minutes per session over the course of 6 months can improve $\dot{V}O_{2max}$ by 15% to 20% in a previously sedentary individual. Resting $\dot{V}O_{2max}$ is either unchanged or slightly increased after training, and submaximal $\dot{V}O_2$ is either unchanged or slightly reduced, representing more efficiency.[4]

Psychologic Benefits of Training

In addition to a myriad of cardiovascular, respiratory, and metabolic improvements that occur after aerobic training, psychologic benefits have been documented, although these effects are less well understood. An overall assessment of the literature indicates that depression, mood, anxiety, psychologic well-being, and perceptions of physical function and well-being improve in response to the performance of physical activity.[2,13] The finding that exercise can decrease symptoms of depression and anxiety is consistent with the fact that individuals who are inactive are more likely to have depressive symptoms than are active individuals. Improvements in depression and mood have been found in populations with and without clinically diagnosed psychologic impairment and in those with good psychologic health, although the literature is less conclusive in this specific area.

A number of factors have been postulated to explain the beneficial effects of aerobic training on psychologic function, including changes in neurotransmitter concentrations, body temperature, hormones, cardiorespiratory function, and metabolic processes as well as improvement in psychosocial factors such as social support, self-efficacy, and stress relief. Further research is needed to verify the potential contribution of changes in these factors to improvement in psychologic function.[2]

Despite the inability to explain why psychologic parameters improve in response to training, the effect on overall quality of life is positive.[14,15] This improvement in quality of life has been demonstrated in individuals with and without disease,[16–19] including patients with coronary heart disease who are obese[20] and elderly,[21] patients with chronic heart failure,[22] patients who have undergone coronary bypass graft surgery,[23] and patients with multiple sclerosis[24] and cancer.[25]

Health-Related Benefits to Exercise

The observed improvement in quality of life in individuals who participate in regular exercise is achieved from quantities of exercise considered to produce health-related (vs fitness-related) benefits. Fitness-related benefits result in significant changes in physical fitness level, as measured by cardiorespiratory endurance and body composition changes. Specific recommendations for fitness-related changes usually include vigorous, continuous activities with a focus on the specific parameters of exercise (intensity, mode, duration, frequency). Health-related benefits can be achieved through the performance of moderate-intensity, intermittent activity with a focus on the accumulated amount of activity performed.[9] Documented health-related benefits from the performance of regular exercise are presented in Table 12-2.[9,11]

Although improvement in fitness level is a worthwhile goal and results in health-related benefits, exercise to achieve health-related benefits appears to be easier for most people to incorporate into their lifestyle and thus provides a valuable exercise option.[26–28] The specific parameters

---

TABLE 12-2 Health-related Benefits from Performance of Regular Exercise

Decreased fatigue
Improved performance in work- and sports-related activities
Improved blood lipid profile
Enhanced immune function
Improved glucose tolerance and insulin sensitivity
Improved body composition
Enhanced sense of well-being
Decreased risk of coronary artery disease, cancer of the colon and breast, hypertension, type 2 diabetes mellitus, osteoporosis, anxiety, and depression

From Pate RR, Pratt M, Blair SN, et al. Physical activity and public health. *JAMA.* 1995;273:402–407 and American College of Sports Medicine. *Resource manual for guidelines for exercise testing and prescription.* 3rd ed. Baltimore: Williams & Wilkins; 1998.

---

necessary to achieve both fitness- and health-related benefits of aerobic exercise are presented later in this chapter.

CLINICAL GUIDELINES

Screening and Supervision of Exercise

Screening

Most individuals, particularly young, healthy clients, can begin a light to moderate exercise program without a medical examination or further testing. However, it is prudent to recommend that before the initiation of an exercise program, all individuals be screened to ensure safety, minimize risks, maximize benefits, and optimize adherence.[11] Preparticipation screening can be self-guided or professionally guided and should include an examination of readiness to participate in exercise, health history (including coronary artery disease [CAD] risk factors), and health behaviors.[29] The ACSM[29] has created an algorithm to delineate who should be medically examined before participation in vigorous exercise (defined as intensity of more than 60% $\dot{V}O_{2max}$).

The ACSM[29] recommends that informed individuals complete the Physical Activity Readiness Questionnaire (PAR-Q)[11,29,30] (Fig. 12-2) and/or the American Heart Association (AHA)/ACSM Health/Fitness Facility Preparticipation Screening Questionnaire.[29] Clients who do not require further medical evaluation include asymptomatic (Table 12-3)[29] women under the age of 55 and men under the age of 45 who have fewer than two CAD risk factors. These coronary risk factors include male family history of CAD at less than 55 years, female family history of CAD at less than 65 years, current or recent smoker (quit in past 6 months), hypertension ($\geq 140/\geq 90$), dyslipidemia (low-density lipoprotein >130 mg/dL, high-density lipoprotein <40 mg/dL, total cholesterol >200 mg/dL), impaired fasting glucose (>120 mg/dL), obesity (body mass index [BMI] >30), and sedentary lifestyle.[29]

Asymptomatic, apparently healthy men and women who are at low risk for CAD may begin a moderate exercise training program (defined as intensity between 40% and 60% $\dot{V}O_{2max}$) and do not need a medical examination or require exercise supervision. Clients who are at moderate or high risk of an untoward event during exercise, including those who answer yes to one of the seven questions on the PAR-Q should seek direction from their physicians before beginning an exercise program.

The clinician should study the client's health history to identify known diseases and symptoms that might indicate the presence of disease and therefore require modification of the exercise prescription. Specific diseases and conditions that should be noted because of their association with CAD

PAR-Q & YOU

(A Questionnaire for People Aged 15 to 69)

 1
Regular physical activity is fun and healthy, and increasingly more people are starting to become more active every day. Being more active is very safe for most people. However, some people should check with their doctor before they start becoming much more physically active.

If you are planning to become much more physically active that you are now, start by answering the seven questions in the box below. If you are between the ages of 15 and 69, the PAR-Q will tell you if you should check with your doctor before you start. If you are over 69 years of age, and you are not used to being very active, check with your doctor.

Common sense is your best guide when you answer these questions. Please read the questions carefully and answer each one honestly.

YES	NO	
_____	_____	1. Has your doctor ever said that you have a heart condition <u>and</u> that you should only do physical activity recommended by a doctor?
_____	_____	2. Do you feel pain in your chest when you do physical activity?
_____	_____	3. In the past month, have you had chest pain when you were not doing physical activity?
_____	_____	4. Do you lose your balance because of dizziness or do you ever lose consciousness?
_____	_____	5. Do you have a bone or joint problem that could be made worse by a change in your physical activity?
_____	_____	6. Is your doctor currently prescribing drugs (for example, water pills) for blood pressure or heart condition?
_____	_____	7. Do you know of *any other reason* why you should not do physical activity?

2 **If you answered YES to any questions:**

Talk to your doctor by phone or in person BEFORE you start becoming much more physicaly active or BEFORE you have a fitness appraisal. Tell your doctor about the PAR-Q and which questions you answered YES.

- You may be able to do any activity you want—as long as you start slowly and build up gradually. Or, you may need to restrict your activities to those which are safe for you. Talk with your doctor about the kinds of activities you wish to participate in and follow his/her advice.

- Find our which community programs are safe and helpful to you.

If you answered NO to all questions:

If you answered NO honestly to all PAR-Q questions, you can be reasonably sure that you can:

- start becoming much more physically active—begin slowly and build up gradually. This is the safest and easiest way to go.

- take part in a fitness appraisal—this is an excellent way to determine your basic fitness so that you can plan the best way for you to live actively.

Delay becoming much more active:

- if you are not feeling well because of temporary illness such as a cold or a fever—wait until your feel better; or

- if you are or may be pregnant—talk to your doctor before you start becoming more active.

3 Please note:

1. If your health changes so that you then answer YES to any of the above questions, tell your fitness or health professional. Ask whether you should change your physical activity plans.

2. Informed Use of the PAR-Q: The Canadian Society for Exercise Physiology, Health Canada, and their agents assume no liability for persons who undertake physical activity, and if in doubt after completing this questionnaire, consult your doctor prior to physical activity.

3. If the PAR-Q is being given to a person before he or she participates in a physical activity program or fitness appraisal, this section may be used for legal or administrative purposes.

I have read, understood and completed this questionnaire. Any questions I had were answered to my full satisfaction

Name _____

Signature _____ Date _____

Signature of Parent _____ Witness _____

or Guardian (for participants under the age of majority)

You are encouraged to copy the PAR-Q but only if you use the entire form.

©Canadian Society for Exercise Physiology *Supported by HealthCanada*
Sociéte Canadienne de Physiologie de L'exercise *Sante Canada*

Figure 12-2 The Physical Activity Readiness Questionnaire.

The Physical Activity Readiness Questionaire (PAR-Q) can be used to screen individuals 15 to 69 years old prior to participation in a moderate intensity exercise program. It was developed to identify those individuals for whom physical activity might be contraindicated or who need further medical evaluation prior to participation in exercise.

TABLE 12-3 Definition of an Asymptomatic Individual

No pain in the chest, neck, jaws, arms or other areas that suggest ischemia
No dyspnea (shortness of breath) at rest or with mild exertion
No dizziness or syncope (loss of consciousness)
No orthopnea (dyspnea at rest or while recumbent)
No ankle edema
No palpitations or tachycardia (unpleasant awareness of forceful or rapid beats)
No intermittent claudication (reproducible ischemic leg pain upon exertion)
No known heart murmur (due to faulty valve or other heart problem)
No unusual fatigue or shortness of breath with usual activities (secondary to cardiovascular, pulmonary, or metabolic disease)

Reprinted with permission from American College of Sports Medicine. *Guidelines for exercise testing and prescription.* 5th ed. Philadelphia: Lippincott, Williams & Wilkins; 2006.

include cardiovascular and respiratory disease, diabetes, obesity, hypertension, and abnormal blood lipid levels.[11]

Also relevant from the client's history are the individual's health behaviors, typically included in the assessment of social habits.[31] Alcohol and drug use, cigarette smoking, diet content, current activity level, and eating disorders should be reviewed because these factors may affect exercise prescription. Other factors that may affect the exercise prescription are medications, personality/behavior, and pregnancy and breast-feeding status.[11]

Supervision

A thorough screening or medical examination is critical for determining which individuals may require supervision during exercise.[29] Apparently healthy individuals do not require supervision during the performance of aerobic exercise, but individuals with two or more risk factors for CAD or who have documented CAD should be supervised during exercise. Supervision is also recommended for clients with cardiorespiratory disease.[29]

Graded Exercise Testing

The development of an appropriate and useful exercise prescription for cardiorespiratory endurance depends on an accurate examination of $\dot{V}O_{2max}$, which is most commonly achieved through the performance of a graded exercise test (GXT). Exercise tests can be maximal, in which clients perform to their physiologic or symptom limit, or submaximal, in which an arbitrary stopping or limiting criterion is used.

Maximal Graded Exercise Tests

The most important characteristics of a maximal GXT are a variable or graded workload that increases gradually and a total test time of 8 to 12 minutes.[29] In addition, individuals undergoing maximal GXT testing are usually monitored with an electrocardiogram (ECG).

The direct measurement of $\dot{V}O_{2max}$ involves the analysis of expired gases, which requires special equipment and personnel and is costly and time consuming.[29] However, $\dot{V}O_2$ can be estimated from prediction equations after the client exercises to the point of volitional fatigue, or it can be estimated from submaximal tests. For most clinicians, maximal exercise testing is not feasible because of the special equipment required and the ECG monitoring, although it is the most accurate test of aerobic capacity. Furthermore, it is recommended that maximal GXT be reserved for research purposes, testing of patients with specific diseases, and evaluation of athletes.[11] Therefore, submaximal testing is most commonly used, especially for low-risk, apparently healthy individuals. Clinicians who wish to conduct maximal GXT are referred to resources provided by the ACSM.[11,29]

Submaximal Graded Exercise Tests

Submaximal exercise tests can be used to estimate $\dot{V}O_{2max}$ because of the linear relationship between HR and $\dot{V}O_2$ and between HR and workload.[11] That is, as workload or $\dot{V}O_2$ increases, HR increases in a linear, predictable fashion. Therefore, $\dot{V}O_{2max}$ can be estimated by plotting HR against workload for at least two exercise workloads and extrapolating to the age-predicted maximum HR (220 − age).[29] The assumptions used for submaximal testing are presented in Table 12-4.

Failure to meet these assumptions fully, which is usually the case, results in errors in the predicted $\dot{V}O_{2max}$. Therefore, $\dot{V}O_{2max}$ measured by submaximal tests is less accurate than that measured by maximal tests. Submaximal tests are

TABLE 12-4 Assumptions for Using Submaximal Testing to Estimate $\dot{V}O_{2max}$

Workloads used are reproducible
Heart rate (HR) is allowed to reach steady state at each stage of the test
Age-predicted maximum HR is uniform (220 − age), with a prediction error of 12% to 15%
A linear relationship exists between HR and oxygen uptake
Mechanical efficiency is the same for everyone ($\dot{V}O_2$ at a given work rate)

Data from American College of Sports Medicine. *Resource manual for guidelines for exercise testing and prescription.* 3rd ed. Baltimore: Williams & Wilkins; 1998; and American College of Sports Medicine. *Guidelines for exercise testing and prescription.* 5th ed. Philadelphia: Lippincott Williams & Wilkins; 2006.

appropriately used to document change over time in response to aerobic training and, given the time and money saved, are clinically useful.

The ACSM[29] provides recommendations for physician supervision during GXT. For women under the age of 55 and men under the age of 45 with no risk factors or symptoms (as defined previously), physician supervision for maximal and submaximal testing is not deemed necessary. Older clients who have two or more risk factors but no symptoms or disease can undergo submaximal testing without physician supervision. Physician supervision during maximal testing is recommended for any individual with two or more risk factors of CAD. Finally, physician supervision is recommended for submaximal and maximal testing of clients with known cardiovascular, pulmonary, or metabolic disease. Therefore, physical therapists (PT) can safely perform submaximal testing of any aged client who is symptom or disease free (as defined by ACSM).[29]

Numerous testing protocols have been published and are available for submaximal exercise testing. Because of the requirement of reproducible workloads, treadmills, bicycle ergometers, and stepping protocols are most commonly used. Test selection should be based on safety concerns; staff familiarity with and knowledge of the testing protocol; equipment availability; and client goals, abilities, and conditions (such as orthopaedic limitations).

Bicycle Ergometer

A common bicycle ergometer test is the Åstrand-Ryhming protocol.[29] This test involves a single 6-minute stage, and workload is based on sex and activity status:

Unconditioned females: 300 to 450 kg/min (50 to 75 W).
Conditioned females: 450 to 600 kg/min (75 to 120 W).
Unconditioned males: 300 to 600 kg/min (50 to 120 W).
Conditioned males: 600 to 900 kg/min (120 to 150 W).

Individuals pedal at 50 revolutions/min, and HR is measured during the fifth and sixth minutes. The two HR measures must be within five beats of each other, and the HR must be between 130 and 170 bpm for the test data to be useful. If the HR is less than 130 bpm, the resistance should be increased by 50 to 120 W and the test continued for another 6 minutes. The test may be terminated when the HR in the fifth and sixth minutes differs by no more than five beats and is between 125 and 170 bpm. The average of the two HRs obtained during the fifth and sixth minutes is calculated, and a nomogram is used to estimate $\dot{V}O_{2max}$.[29] The value determined from the nomogram is multiplied by a correction factor to account for the age of the client (Fig. 12-3; Table 12-5).

For example, an unconditioned 40-year-old woman performed the test at a resistance of 75 W (450 kg/min) and attained a HR in the fifth minute of 150 bpm and a HR in the sixth minute of 154 bpm. Thus, the average HR used in the nomogram (Fig. 12-3) is 152 bpm. To use the nomogram, place the left end of a straightedge along the line for women with a pulse rate of 152 bpm (left side of the figure). The right end of the straightedge is now lined up at the appropriate workload for this woman: 450 kg/min. The point at which the straightedge crosses the $\dot{V}O_{2max}$ line indicates the client's estimated $\dot{V}O_{2max}$: 2.0 L/min. The estimated $\dot{V}O_{2max}$ (2.0 L/min) is then corrected for age by multiplying by 0.83 (Table 12-5) to yield a $\dot{V}O_{2max}$ of 1.66 L/min for this client.

Treadmill

Submaximal treadmill tests are also used to estimate $\dot{V}O_{2max}$.[29] A single-stage submaximal treadmill test was developed for testing low-risk clients. The test involves beginning with a comfortable walking pace between 2.0 and 4.5 miles per hour (mph) at 0% grade for a 2- to 4-minute warmup designed to increase the HR to within 50% to 75% of the age-predicted (220 − age) maximum HR, followed by 4 minutes at 5% grade at the same self-selected walking speed. HR is measured at the end of the 4-minute stage, and $\dot{V}O_{2max}$ is estimated using the following equation:

$$\dot{V}O_{2max} \text{ (mL/kg/min)} = 15.1 + (21.8 \times \text{speed [mph]})$$
$$\times (0.327 \times \text{HR [bpm]}) - (0.263 \times \text{speed} \times \text{age [years]})$$
$$+ (0.00504 \times \text{HR} \times \text{age}) + (5.98 \times \text{sex})$$

Sex is given a value of 0 for females and 1 for males.

Step

Step tests were developed to test large numbers of individuals expeditiously, and they represent another mode of submaximal exercise testing. Several protocols have been developed, but only one is presented here.[32] The Queens College Step Test requires a 16.25-inch step (similar to the height of a bleacher).[32,33] Individuals step up and down to a four-count rhythm:

Count 1: client places one foot on the step.
Count 2: client places the other foot on the step.
Count 3: the first foot is brought back to the ground.
Count 4: the second foot is brought down.

A metronome helps maintain the prescribed stepping beat. Females step for 3 minutes at a rate of 22 steps/min, and males step for 3 minutes at a rate of 24 steps/min. After 3 minutes a recovery 15-second pulse is measured, starting 5 seconds into recovery, while the client remains standing. The pulse rate obtained is converted to bpm by multiplying by four. This value is

Figure 12-3 The Åstrand-Rhyming nomogram is used to calculate aerobic capacity ($\dot{V}O_{2max}$) from pulse rate during submaximal work. Knowledge of the pulse rate, sex, and work load of a client allows the clinician to determine absolute $\dot{V}O_{2max}$. $\dot{V}O_{2max}$ values obtained from the nomogram should be adjusted for age by a correction factor (Table 12-5).

TABLE 12-5 Correction Factor for Age for Åstrand-Rhyming Nomogram

Age	Correction Factor
15	1.12
25	1.00
35	0.87
40	0.83
45	0.78
50	0.75
55	0.71
60	0.68
65	0.65

Reprinted with permission from American College of Sports Medicine. *Guidelines for exercise testing and prescription.* 5th ed. Philadelphia: Lippincott Williams & Wilkins; 2006.

termed the recovery HR. The following equations are then used to estimate $\dot{V}O_{2max}$:

Females: $\dot{V}O_{2max}$ (mL/kg/min) $= 65.81 - (0.1847$
$- $ recovery HR [bpm])

Males: $\dot{V}O_{2max}$ (mL/kg/min) $= 111.33 - (0.42$
$\times$ recovery HR [bpm])

Field

Field tests refer to exercise testing protocols that are derived from events performed outside, or "in the field." These tests are submaximal tests and, like the step test, are more practical for testing large groups of people. Field tests are appropriate when time and equipment are limited and for examining individuals over the age of 40. Although a variety of field tests exist, only the Cooper 12-minute test and the 1-mile walk test are presented.[33]

In the Cooper 12-minute test, individuals are instructed to cover the most distance possible in 12 minutes, preferably by running, although walking is acceptable. The distance covered in 12 minutes is recorded and $\dot{V}O_{2max}$ is estimated according to the following equation:

$\dot{V}O_{2max}$ (mL/kg/min) $= 35.97 \times$ (total miles run) $- 11.29$

The 1-mile walk test is another option in the submaximal field test category.[34] Individuals walk 1 mile as fast as possible, without running. The average HR for the last 2 minutes of the walk is recorded by a HR monitor. If a HR monitor is not available, a 15-second pulse can be measured immediately after the test is completed. $\dot{V}O_{2max}$ is estimated from the following equation:

$\dot{V}O_{2max}$ (mL/kg/min) $= 132.85 - (0.077$
$\times$ body weight [pounds]) $- (0.39 \times$ age [years])

$+ (6.32 \times$ sex) $- (3.26 \times$ elapsed time [minutes])
$- (0.16 \times$ HR [bpm])

Sex is scored 0 for females and 1 for males.

Monitoring

All clients should be closely monitored during exercise test performance. Vital signs should be examined before, during each stage or workload of the test, and after the test for 4 to 8 minutes of recovery.[11] In addition, a rating of perceived exertion (RPE) is commonly used to monitor exercise tolerance.[35] RPE refers to the "degree of heaviness and strain experienced in physical work as estimated according to a specific rating method"[35] and indicates overall perceived exertion. The Borg RPE Scale is shown in Table 12-6.[35] In addition, individuals should be monitored for signs and symptoms of exercise intolerance. The guidelines for stopping an exercise test are presented in Table 12-7.[29]

Summary—Graded Exercise Testing

Exercise testing serves several important functions. Maximal testing can be used to screen for the presence of CAD and to directly measure $\dot{V}O_{2max}$ in situations that require accuracy (research, athletic performance). Submaximal exercise testing is less accurate than maximal testing but is useful for establishing a baseline before initiating an exercise training program, for documenting improvement as a response to training, for motivating a client to adopt an exercise habit, and for formulating an exercise prescription based on physiologic parameters specific to the client.

TABLE 12-6 Rating of Perceived Exertion

Rating	Description
6	
7	Very, very light
8	
9	Very light
12	
11	Fairly light
12	
13	Somewhat hard
14	
15	Hard
16	
17	Very hard
18	
19	Very, very hard
20	

Reprinted with permission from American College of Sports Medicine. *Guidelines for exercise testing and prescription.* 5th ed. Philadelphia: Lippincott Williams & Wilkins; 2006.

TABLE 12-7 Guidelines for Cessation of an Exercise Test in a Typical Physical Therapy Clinic

---

Onset of angina or angina-like symptoms

Significant drop (20 mm Hg) in systolic blood pressure (SBP) or failure of SBP to rise with increase in exercise intensity

Excessive rise in SBP >260 mm Hg or diastolic BP >115 mm Hg

Signs of poor perfusion: lightheadedness, confusion, ataxia, pallor, cyanosis, nausea, cold or clammy skin

Failure of heart rate to increase with increased exercise intensity

Noticeable change in heart rhythm via palpation or auscultation

Client asks to stop

Physical or verbal manifestations of severe fatigue

Failure of the testing equipment

Based on information from the American College of Sports Medicine. *Guidelines for exercise testing and prescription.* 7th ed. Philadelphia: Lippincott Williams & Wilkins; 2006.

TECHNIQUES: EXERCISE PRESCRIPTION

An individualized exercise prescription has five components: intensity, duration, frequency, mode, and progression of activity. When possible, the exercise prescription should be based on an objective examination of the client's response to exercise. A primary objective of an exercise prescription is to assist in the adoption of regular physical activity as a lifestyle habit; thus, the PT and PTA should take into consideration the behavioral characteristics, personal goals, and exercise preferences of the client.[29] Furthermore, the exercise prescription should function to improve physical fitness, reduce body fat, and improve cardiorespiratory endurance, depending on the specific goals of the individual. The PT and PTA should recognize that a thorough exercise prescription should include activities that address all elements of health-related physical fitness (cardiorespiratory endurance, body composition, muscular endurance, strength, and flexibility); however, this chapter focuses only on cardiorespiratory endurance.

Intensity

Exercise intensity indicates how much exercise should be performed or how hard the client should exercise and is typically prescribed on the basis of maximal HR (HR_{max}), $HR_{reserve}$, $\dot{V}O_{2max}$, or RPE. Prescribing exercise intensity using HR is considered the preferred method because of the correlation between HR and stress on the heart and because it is easy to monitor during exercise.[4] This is especially true with young healthy clients or individuals who are not taking medications that affect their HR. One method of prescribing exercise is to use a percentage of HR_{max}, either directly determined by a GXT or estimated on the basis of the age-predicted maximum HR (220 − age). The training range should be between 64% to 70% and 94% of HR_{max}.[29]

A second method for prescribing exercise involves the use of the $HR_{reserve}$, or the Karvonen formula:

$$HR_{reserve} = (HR_{max} - HR_{rest}) \times (training\ range) + HR_{rest}$$

Training range is a value between 0.40 to 0.50 and 0.94, selected by the PT.

The Karvonen method is preferable as percent HR values correspond directly to percent $\dot{V}O_{2max}$ values. If exercise is prescribed based on $\dot{V}O_{2max}$, 50% to 85% is also used as a training range. If RPE is the base, the prescribed exercise intensity is within the range of 12 to 16 (Table 12-6). The RPE is especially useful for prescribing intensity for individuals who are unable to take their pulse or when HR is altered because of the influence of medication. The use of RPE should be considered an adjunct to monitoring HR in all other individuals.[29]

Selection of an appropriate training range, as opposed to a specific training value, has been recommended to provide greater flexibility in the exercise prescription while ensuring that a training response will be achieved.[4] For example, a client who is starting out on an exercise program might be given a target HR at the lower end of the range (e.g., between 64% and 70% of HR_{max}), instead of being told to keep the target HR at 90% of HR_{max}. Health-related benefits can be realized at lower intensities, and thus lower intensities may be appropriate if the goal of exercise is to improve health instead of fitness.[36]

Duration

The length of time spent exercising is described by the component of duration. The optimal duration recommended for aerobic training is between 20 to 60 minutes per exercise session.[4,29] For individuals who are unable to perform 20 minutes of continuous exercise, discontinuous exercise can be prescribed. That is, several 12-minute bouts can be performed, for example, until the client can tolerate 20 to 30 minutes of continuous exercise. Duration can be progressed up to 60 minutes of continuous activity.[29]

Duration should also include warmup (5 to 15 minutes) and cooldown (5 to 12 minutes) activities in addition to the aerobic component. The warmup slowly increases the HR and respiratory rate and will reduce muscle soreness. The warmup can include gentle stretching activities and low-intensity training using the mode selected for aerobic conditioning.[4] An appropriate cooldown can be accomplished by gradually reducing the intensity of the endurance activity and continuing beyond the duration of the training period at a low level. Stretching activities are also appropriate as part of the cooldown and enhance flexibility.

Frequency

A second time-related component of exercise prescription is frequency, or how often exercise should be performed. The optimal frequency for most individuals is three to five times per week.[4,29] Clients who are fairly fit should begin a program at three to four times per week and progress to five times. Individuals with low functional capacities can perform daily or twice-daily exercise because the total amount of exercise (considering intensity, duration, and frequency) is low.[29]

The PT and PTA should consider the interaction of intensity, duration, and frequency for clients who are not capable of meeting the minimal criteria. These factors are also important for clients who exceed the suggested limits of exercise because of the increased risk for musculoskeletal injury as a result of overtraining.

Mode

The question of which activity to perform is addressed by the component of mode in the exercise prescription. Generally, the greatest improvement in aerobic capacity is achieved through rhythmic activities that involve large muscle groups, such as walking, running, hiking, cycling, rowing, and swimming.[29] A wide variety of activities can be prescribed to improve cardiorespiratory endurance, but it has been suggested that unfit individuals start out with activities that can be maintained at a constant intensity, such as cycling and treadmill walking. Once a basic level of fitness has been obtained, activities with variable intensity, such as team and individual sports and dancing, can be prescribed.[4,29]

Consideration should also be given to potential orthopaedic stresses produced by the selected mode.[29] For example, an obese client might reap greater benefits and a decreased risk of injury with a nonweight-bearing activity (cycling, water aerobics) than with a weight-bearing activity (walking, running). Individuals are more likely to engage in activities they enjoy and have access to; fortunately, there is a wide variety of modes available to enhance compliance with the exercise prescription.

Figures 12-4 to 12-10 illustrate aerobic activities commonly performed on equipment that meet the criteria for appropriate exercise. These exercises involve large muscle groups; are appropriate for enhancing cardiovascular fitness if proper guidelines for intensity, duration, and frequency are followed; and can be used in a clinical setting. The purpose of each activity is to increase aerobic capacity. The client should be able to perform the exercise at a level based

on previous activity and tolerance to stress. Compliance is enhanced if the client finds the exercise enjoyable. The procedure for each exercise is based on the intensity, duration, frequency, and progression that the PT prescribes for the client. The client is thus provided with an individualized exercise prescription and treatment plan for safely and efficiently increasing aerobic capacity.

Progression

The final component of the exercise prescription is progression, or how the program changes over time. An aerobic exercise program may progress through a series of stages: initiation, improvement, and maintenance.

Initial Stage

The initial stage is designed to enable the individual to slowly adapt to the exercise program and lasts 1 to 6 weeks.[12,29] The parameters of the prescription are set at low ranges so that exercise is prescribed at 40% to 60% of $HR_{reserve}$ or $\dot{V}O_{2max}$ (RPE of 11 to 12), duration is set between 15 and 30 minutes per session, and frequency is prescribed for three to four times per week on nonconsecutive days. Individuals who are not experienced with exercise or who have lower aerobic capacities should begin at the low end of the ranges provided (e.g., 40% of $HR_{reserve}$, 15 minutes per session, three times per week). Clients who have experience with exercise or who have higher aerobic capacities can begin at the higher end of the ranges.

Improvement Stage

Progression to the improvement stage is recommended when the client can perform the exercise prescription independently at a frequency of five to six sessions per week for a duration of 30 to 40 minutes per session for 2 weeks without signs of musculoskeletal overuse or excessive fatigue.[11] Progression continues during the improvement stage but at a faster rate than in the initiation stage.[29] This stage lasts 4 to 8 months and involves increases in intensity to the higher ranges (50% to 85% $HR_{reserve}$ or $\dot{V}O_{2max}$) and consistent increases in duration to 20 to 30 minutes continuously.

Duration should be increased up to 20% per week until clients are able to complete 20 to 30 minutes of moderate- to vigorous-intensity exercise. Frequency can then be increased until a frequency goal is reached. Thereafter, intensity can be increased no more than 5% of $HR_{reserve}$ every sixth session.[29] Interval training in which one higher-intensity session per week is added or using extended higher-intensity work intervals are very helpful in gaining increases in aerobic capacity during this stage of training.[29]

Although these general guidelines are helpful, the client's objective and subjective training responses should

Figure 12-4	Recumbent bicycle.

ADVANTAGES: Seat is more comfortable than that of a traditional bicycle; back support provides a more upright spine posture; relatively quiet to operate; easy to monitor/measure vital signs during use; safer than a traditional bicycle due to a wider base of support and ease of mounting and dismounting.[11]

DISADVANTAGES: Local muscle fatigue in the lower extremities may limit performance; difficult to elevate heart rate to target range due to the more supine position required on the recumbent bicycle compared with a traditional bicycle or other modes of upright exercise.

FIT: Seat position should be adjusted to allow 15 to 20 degrees of knee flexion when the lower extremity is in the most outstretched position on the pedal and the ankle is at 90 degrees of dorsiflexion. (Courtesy of Lifefitness, Franklin Park, IL)

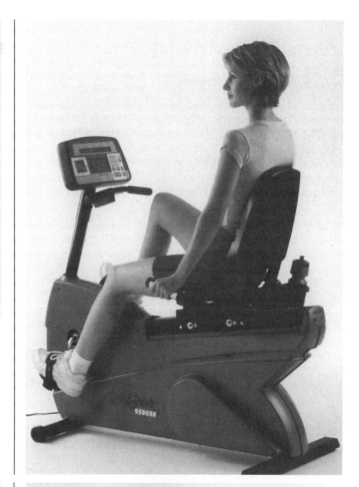

Figure 12-5	Stationary bicycle.

ADVANTAGES: Allows nonweight-bearing exercise, no impact.

Relatively quiet to operate; easy to monitor/measure vital signs during use; requires little time/effort for habituation.

DISADVANTAGES: Local muscle fatigue in the lower extremities may limit performance; difficult to elevate heart rate to target range due to muscle fatigue limitation; not all clients are familiar with or experienced with bicycling; no weight bearing achieved.

FIT: Seat position should be adjusted to allow 15 to 20 degrees of knee flexion when the foot is in the lowest position on the pedal and the ankle is in 90 degrees of dorsiflexion. (Courtesy of Lifefitness, Franklin Park, IL)

Figure 12-6   Nu-Step recumbent stepper.

ADVANTAGES: Large seat provides a comfortable form of sitting activity; motion of stepping is familiar to most clients so habituation is minimal; provides low-impact form of activity; safer than a traditional stair climber due to a wider base of support and ease of mounting and dismounting; utilizes all four limbs so is considered a total body exercise, and clients can easily achieve target heart rate.

DISADVANTAGES: No weight bearing achieved; may be difficult to measure vital signs due to involvement of upper extremities during exercise.

FIT: Seat should be adjusted to allow slight knee flexion when lower extremity is in most extended position. (Courtesy of Lalonde & Co, Ann Arbor, MI)

Figure 12-7   Stair climber.

ADVANTAGES: The motion of stepping is familiar to most clients so habituation is minimal; provides weight bearing; provides a low-impact form of activity; occupies less space than most other types of equipment.

DISADVANTAGES: May aggravate or cause knee problem due to stress on knee joints; posture on the equipment should be carefully scrutinized due to tendency for users to adopt poor postures and rely too much on upper extremities for support; somewhat difficult to mount; requires good balance. (Courtesy of Lifefitness, Franklin Park, IL)

Figure 12-8 Treadmill.

ADVANTAGES: Walking/running are familiar activities for most clients so habituation is minimal; provides weight bearing; uses large lower-extremity muscles that require less energy, enabling heart rate to be elevated and kept in target range without local muscle fatigue; easy to adjust intensity (speed and/or elevation).

DISADVANTAGES: Weight-bearing exercise may be difficult for obese clients or for those with orthopaedic limitations; requires a lot of space; expensive; difficult to monitor/measure vital signs when clients walk fast or run; tends to makes significant noise when in use (making it difficult to hear blood pressure). (Courtesy of Lifefitness, Franklin Park, IL)

Figure 12-9 Total-body system.

ADVANTAGES: Utilizes all four limbs so is considered a total-body exercise, and clients can easily achieve target heart rate; low impact.

DISADVANTAGES: Requires greater coordination than other modes of activity so takes client longer to habituate; requires greater floor space than other pieces of equipment; difficult to monitor/measure vital signs due to involvement of upper extremities during exercise; difficult to mount/dismount. (Courtesy of Lifefitness, Franklin Park, IL)

most heavily influence training progression.[11] Signs and symptoms of inappropriately paced progression include inability to complete an exercise session, decreased interest in training, increased HR and RPE values at the same workload, and increased complaints of aches and pains.[37]

Adjustments in the rate of progression should be made for the elderly and deconditioned because of their increased time required for adaptation.[29] Together, the initial and improvement stages may take up to 8 or 9 months and result in a 5% to 30% increase in aerobic capacity.[11,36]

| Figure 12-10 | Upper-body ergometer. |

ADVANTAGES: Eliminates lower extremities for those with significant lower-extremity impairments, while providing a mechanism to perform aerobic exercise; easy to mount/dismount; relatively quiet to operate.

DISADVANTAGES: Local muscle fatigue limits performance; lower heart rates are achieved due to the use of smaller muscles; unfamiliar for most clients so requires greater habituation time; difficult to monitor/measure vital signs during activity.

FIT: Seat should be adjusted to allow slight elbow flexion during maximum upper-extremity extension while back maintains contact with seat; seat height should be adjusted so that client shoulder height is even with axis of arm crank. (Courtesy of Henley Healthcare, Sugar Land, TX.)

Maintenance Stage

During the maintenance stage of training further improvement in aerobic capacity is minimal and the focus is on maintaining aerobic fitness above the 50th percentile.[29] Additionally, clients should be encouraged to diversify their exercise mode and begin to enjoy exercise as a lifetime habit.[11] It is important to realize that fitness level will decrease about 50% within 4 to 12 weeks if a maintenance program is not performed, indicating the importance of prescribing activities that are similar in energy cost to the activities performed during the improvement stage.

Activity diversification is therefore suggested to decrease boredom and increase enjoyment, decrease the potential for overuse injuries, add competition to the program, if desired, and explore new interests.[11,28] For example, a client who was new to exercise and began a training program with treadmill walking or with a cycling program, because of the ability to carefully control and monitor workload, could participate in water exercise or soccer during the maintenance stage. Additional physical activities can substitute for activities performed in the earlier stages so that the total training volume stays the same to maintain aerobic conditioning. Individuals training for competition, which usually occurs during the maintenance stage, can diversify training on noncompetition days to decrease overuse, rotate muscle groups to spread out stresses, and maintain cardiovascular fitness.[11]

It is also appropriate to review training goals, repeat exercise testing, and establish new goals during the maintenance stage so that the participant will be more likely to continue exercising as a regular habit. The documented success of programs designed to encourage the adoption of a regular exercise habit is similar to the success of changing other health-related behaviors, such as cessation of smoking and weight reduction. Approximately 50% of clients who initiate such health-related behaviors reach the maintenance stage.[38]

Compliance

Factors that best predict exercise dropout (or noncompliance) are related to the client, program, and other characteristics. Personal characteristics that predict dropout are smoking, sedentary leisure time, sedentary occupation, type A personality, blue-collar occupation, overweight or overfat, poor self-image, depression, anxiety, and a poor credit rating.[39] Program factors that predict dropout include inconvenient time or location, excessive costs, high intensity, lack of variety, solo participation, lack of positive feedback, inflexible goals, and poor leadership. Additional factors that have been identified to predict dropouts are lack of spouse support, inclement weather, excessive job travel, injury, medical problems, and job change or move. These factors in sum indicate that the PT and PTA should develop specific strategies to enhance compliance with the exercise prescription.[40] Table 12-8 lists some of these strategies.

The use of behavior change theories to enhance the adoption of exercise has recently received increased attention in the literature, specifically the application of the "stages of change" model.[28,39,41,42] The model posits that individuals cycle along a continuum of behavioral change from precontemplation (no intention to make a change) to contemplation (considering a change) to preparation

---

TABLE 12-8 Suggested Strategies for Enhancing Compliance with Exercise Prescriptions

Minimize musculoskeletal injuries by adhering to principles of exercise prescription

Encourage group participation or exercising with a partner

Emphasize variety of modes of activities and enjoyment in the program

Incorporate behavioral techniques and base prescription on theories of behavior change

Use periodic testing to document progress

Give immediate feedback to reinforce behavior changes

Recognize accomplishments

Invite client's partner to become involved and support training program

Ensure that exercise leaders are qualified and enthusiastic

Reprinted with permission from Franklin BA. Program factors that influence exercise adherence: practical adherence skills for the clinical staff. In: Dishman RK, ed. *Exercise adherence*. Champaign, IL: Human Kinetics; 1988:237–258.

(beginning to make changes) to action (actively engaging in the new behavior) to maintenance (sustaining the change over time).[42] Researchers have shown that pre-exercise identification of the client's stage can be used to target an intervention approach that will enhance movement toward maintenance.[42] Assessment of the stage is easily accomplished via a five-item questionnaire; one item represents each stage (Table 12-9).

Once the stage is identified, the intervention can be tailored to enhance compliance and movement toward maintenance. For example, an individual in the contemplation stage is not quite ready for an exercise prescription. Efforts in this stage should focus on providing information about the costs and benefits of exercise, strategies to increase activity within the present lifestyle, and the social benefits of activity. Clients in the preparation stage benefit most from a thorough examination and exercise prescription. Clients in the action or maintenance stage benefit from learning about strategies to prevent relapse, making

exercise enjoyable, and diversifying the exercise prescription to include more variety. Given the difficulty most people encounter when changing health-related behaviors, it seems prudent to use documented behavior change theories when possible, such as the stages of change model.

Summary—Exercise Prescription

A scientifically based exercise prescription includes the elements of intensity, duration, frequency, mode, and progression. The program is individualized, based on objective data obtained from a thorough examination and on psychosocial factors unique to the client. Compliance with an exercise prescription is most likely achieved when the prescription meets the needs and goals of the individual and is based on recognized scientific principles and theoretic models.

TABLE 12-9 Questionnaire to Determine the Stage of Change of a Client

Stage	Question
Precontemplation	"I presently do not exercise and do not plan to start exercising in the next 6 months"
Contemplation	"I presently do not exercise, but I have been thinking about starting to exercise within the next 6 months"
Preparation	"I presently get some exercise but not regularly"
Action	"I presently exercise on a regular basis, but I have begun doing so only within the past 6 months"
Maintenance	"I presently exercise on a regular basis and have been doing so for longer than 6 months"

Reprinted with permission from Marcus BH, Simkin LR. The stages of exercise behavior. *J Sports Med Phys Fitness*. 1993;33:83–88.

CASE STUDY 1

PATIENT INFORMATION

A 46-year-old woman presented with a right medial meniscus repair via arthroscopy 10 weeks ago. Review of history revealed hypercholesterolemia for 1 year and hysterectomy 4 years ago. The patient was currently taking 30 mg of atorvastatin (cholesterol-lowering medication) once a day. Initially, the patient was treated immediately after the surgery for knee rehabilitation; the knee pain had resolved, and she was discharged with all goals achieved. Now that her knee pain was resolved, her goals were to start exercising again for the purposes of decreasing cholesterol, staying healthy, and decreasing body weight (she would like to lose 20 pounds).

Health history examination revealed no family history of CAD, no smoking/alcohol/drug use, and no eating disorders. She was presently consuming a low-fat diet since her diagnosis of hypercholesterolemia. Physical examination by the PT revealed a height of 5 feet, 4 inches (1.65 meters), weight of 160 pounds (72.7 kg), BMI of 27 kg/m^2. Resting vital signs were HR of 86, BP of 132/80, and RR of 16. Right knee had 0-degree extension, 120-degree flexion, 5/5 hamstrings, 4+/5 quadriceps, and hips and ankles within normal limits for range of motion (ROM) and strength bilaterally. Gait was without deviation. Pain was 0/10 except after significant walking/standing, which she rated as a 2/10. She had returned to work full time and was independent in activities of daily living. The patient completed the PAR-Q and answered "yes" to questions 5 and 6 (Fig. 12-2).

LINKS TO
GUIDE TO PHYSICAL THERAPIST PRACTICE

The primary pattern from the *Guide to Physical Therapist Practice* that applies to this Patient is Pattern 4J: impaired joint mobility, motor function, muscle performance, and ROM associated with bony or soft tissue surgical procedures.[31] Meniscal repairs are included within this pattern, which lists aerobic endurance activities under specific direct interventions. A secondary pattern for this patient would be Pattern 6A: primary prevention/risk factor reduction for cardiopulmonary disorders; since this patient has hypercholesterolemia, a risk factor for CAD. Aerobic conditioning activities are also included as a specific direct intervention in Pattern 6A.

INTERVENTION

This patient returned under her previous prescription for knee rehabilitation. Due to the patient's age and sex, PAR-Q results, and presence of one (hypercholesterolemia) and possibly two (sedentary lifestyle) risk factors for CAD, the referring physician was contacted to discuss whether or not the patient required further medical screening prior to commencing an exercise program. After a discussion with the patient's primary care physician, it was determined that the patient should undergo a submaximal GXT with supervision and monitoring, followed by 1 week of supervised exercise training. If the patient was symptom free during the supervised exercise period, an independent exercise program would be prescribed.

Since the patient was 10 weeks after surgery and an unconditioned individual, the Åstrand-Rhyming bicycle ergometer submaximal GXT was selected and administered to the patient. She completed 6 minutes of exercise at a workload of 450 kg/min (as recommended for unconditioned women) with a resulting HR at both the fifth and sixth minute of 130 bpm. Using the nomogram in Figure 12-3 and plotting a line from a HR of 130 (for women) and a work load of 450 kg/min (for women), the line falls on a $\dot{V}O_{2max}$ estimate of 2.8 L/min. Using the correction factor for her age of 0.78 (Table 12-5), the adjusted $\dot{V}O_{2max}$ estimate for the patient was 2.2 L/min. Converting her absolute $\dot{V}O_{2max}$ to relative $\dot{V}O_{2max}$ {2.2 L/min × 1,000 mL/L − 72.7 kg [weight of patient] = 30.3 mL/kg/min} resulted in a predicted relative $\dot{V}O_{2max}$ of 30.3 mL/kg/min. According to Table 12-10, which shows the normal $\dot{V}O_{2max}$ values by adjusted age and sex, the patient fell within the normal range (32 ± 21 mL/kg/min).

According to the stages of change model, this patient was in the preparation stage, indicating that she was ready to adopt a regular exercise habit and was ready for an exercise prescription for guidance. According to recent guidelines, a BMI of 27 kg/m^2 classified the patient as overweight (BMI <25 = normal, 25 to <30 = overweight, 30 or more = obese).[45] Given her overweight status and the patient's goals, a lower-intensity, longer-duration program was thought to

TABLE 12-10 Normal Values of $\dot{V}O_{2max}$ (mL/kg/min) Uptake at Different Ages by Sex

Age	Male	Female
20–29	43 (± 22)	36 (± 21)
30–39	42 (± 22)	34 (± 21)
40–49	40 (± 22)	32 (± 21)
50–59	36 (± 22)	29 (± 22)
60–69	33 (± 22)	27 (± 22)
70–79	29 (± 22)	27 (± 22)

Reprinted with permission from American College of Sports Medicine. *Resource manual for guidelines for exercise testing and prescription.* 3rd ed. Baltimore: Williams & Wilkins; 1998.

be an appropriate prescription to decrease the risk of musculoskeletal injury and maximize weight loss. A recommended goal for weight loss was 1 to 2 pounds per week[11] through nutrition changes and exercise. Since she had already adopted a low-fat diet, the exercise program was thought to assist in her goal to lose weight.

Because she reported knee pain after walking, the exercise program was initially prescribed on the bicycle. The PT established a program to be progressed to walking as her knee and fitness level allowed and asked a PTA to assist with interventions. The initial prescription was as follows:

Intensity: Using the Karvonen equation and 40% to 60% as the beginning HR range, the following target HR range was calculated:

Target HR at 40% $HR_{reserve} = ([HR_{max} - HR_{rest}] \times 0.4) + HR_{rest} = ([174 - 86] \times 0.4) + 86 = 121$ bpm

Target HR at 60% $HR_{reserve} = ([HR_{max} - HR_{rest}] \times 0.6) + HR_{rest} = ([174 - 86] \times 0.6) + 86 = 139$ bpm

Training HR range was set at 121 to 139 bpm. Referring back to her submaximal GXT, the workload required to achieve the training HR range could be determined. The patient achieved a HR of 135 bpm at a workload of 450 kg/min of resistance on the bicycle ergometer. Therefore, initial workload was set at that level and the HR monitored to determine whether resistance should be increased or decreased. The RPE was also to be used to monitor intensity at an initial level of 12 to 13.

Duration: Following a warmup of 5 minutes of gentle ROM and stretching exercises and 5 minutes of no load on the bicycle, the patient was to pedal for 15 to 20 minutes, increasing 5 minutes per week to the goal of 30 to 40 minutes. The patient concluded the exercise training portion with 3 minutes of cooldown on the bike at no load and 5 to 10 minutes of stretching.

Frequency: The patient exercised three times per week the first week in the clinic where she could be supervised, progressing to five times per week, as tolerated.

Mode: Stationary bicycle ergometer (Fig. 12-5).

The initial goals of the program were to become independent in pulse taking and monitoring of exercise, perform the exercise prescription independently, and progress to exercising at 450 kg/min for 35 to 40 minutes four to five times per week by the fourth week. The PTA documented that the patient was independent in pulse taking and the home exercise program. The PTA also noted that the patient was able to perform aerobic conditioning with a perceived exertion of 11 and a HR of 110 bpm after 20 minutes on the stationary bicycle.

PROGRESSION

THREE TO FOUR WEEKS AFTER INITIAL EXAMINATION

The patient experienced no signs or symptoms of exercise intolerance during the first week of supervised exercise and was able to complete the exercise as prescribed. She was given a home program and returned for re-examination after the fourth week, at which time she was exercising on the bicycle at 450 kg/min for 35 minutes continuously four to five times per week. The program was modified by increasing the training HR range to 60% to 70% of $HR_{reserve}$, or 139 to 147 bpm (RPE = 13–14). This intensity required the patient to set a higher workload on the bicycle (500–600 kg/min). The duration was decreased to 20 minutes initially to offset the increase in intensity, and she was instructed to increase the duration by 5 minutes per week until she reached 40 minutes. The frequency was continued at three to five times per week. The PTA continued to work with the patient, noting an increase in duration to 40 minutes with the stationary bicycle.

THREE MONTHS AFTER INITIAL EXAMINATION

The patient had successfully completed the training program on the bicycle over the previous 2 months and was currently exercising three to five times per week at 500 to 600 kg/min for 40 minutes. The PTA reported that the patient was spending approximately 1 hour exercising three to five times per week as a result of the aerobic training and wished to maintain the time frame. The PTA instructed the patient to add walking to her program now on alternate days to increase overall energy expenditure. The patient was told to use HR as a guide and to start out walking 20 minutes fast enough to elicit a HR in the training range of 139 to 147 bpm or RPE = 13 to 14. The patient was instructed to increase duration by no more than 5 minutes per week. The patient was scheduled for a return examination in 3 months, when a repeat GXT would be performed to examine progress.

SIX MONTHS AFTER INITIAL EXAMINATION

At the 6-month re-examination the patient weighed 146 pounds (66.36 kg) and her resting HR was 78 bpm. She had been exercising 5 to 6 days per week, 3 days on the bicycle and 2 to 3 days walking. She was able to increase her target HR into the prescribed range by cycling at 600 kg/min and by walking as fast as she could. A follow-up submaximal test was performed at the 6-month re-examination. The Åstrand Rhyming bicycle ergometer protocol was repeated. This time the patient completed 6 minutes of exercise at a workload of 600 kg/min with a resulting HR at both the fifth and sixth minutes of 138 bpm. Using the nomogram in Figure 12-3 and plotting a line from a HR of 138 (for women) and a work load of 600 kg/min (for women), the line falls on a $\dot{V}O_{2max}$ estimate of 3.0 L/min. Using the correction factor for her age of 0.78 (Table 12-5), the adjusted $\dot{V}O_{2max}$ estimate for the patient was 2.3 L/min. Converting her absolute $\dot{V}O_{2max}$ to relative $\dot{V}O_{2max}$ (2.3 L/min × 1,000 mL/L − 66.36 kg [new weight of patient] = 35.2 mL/kg/min) resulted in a predicted relative $\dot{V}O_{2max}$ = 35.2 mL/kg/min. The patient's predicted $\dot{V}O_{2max}$ had increased approximately 15% over the 6-month training period and she had lost approximately 15 pounds.

OUTCOMES

The PTA worked with the patient to help her with strategies to reinforce the adoption of regular exercise. The patient revealed her intention to continue exercising regularly. She had established a relationship with a neighbor with whom she walked and she was satisfied using the stationary bicycle because it was at home and convenient. A new exercise prescription was given to the patient by the PT using an intensity of 70% to 80% $HR_{reserve}$ (145–155 bpm), which would require a resistance of between 600 and 750 kg/min on the bicycle ergometer. The patient had achieved the initial goals set, although she had lost 15 pounds instead of her goal to lose 20; but she was confident that with continued exercise she would lose another 5 pounds and maintain her weight at that level.

SUMMARY—AN EFFECTIVE PT–PTA TEAM

This case study demonstrates components of an effective working relationship of the PT and PTA. The documentation that was performed was effective and created effective communication of the treatment of the patient. The PTA should document any data collections that are done such as the RPE and HR. The PTA in this situation could have assisted the PT with the submaximal GXT testing and also gathered other critical information about the patient's cardiovascular fitness throughout treatment.

Cardiac Rehabilitation

Estimates for the year 2002 (the last year for which estimates are available) were that more than 70 million Americans would have one or more forms of CVD.[43] Since 1900 (with the exception of 1918) CVD has been the leading cause of death in America.[43] In 2002 CVD accounted for 38.0% of all deaths in the United States.[43] Coronary heart disease (myocardial infarction, other acute ischemic coronary heart disease, angina pectoris, atherosclerotic CVD, and all other forms of heart disease) accounts for the majority of these deaths and is the single largest killer of American men and women.[43] Atherosclerotic disease is a progressive process in which lipids, macrophages, T lymphocytes, smooth muscle cells, extracellular matrix, and calcium accumulate in the intimal layer of arteries. This accumulation causes a thickening and narrowing of the vessel lumen.[44] Over time this process continues and the developing atheroma is covered by a fibrous cap. Eventually the atheroma can develop into an aneurysm, grow

large enough to occlude the vessel or rupture and cause occlusion. This process can affect coronary, cerebral, peripheral vascular, aortic, renal, and other blood vessels.

PTAs treat patients with atherosclerotic disease everyday. It is extremely likely that the adult physical therapy patient, regardless of reason for referral, has atherosclerotic disease. While much attention is paid to the care of orthopaedic and neurologic patients, greater attention must be paid to treating patients with atherosclerotic disease. As stated so eloquently by Falkel,[45] "no one ever died of a sprained ankle." The focus of this section is to present basic principles of cardiac rehabilitation. The PTA should be aware that the low-intensity exercise guidelines described below can and should be used for any patient for whom the risk of exercise is either uncertain or moderate to high.

In the United States in the early 1900s myocardial infarction patients were almost completely immobilized with bed rest for at least 6 to 8 weeks.[46] In fact, patients were prevented from climbing stairs for at least 1 year and most patients never returned to work or normal living.[46]

This trend continued until the 1940s when Levine encouraged patients to sit in a chair for 1 to 2 hours per day, beginning the first day after a myocardial infarction. By the mid-1960s and early 1970s pioneers such as Wenger, Hellerstein, Pifer, DeBusk, Acker, and Zohman studied and promoted early mobilization following myocardial infarction.[46] Their views were unique and completely opposite conventional medical practice. Because of their common sense, wisdom, and tenacity, as well as the eventual support of other organizations, (American Heart Association [AHA], American College of Sports Medicine [ACSM], and American Association of Cardiovascular and Pulmonary Rehabilitation [AACVPR]), the morbidity and mortality of many patients with cardiac diseases have been positively affected. These organizations have published guidelines for developing and maintaining safe and efficacious cardiac rehabilitation programs.[29,47,48] Unfortunately, representation from the American Physical Therapy Association is absent from the authorship of these authoritative texts and position papers.

SCIENTIFIC BASIS

Two research groups[49,50] performed meta-analysis of randomized, controlled studies to determine if cardiac rehabilitation programming had a beneficial effect on the participants. These studies involved almost 9,000 patients. Most of the patients in these studies participated in supervised exercise training for 2 to 6 months followed by unsupervised exercise. Researchers reported that cardiac rehabilitation program participants die at a lower rate following cardiac rehabilitation than do nonparticipants. Although participant and nonparticipant groups may both suffer reinfarction at a similar rate, nonparticipants in cardiac rehabilitation are more likely to die from that event.[49,50] Therefore, a regular exercise program may play an important role in the survival of a person who has had an infarction following cardiac rehabilitation. Although this phenomenon cannot be easily explained, enhanced survival may occur due to an enhanced electrical stability, reduced ventricular fibrillation, or reduced myocardial damage.

In addition, other submaximal exercise benefits of cardiac rehabilitation include a reduction in exercise HR, SBP, ischemic response, and rate–pressure product. Other benefits noted following cardiac rehabilitation include increases in the rate–pressure product at the onset of angina, peak oxygen consumption, quality of life, and exercise capacity.[51,52] Exercised patients have fewer cardiac events and hospital readmissions.[51] Significant reductions in risk factors also occur following comprehensive cardiac rehabilitation and include reductions in serum cholesterol, triglycerides, and low-density lipoprotein cholesterol, as well as increases in high-density lipoprotein cholesterol and significantly slower progression in coronary stenoses.[52,53] While comprehensive cardiac rehabilitation programs have been shown to benefit patients in the areas of smoking cessation, weight loss, resting BP and symptomology, more

randomized, controlled research trials need to be conducted related to these important issues.[54]

Cardiac Rehabilitation Defined

The term cardiac rehabilitation refers to "coordinated, multifaceted interventions designed to optimize a cardiac patient's physical, psychological, and social functioning, in addition to stabilizing, slowing, or even reversing the progression of the underlying atherosclerotic processes, thereby reducing morbidity and mortality."[55] Thus, cardiac rehabilitation/secondary prevention programs currently include baseline patient assessments, nutritional counseling, aggressive risk factor management (i.e., lipids, hypertension, weight, diabetes, and smoking), psychosocial and vocational counseling, and physical activity counseling and exercise training. In addition, the appropriate use of cardioprotective drugs that have evidence-based efficacy for secondary prevention is included.[48]

Patients who participate in cardiac rehabilitation programs include individuals who have had a recently diagnosed myocardial infarction or stable angina pectoris or have undergone coronary artery bypass graft surgery or angina. Other patients include those who have undergone percutaneous coronary artery balloon angioplasty/stents, arthrotomy, or heart transplantation (or candidates). Patients who have stable heart failure, peripheral arterial disease with claudication, or other forms of heart disease may also participate. Patients who have undergone other cardiac surgical procedures such as valvular repair or replacement are obvious candidates for cardiac rehabilitation.

Although individuals with the aforementioned surgical repairs or pathologies are clearly in need of a formal, supervised cardiac rehabilitation program, insurance reimbursement varies. The cost of cardiac rehabilitation should be discussed with the patient and family and permission from their insurance company should be sought upon referral.

Provision of Cardiac Rehabilitation

Historically a number of types of professionals have been involved in providing cardiac rehabilitation services. One of the most important personnel is the medical director, who may be a cardiothoracic surgeon, cardiologist, internist, emergency physician, or other physician with a specific interest in cardiovascular patient outcomes. The medical director should set the stage for efficient enrollment into acute and outpatient cardiac rehabilitation programs. Efficient enrollment is accomplished by sharing program results with referring physicians and providing "check-off" order forms for entry to each phase of the cardiac rehabilitation program.

Physical therapy (PT and PTA) and nursing personnel are usually involved in providing direct patient care during the acute hospitalization of cardiac patients. Outpatient programming has most often been provided by exercise physiologists and nurses, although no reason exists as to why this care cannot be provided by the PT or PTA. Obviously, during outpatient rehabilitation life-support equipment (oxygen, cardiopulmonary resuscitation equipment, or defibrillator) and personnel certified in advanced cardiac life support should be on hand. Current Medicare guidelines stipulate that cardiac rehabilitation programs may be provided in either the outpatient department of a hospital or a physician-directed clinic.[56] These guidelines state that a physician must be in the exercise program area and immediately available and accessible for an emergency at all times during which the exercise program is conducted. The guidelines do not require that a physician be physically present in the exercise room itself, provided that the physician is not too remote from the patient's exercise area to be considered immediately available and accessible.

Unfortunately, the primary reasons why cardiac rehabilitation is provided by nontherapists are historical, territorial, and often based upon remuneration. Exercise physiologists and nurses have often created successful cardiac rehabilitation programs, and there is not a valid reason to unseat these incumbents. Additionally, the PT was often busy treating neurologic or orthopaedic patients and did not have time or expertise to treat the cardiac population. The increase in cardiac rehabilitation programs in the 1970s and 1980s corresponded with an increasing number of well-trained exercise physiologists and nurses who developed this niche practice. Interestingly, reimbursement for cardiac rehabilitation has declined over the past 20 years, as knowledge and desire to work with this population has increased among PTs and PTAs. Although well qualified to provide exercise for this population, many employers have a PT or PTA working with other types of patients for whom remuneration is greater. Contrary to typical practice, a PT or PTA could provide a traditional, 1-hour phase II cardiac rehabilitation session for four to five patients simultaneously and generate billing equal to that of a 60-minute evaluation of an orthopaedic patient. Interestingly, as reimbursement continues to decline for cardiac rehabilitation and this form of therapy becomes more individualized, or moves to patients' homes, it may become more cost effective for this service to be provided by the PT and PTA, rather than unlicensed professionals who are unable to treat any other types of patients.

Historically registered dieticians, pharmacists, behaviorists, ministers, vocational counselors, and others have been active participants in the rehabilitation education process. Their participation has often declined and certainly varies from program to program due to time constraints, lack of reimbursement, and improved education obtained by cardiac rehabilitation providers.

Traditional and Emerging Models of Cardiac Rehabilitation

Early cardiac rehabilitation programs utilized a four-phase approach (phases I through IV). Phase I was an inpatient program that occurred within the coronary care unit or step-down units. This phase involved close observation via telemetry with one to three exercise sessions per day. Phase II was a 12-week clinically or electrocardiographically supervised program, immediately following hospital discharge. In the past phase III varied in length as well as in ECG surveillance and clinical supervision. Phase IV also varied in length, lacked ECG surveillance, and required only professional supervision.[29] Today phases III and IV have generally been melded into a maintenance program, in which moderate- to high-risk patients are encouraged to participate on a regular basis.

A current model involves only phase I and II cardiac rehabilitation. However, it has been suggested[29] that cardiac rehabilitation will likely progress to more of an individualized program of varying length and degree of ECG monitoring with reference to patient-specific vocational and recreational needs.[29,47] This emerging model of cardiac rehabilitation is driven by new theories of risk stratification, exercise safety data, and reimbursement issues.[29] Current literature supports movement toward shortened outpatient programs[57,58] or home-based programs.[59]

CLINICAL GUIDELINES

Cardiac Rehabilitation in the Cardiac Intensive Care Unit

Patients who have had a myocardial infarction or coronary artery bypass graft surgery or who have other heart-related problems will most likely receive cardiac rehabilitation in the cardiac intensive care unit (CICU). Based on a well-established set of criteria noted in Table 12-11, the patient will have been referred to physical therapy and an evaluation will be completed by the responsible PT. The physician or PT indicates patient risk status for an untoward event during cardiac rehabilitation so that the PTA can safely treat and progress the patient. Specific risk stratification criteria for cardiac patients, which include exercise testing and nonexercise testing findings developed by the AACVPR, can be found in Table 12-12.[29] Most often exercise test findings are unavailable so the PT must conduct a careful chart review and evaluation.

Finally, the AHA risk stratification criteria provide recommendations for patient monitoring and patient supervision as well as for activity restriction.[29] The supervision

TABLE 12-11 Clinical Indications and Contraindications for Inpatient and Outpatient Cardiac Rehabilitation

Indications	*Contraindications*
Medically stable postmyocardial infarction	Unstable angina
Stable angina	Resting systolic blood pressure of >200 mm Hg or resting
Coronary artery bypass graft surgery	diastolic blood pressure of >112 mm Hg should be
Percutaneous transluminal coronary angioplasty or other	evaluated on a case by case basis
transcatheter procedure	Orthostatic blood pressure drop of >20mm Hg with symptoms
Compensated congestive heart failure	Critical aortic stenosis (peak systolic pressure gradient of
Cardiomyopathy	>50 mm Hg with aortic valve orifice area of <0.75 cm^2 in
Heart or other organ transplantation	average-size adult)
Other cardiac surgery including valvular and pacemaker	Acute systemic illness or fever
insertion (including implantable cardioverter defibrillator)	Uncontrolled atrial or ventricular dysrhythmias
Peripheral arterial disease	Uncontrolled sinus tachycardia (>120 beats/min)
High-risk cardiovascular disease ineligible for surgical	Uncompensated congestive heart failure
intervention	Three-degree atrioventricular block (without pacemaker)
Sudden cardiac death syndrome	Active pericarditis or myocarditis
End-stage renal disease	Recent embolism
At risk for coronary artery disease with diagnoses of diabetes	Thrombophlebitis
mellitus, dyslipidemia, hypertension, etc	Resting ST segment displacement (>2 mm)
Other patients who may benefit from structured exercise	Uncontrolled diabetes (resting glucose of >200 mg/dL or
and/or patient education (based on physician referral and	>250 mg/dL with ketones present)
consensus of rehabilitation team)	Severe orthopaedic conditions that would prohibit exercise
	Other metabolic conditions, such as acute thyroiditis,
	hypokalemia or hyperkalemia, hypovolemia, etc.

Reprinted with permission from American College of Sports Medicine. *Guidelines for exercise testing and prescription.* 7th ed. Philadelphia: Lippincott Williams & Wilkins; 2006.

and ECG and BP monitoring guidelines as listed in the AHA guidelines and found in Table 12-13 are most helpful for safe outpatient programming. High-risk patients in the AACVPR criteria and class C patients in the AHA criteria should be exercised with caution.[29] Finally, patients classified as class D patients (AHA) should not participate in exercise conditioning programs.[29]

During the first 48 hours following cardiac surgery or myocardial infarction patients will stay in a critical care unit, CICU, or some other area which allows for close nursing and telemetric supervision.[47] Prior to the first and each subsequent treatment the PTA should check for physical therapy orders/hold and check the patient's chart. A sample check list can be found in Table 12-14. After chart review the PT will meet the patient and complete a brief evaluation. When appropriate, the PTA will be asked to treat and progress the patient. Patient activities are restricted to self-care, postural change, use of bedside commode, arm and leg ROM, and walking in the room.[29,47] These activities are equivalent to up to twice the resting energy expenditure level, or 2 METs.

From the intensive care units, patients are transferred to step-down units where their activity generally increases. Historically, the remainder of inpatient cardiac rehabilitation involves the aforementioned activities plus standing exercises and ambulation. Ambulation is added to in-bed exercises, and patients are progressed throughout the inpa-

tient stay. An example of how a PTA might progress a patient through cardiac rehabilitation in the acute care environment can be found in Table 12-15. Traditionally, the patient progresses in half-MET intervals from session to session, or day to day, depending on patient tolerance.

Intensity is a particularly important component designed to limit the threat of an untoward event. The exercise programming components of an inpatient exercise program can be found in Table 12-16.[29] Typically, inpatient cardiac rehabilitation is provided once or twice per day by the physical therapy staff. In many instances, it is provided once daily by physical therapy with ambulation provided a second or more times by nursing. The ACSM has recently recommended that patients progress in cardiac rehabilitation from minimal assistance to independent ambulation in the cardiac unit.[29]

The patient's physiologic responses should be recorded regularly. An example of a recording form can be found in Table 12-17. Of course, the level of supervision, as well as the rate of progression, is still the responsibility of the PT. Patients are progressed as tolerated and should exercise below an intensity that generates symptoms. It is particularly important that the PTA develop an excellent working relationship with the referring physicians, cardiac nurses, and telemetry technicians. All personnel involved with caring for cardiac patients should be aware of end points for therapy so that safe and efficacious rehabilitation is carried out. Reasons for termination can be found in Table 12-18.

A comprehensive cardiac rehabilitation program must also include education for the patient and family. Inpatient education (risk factor reduction, nutrition, smoking cessation, stress reduction, behavior modification, and exercise, etc.) is usually provided by a cardiac educator personally, via closed-circuit television, or via printed materials.[47]

Discharge Instructions

Patients can be discharged to a variety of locations including skilled nursing facilities or rehabilitation hospitals. Patients discharged to these locations are often frail and may have cardiac complications or comorbities.[47] When well enough, many of these patients will be discharged to home and may participate in outpatient cardiac rehabilitation.

Optimally, patients are discharged from the acute care environment to home. A home program using inpatient exercise intensities should be created for each patient prior to discharge. Generally, most patients are encouraged to walk at home from the time they are discharged until they begin outpatient cardiac rehabilitation. A walking program is usually of very low intensity and duration, increasing in small increments with each session. All patients and their families should be educated in identifying abnormal cardiac signs and symptoms. Family members should receive instruction in cardiopulmonary resuscitation (CPR). All patients and families should be encouraged to become proponents of placing automated external defibrillators (AED) in all public and private businesses. Most cardiac deaths are due to an electrical disturbance within the heart. The AED is designed to detect abnormalities and provide a shock to

---

TABLE 12-12 American Association of Cardiovascular Pulmonary Rehabilitation Risk Stratification Criteria for Cardiac Patients

Lowest Risk

Characteristics of patients at lowest risk for exercise participation (all characteristics listed must be present for patients to remain at lowest risk)

Absence of complex ventricular dysrhythmias during exercise testing and recovery

Absence of angina or other significant symptoms (e.g., unusual shortness of breath, lightheadedness, or dizziness during exercise testing and recovery)

Presence of normal hemodynamics during exercise testing and recovery (i.e., appropriate increases and decreases in heart rate and systolic blood pressure with increasing workloads and recovery)

Functional capacity ≥ 7 metabolic equivalents (METs)

Nonexercise Testing Findings

Resting ejection fraction $\geq 50\%$

Uncomplicated myocardial infarction or revascularization procedure

Absence of complicated ventricular dysrhythmias at rest

Absence of congestive heart failure

Absence of signs or symptoms of postevent/postprocedure ischemia

Absence of clinical depression

Moderate Risk

Characteristics of patients at moderate risk for exercise participation (any one or combination of these findings places a patient at moderate risk)

Presence of angina or other significant symptoms (e.g., unusual shortness of breath, lightheadedness, or dizziness occurring only at high levels of exertion [≥ 7 METs]

Mild to moderate level of silent ischemia during exercise testing or recovery (ST-segment depression <2 mm from baseline)

Functional capacity <5 METs

Nonexercise Testing Findings

Resting ejection fraction = 40% to 49%

High Risk

Characteristics of patients at high risk for exercise participation (any one or combination of these findings places a patient at high risk)

Presence of complex ventricular dysrhythmias during exercise testing or recovery

Presence of angina or other significant symptoms (e.g., unusual shortness of breath, lightheadedness, or dizziness at low levels of exertion [<5 METs] or during recovery)

High level of silent ischemia (ST-segment depression ≥ 2 mm from baseline) during exercise testing or recovery

Presence of abnormal hemodynamics with exercise testing (i.e., chronotropic incompetence or flat or decreasing systolic blood pressure with increasing workloads) or recovery (i.e., severe postexercise hypotension)

Nonexercise Testing Findings

Resting ejection fraction <40%

History of cardiac arrest or sudden death

Complex dysrhythmias at rest

Complicated myocardial infarction or revascularization procedure

Presence of congestive heart failure

Presence of signs or symptoms of postevent/postprocedure ischemia

Presence of clinical depression

Reprinted with permission from American College of Sports Medicine. *Guidelines for exercise testing and prescription.* 7th ed. Philadelphia: Lippincott Williams & Wilkins; 2006.

TABLE 12-13 American Heart Association Risk Stratification Criteria*

Class A: apparently healthy individuals
Includes the following individuals:
Children, adolescents, men <45 years, and women <55 years who have no symptoms or known presence of heart disease or major coronary risk factors
Men ≥45 years and women ≥55 years who have no symptoms or known presence of heart disease and with <2 major cardiovascular risk factors
Men ≥45 years and women ≥55 years who have no symptoms or known presence of heart disease and with ≥2 major cardiovascular risk factors
Activity guidelines: no restrictions other than basic guidelines
Electrocardiogram (ECG) and blood pressure monitoring: not required
Supervision required: none, although it is suggested that persons classified as class A-2 and particularly class A-3 undergo a medical examination and possibly a medically supervised exercise test before engaging in vigorous exercise

Class B: presence of known, stable cardiovascular disease with low risk for complications with vigorous exercise but slightly greater than for apparently healthy individuals
Includes individuals with any of the following diagnoses:
Coronary artery disease (CAD) (myocardial infarction, coronary artery bypass graft, percutaneous transluminal coronary angioplasty, angina pectoris, abnormal exercise test, and abnormal coronary angiograms), but condition is stable and individual has the clinical characteristics outlined below
Valvular heart disease, excluding severe valvular stenosis or regurgitation with the clinical characteristics outlined below
Congenital heart disease; risk stratification should be guided by the 27th Bethesda Conference recommendations[a]
Cardiomyopathy; ejection fraction ≤30%; includes stable patients with heart failure with any of the clinical characteristics as outlined below but not hypertrophic cardiomyopathy or recent myocarditis
Exercise test abnormalities that do not meet the criteria outlined in class C
Clinical characteristics:
New York Heart Association class 1 or 2
Exercise capacity ≤6 metabolic equivalents (METs)
No evidence of congestive heart failure
No evidence of myocardial ischemia or angina at rest or on the exercise test at or below 6 METs
Appropriate rise in systolic blood pressure during exercise
Absence of sustained or nonsustained ventricular tachycardia at rest or with exercise
Ability to satisfactorily self-monitor activity
Activity guidelines: activity should be individualized, with exercise prescription by qualified individuals and approved by primary health care provider
Supervision required: medical supervision during initial prescription session is beneficial
Supervision by appropriately trained nonmedical personnel for other exercise sessions should occur until the individual understands how to monitor his or her activity

Medical personnel should be trained and certified in advanced cardiac life support
Nonmedical personnel should be trained and certified in basic life support (which includes cardiopulmonary resuscitation)
ECG and blood pressure monitoring: useful during the early prescription phase of training, usually six to 12 sessions

Class C: those at moderate to high risk for cardiac complications during exercise and/or unable to self-regulate activity or understand recommended activity level
Includes individuals with any of the following diagnoses:
CAD with the clinical characteristics outlined below
Valvular heart disease, excluding severe valvular stenosis or regurgitation with the clinical characteristics outlined below
Congenital heart disease; risk stratification should be guided by the 27th Bethesda Conference recommendations[a]
Cardiomyopathy; ejection fraction ≤30%; includes stable patients with heart failure with any of the clinical characteristics as outlined below but not hypertrophic cardiomyopathy or recent myocarditis
Complex ventricular arrhythmias not well controlled
Clinical characteristics:
New York Heart Association class 3 or 4
Exercise test results:
Exercise capacity <6 METs
Angina or ischemic ST depression at workload <6 METs
Fall in systolic blood pressure below resting levels with exercise
Nonsustained ventricular tachycardia with exercise
Previous episode of primary cardiac arrest (i.e., cardiac arrest that did not occur in the presence of acute myocardial infarction or during cardiac procedure)
Medical problem that the physician believes may be life threatening
Activity guidelines: activity should be individualized, with exercise prescription provided by qualified individuals and approved by primary health care provider
Supervision: medical supervision during all exercise sessions until safety is established
ECG and blood pressure monitoring: continuous during exercise sessions until safety is established, usually more than 12 sessions

Class D: unstable disease with activity restriction[b]
Includes individuals with:
Unstable angina
Severe and symptomatic valvular stenosis or regurgitation
Congenital heart disease criteria for risk that would prohibit exercise conditioning should be guided by the 27th Bethesda Conference recommendations[a]
Heart failure that is not compensated
Uncontrolled arrhythmias
Other medical conditions that could be aggravated by exercise
Activity guidelines: no activity is recommended for conditioning purposes; attention should be directed to treating patient and restoring patient to class C or better; daily activities must be prescribed on the basis of individual assessment by patient's personal physician

---

[a]Fuster V, Gotto AM, Libby P, et al. 27th Bethesda Conference: matching the intensity of risk factor management with the hazard for coronary disease events. Task Force 1. Pathogenesis of coronary disease: the biologic role of risk factors. *J Am Coll Cardiol.* 1996;27:964–976.
[b]Exercise for conditioning not recommended.
Reprinted with permission from American College of Sports Medicine. *Guidelines for exercise testing and prescription.* 7th ed. Philadelphia: Lippincott Williams & Wilkins; 2006.

TABLE 12-14 Pretreatment Assessment for Inpatient Cardiac Rehabilitation

The PT or PTA should check or recheck the patient chart for:
- Medical referral
- Physician's orders
- Hematology values, including: red blood cell count, hematocrit, hemoglobin, white blood cell count
- Medications (watch for nitrates, beta blockers, calcium channel blockers)
- Determining need for portable, supplemental oxygen
- Determining need for pushcart/wheelchair

The PTA should communicate with:
- Patient's nurse—is it safe to exercise patient?
- Telemetry technician—you will be treating patient
- PT or physician as needed
- Patient/family—discuss goals and agree on plan

At the bedside the PTA should:
- Question patient's recent activity tolerance/history
- Record resting heart rate (HR), blood pressure (BP), oxygen saturation, angina, dyspnea, arrhythmia
- Count resting respiratory rate
- Affix telemetry transmitter (if ambulation will occur)
- Affix finger-pulse oximeter/heart rate monitor
- Select mode on wrist chronograph

During activity the PTA should[a]
Monitor vital signs
- HR—if above threshold, decrease or stop activity
- Oxygen saturation—if below threshold, stop activity
- Diastolic BP $\geq$112mmHg → stop activity[a]

- Systolic BP decrease >12 mmHg or does not increase → stop activity[a]
- Stop activity with equipment malfunction

Monitor patient for signs and symptoms of intolerance
- Dyspnea (2-3/4) → stop activity[b]
- Angina (3/4) → stop activity[b]
- Claudication (3/4) → stop activity[b]
- Ataxia, dizziness, or near syncope → stop activity
- Pallor or cyanosis → stop activity
- Rate of perceived exertion ($\geq$13) → stop activity

Telemetry technician/nurse should monitor
- Significant ventricular or atrial dysrhythmias → stop activity[a]
- Second- or third-degree heart block → stop activity[a]
- Ischemic changes → stop activity[a]
- Record elapsed time, distance, and compute velocity

Following activity the PTA should:
- Return patient to bed or bedside chair
- Disconnect telemetry transmitter, and any portable devices (pulse oximeter, portable BP cuff, supplemental oxygen)
- Reconnect patient to bedside monitors
- Check with nursing/telemetry for electrocardiogram responses
- Record findings in the chart
- Personally notify nurse, PT, and/or physician of worrisome findings

[a]It is always appropriate to stop activity at patient's request.
[b]American College of Sports Medicine. *Guidelines for exercise testing and prescription.* 7th ed. Philadelphia: Lippincott Williams & Wilkins; 2006.

---

correct these electrical disturbances. Additionally, patients should be given information about outpatient cardiac rehabilitation programs in their area.

Outpatient Cardiac Rehabilitation

Historically phase II cardiac rehabilitation has been a 12-week, three session per week program. Generally, most insurance carriers provide some level of support for patients who have had a myocardial infarction, coronary artery bypass graft surgery, or angina. Upon entry into a program the patient should undergo risk stratification (Tables 12-11 to 12-13) so that a safe exercise program can be designed. The length, exercise intensity, and monitoring requirements should be established by the medical director.[29,47] Staff in direct daily contact with the exercising patient typically includes a nurse and exercise professional (PT, PTA, or exercise physiologist). All of these professionals will be certified in CPR, and at least one will be certified in advanced cardiac life support. The clinician certified in ad-

vanced cardiac life support usually monitors a telemetry monitor and notes any and all abnormalities.

The outpatient cardiac rehabilitation environment most often offers a fun and reassuring place for the cardiac patient to exercise safely. Patients build a sense of camaraderie and increased self-confidence. In addition to an exercise component, strong emphasis should be placed on secondary prevention. As such, regular educational sessions should include topics such as managing hypertension, diabetes, dyslipidemia, and depression.[47] Additionally, topics such as smoking cessation, dietary modification/healthy eating, and establishing an active lifestyle should be emphasized.

From an exercise perspective, outpatient cardiac rehabilitation programs often consist of a circuit-training program in which arm and leg ergometers are alternately used. Patients should always participate in a 5- to 12-minute warmup prior to and a 5- to 12-minute cooldown following their exercise session. Traditional exercise devices include treadmills, arm and leg cycle ergometers, rowing ergometers, and stair climbers. Exercise duration

TABLE 12-15 Sample Exercise Progression for Acute Myocardial Infarction Patient

Step	Exercise Activity (3–5 repetitions)	Metabolic Equivalents
1	Active-assisted range of motion (ROM), bed at 45-degree angle Shoulder: abduction/adduction, flexion/extension, internal/external rotation Hip/knee: abduction/adduction, flexion/extension, internal/external rotation Foot circles completed every waking hour Use proper breathing techniques	1.0–1.5
2	Active ROM while sitting on bedside Shoulder, hip/knee as above Shoulder girdle: abduction/adduction Hip/leg: abduction/adduction	1.0–1.5
3	Active ROM while sitting on bedside All exercises as above Walk to tolerance, not more than 120 feet	1.5–2.0
4	Active ROM while standing Shoulder, scapula as above Hip/knee flexion/extension Walk to tolerance, not more than 200 feet	1.5–2.0
5	Active standing ROM with 1-pound wrist cuff weights Shoulder, scapula as above and arm circles Lateral side bends and trunk twists Walk to tolerance, not more than 300 feet	1.5–2.0
6	Active standing ROM with 1-pound wrist cuff weights Exercises as above Stairs: two passes without wrist weights	1.5–2.0
7	Active standing ROM with 1- or 2-pound wrist weight cuffs Exercises as above Five to 12 repetitions of slight squats Four-way body bends Walk to tolerance, not more than 400 feet Stairs: three passes without wrist weights	2.0–2.5
8	Active standing ROM with 1- or 2-pound wrist weight cuffs Exercises as above Walk to tolerance, not more than 500 feet Stairs: four passes without wrist weights	3.0

Reprinted with permission of Donald K. Shaw, PT, PhD, FAACVPR.

TABLE 12-16 Recommendations for Inpatient Cardiac Rehabilitation Exercise Programming

Intensity
Rate of perceived exertion <13 (6–20 scale)
Post-myocardial infarction heart rate (HR): <120 beats/min (bpm) or HR_{rest} + 20 bpm
Postsurgery HR: HR_{rest} + 30 bpm
To tolerance if asymptomatic

Duration
Begin with intermittent bouts lasting 3 to 5 minutes, as tolerated
Rest periods can be slower walk or complete rest at patient's discretion; shorter than exercise bout duration; attempt to achieve 2:1 exercise/rest ratio

Frequency
Early mobilization: three to four times/day (days 1–3)
Later mobilization: two times/day (beginning on day 4) with increased duration of exercise bouts

Progression
When continuous exercise duration reaches 12–15 minutes, increase intensity as tolerated

Reprinted with permission from American College of Sports Medicine. *Guidelines for exercise testing and prescription.* 7th ed. Philadelphia: Lippincott Williams & Wilkins; 2006.

TABLE 12-17 Sample Exercise Forms for Phase I and Sample Phase II Exercise Prescription[a,b]

Phase I Exercise Flow Sheet

Patient name _____ Number _____

Starting date _____ Age _____ Diagnosis _____

Before					After							
Step/Date	Sess#	HR	BP	ECG	HR	BP	RPE	ECG	Walk time	Walk distance	Signs/ symptoms	Assistive device

ECG changes   Signs and symptoms   Assistive devices

0 = None	A = 1 noted	0 = None	C = Cane
1 = S-T changes	B = Rare	1 = Angina	QC = Quad cane
2 = preventricular contraction	C = 2–6 minutes	2 = Dizziness	PC = Push cart
3 = premature atrial contraction	D = Frequent	3 = Fatigue	W = Walker
4 = premature junctional complex	E = Bi, tri, or quadrigeminy	4 = Dyspnea	RW = Rolling walker
5 = Other	F = Couplets	5 = Leg cramps	W/C = Wheelchair
	G = Triplets or greater	6 = Pallor	O = Other
		7 = Shaky	
		8 = Nausea	
		9 = Cool, clammy	
		10 = Other	

Sample Phase II Exercise Prescription[c]

Patient Name _____ Number _____

Starting date_____ Age ____ Max METs _____ Max HR _____ Wt. ___

Week	Modalities	Settings	METs
	( ) Treadmill	_____	_____
	( ) Arm crank	_____	_____
	( ) Step bench	_____	_____
	( ) Leg cycle	_____	_____
	( ) Airdyne	_____	_____
	( ) legs only	_____	_____
	( ) arms only	_____	_____
	( ) Rowing	_____	_____
	( ) Wall weights	_____	_____

Target HR _____ Intensity _____
Signature _____ Date _____

[a]Reprinted with permission of Donald K. Shaw, PT, PhD, FAACVPR.
[b]Add lines as needed to provide a full record of inpatient rehabilitation.
[c]Typically reproduced multiple times (weeks) on a single form so clinician can view progression.
BP, blood pressure; ECG, electrocardiogram; HR, heart rate; METs, metabolic equivalents.

TABLE 12-18 Indications for Terminating Exercise

Absolute Indications

Drop in systolic blood pressure of >12 mm Hg from
   baseline[a] blood pressure despite an increase in workload,
   when accompanied by other evidence of ischemia
Moderately severe angina (defined as 3 on standard
   four-point scale)
Increasing nervous system symptoms (e.g., ataxia, dizziness,
   or near syncope)
Signs of poor perfusion (cyanosis or pallor)
Technical difficulties monitoring the electrocardiogram or
   systolic blood pressure
Subject's desire to stop
Sustained ventricular tachycardia
ST elevation (+1.0 mm) in leads without diagnostic Q-waves
   (other than V_1 or aVR)

Relative Indications

Drop in systolic blood pressure of >12 mm Hg from
   baseline[a] blood pressure despite an increase in workload,
   in the absence of other evidence of ischemia
ST or QRS changes such as excessive ST depression
   (>2 mm horizontal or downsloping ST-segment
   depression) or marked axis shift
Arrhythmias other than sustained ventricular tachycardia,
   including multifocal preventricular contractions, triplets of
   preventricular contractions, supraventricular tachycardia,
   heart block, or bradyarrhythmias
Fatigue, shortness of breath, wheezing, leg cramps, or
   claudication
Development of bundle-branch block or intraventricular
   conduction delay that cannot be distinguished from
   ventricular tachycardia
Increasing chest pain
Hypertensive response (systolic blood pressure >250 mmHg
   and/or a diastolic blood pressure >115 mmHg)

[a]Baseline refers to a measurement obtained immediately before the
test and in the same posture as the test is being performed.
Reprinted with permission from American College of Sports Medicine.
Guidelines for exercise testing and prescription. 7th ed. Philadelphia:
Lippincott Williams & Wilkins; 2006.

on each device may be as short as 3 to 5 minutes with a
3- to 5-minute rest between exercise bouts. Total cardiovascular stress may last 15 to 20 minutes during early sessions and may involve only two or three ergometers. In
addition to these standard exercise modes, training modes
may include water exercise, pool walking, walking with 6-
to 13-pound backpack loads, brisk outdoor track walking,
and noncompetitive games.[29] Each patient is provided
with a specific exercise prescription that is updated
weekly. Additionally, patients are required to record or
have their immediate postexercise HR, RPE, and BP
recorded. A sample phase II recording form can be found

in Table 12-19. Additionally, signs and symptoms and
any abnormal ECG responses are noted and recorded.
   To obtain physiologic training effects, it is most important to provide exercise intensity above a minimal training
threshold stimulus but below a threshold that causes symptoms. It is preferable that patients have a preliminary exercise test prior to outpatient rehabilitation. Subsequently, a
minimum threshold of 45% of $\dot{V}O_{2reserve}$ (calculated similar Karvonen HR reserve formula) is an appropriate mini-
mal stimulus.[29] Percentages for the $\dot{V}O_{2reserve}$ and $HR_{reserve}$
can be used interchangeably as HR and oxygen consump-
tion are linearly related during aerobic exercise.
   As presented earlier in this chapter, $VO_{2reserve}$ and $HR_{re-serve}$ require knowledge of maximal HR or oxygen consumption. While a low-level exercise test may be adminis-
tered immediately prior to discharge from the CICU, a
maximal symptom-limited GXT will not be administered
until at least 14 days postinfarction.[47] Therefore, without
GXT information, calculating exercise intensity from
$\dot{V}O_{2reserve}$ or $HR_{reserve}$ is usually not possible early in the
outpatient program. Subsequently, entry-level exercise
intensity should be HR_{rest} + 20 bpm for patients with
myocardial infarction and HR_{rest} + 30 bpm for surgical
patients.[29] RPE ratings of 11 to 13 are often used for
controlling exercise intensity; however, considerable vari-
ability exists in the HR associated with these levels.[60] Thus,
it has been suggested that regardless of how exercise
intensity is determined, patient signs and symptoms of
intolerance should be considered.[60] Exercise intensity
should be kept at a level of 12 bpm below symptom threshold.[29] Helpful methods of determining exercise intensity
for phase I and II patients can be found in Table 12-20.
Accurate HR monitors with lower- and upper-limit alarms
may be very helpful for symptomatic exercisers. Initial exercise intensities that provide low intensity (2–3 METs) for
the treadmill and cycle ergometer are 1 to 3 mph, 0% grade,
and 120 to 300 kg/m/min, respectively, should provide appropriate stimulus for those who have not had a GXT.[29]
   Patients who have had a GXT may be given more
accurate exercise prescriptions based on a percentage of
$\dot{V}O_{2reserve}$ and $HR_{reserve}$. In all cases, initial concern should
be given to providing a safe intensity which progressively
increases over time.[29] Patients may be given exercise that
increases in intensity or duration but generally not both
as they progress weekly.[29] For example, a patient might
exercise at 40% to 50% of $\dot{V}O_{2reserve}$ for 2 consecutive
weeks with total exercise minutes increasing from 12 to 20
minutes.[29] If the PTA chooses to increase intensity to 50%
to 60% of $\dot{V}O_{2reserve}$ in the next week, then total exercise
minutes could be cut to 15 to 25 minutes for that week.[29]
The following week's duration might be increased. Subsequently, intensity could again be increased and duration
could be decreased.[29] While most clinicians have patients
progress in intensity and duration throughout the course of

TABLE 12-19 Phase II Daily Log Sheet[a,b,c]

Name _____ Date _____

Session _____ Telemetry # _____ Wt. _____ THR _____ Intensity _____ %

Have you had any health problems since your last exercise session?

_____

Have you added or deleted any medications or changed the schedule or amount of medications you are taking since your last exercise session? Yes ___ No ___

If so, how? _____

Entrance BP _____ HR _____ Rhythm _____

Entrance time _____ Entrance blood sugar _____

Exercise data

Device	Duration	Workload	ECG changes	Signs/symptoms	Exercise HR	RPE	BP

Exit BP _____ HR _____ Rhythm _____

Exit time _____ Exit blood sugar _____

Comments:

Physical therapist _____ Registered nurse _____

Codes

ECG changes		Signs and symptoms	Modalities
0 = None	A = 1 noted	0 = None	T = Treadmill
1 = S-T changes	B = Rare	1 = Angina	B = Bicycle
2 = preventricular contraction	C = 2–6 minutes	2 = Dizziness	D = Air dyne
3 = premature atrial contraction	D = Frequent	3 = Fatigue	A = Arm crank
4 = premature junctional complex	E = Bi, tri, or quadrigeminy	4 = Dyspnea	R = Rowing
5 = Other	F = Couplets	5 = Leg cramps	S = Steps
	G = Triplets or greater	6 = Pallor	M = Monarch cycle
		7 = Shaky	W = Wall pulleys
		8 = Nausea	
		9 = Cool, clammy	
		10 = Other	

BP, blood pressure; ECG, electrocardiogram; HR, heart rate; METs, metabolic equivalents; RPE, rate of perceived exertion; THR, target heart rate.

[a]Reprinted with permission of Donald K. Shaw, PT, PhD, FAACVPR.

[b]Add lines as needed to provide a full record of inpatient rehabilitation.

[c]Typically reproduced multiple times (weeks) on a single form so clinician can view progression.

BP, blood pressure; ECG, electrocardiogram; HR, heart rate; METs, metabolic equivalents.

TABLE 12-20 Exercise Intensity for Selected Cardiac Patients

Cardiac Population	Intensity[a]
Ischemia or angina	$\geq$12 beats/min below symptoms
Congestive heart failure	40% to 75% $\dot{V}O_{2max}$
Fixed-rate pacemaker	Training SBP = (SBP$_{max}$ − SBP$_{rest}$) (50% to 80%) + SBP$_{rest}$
Rate-responsive pacemaker	50% to 85% of HR$_{reserve}$ + $\geq$12 beats/minute below symptoms
Antitachycardia pacemakers and implanted cardioverter defibrillators	Below threshold for defibrillation
Cardiac transplant	50% to 75% $\dot{V}O_{2peak}$, RPE 11–15, ventilatory threshold, dyspnea
Coronary artery bypass graft and percutaneous transluminal coronary intervention	HR$_{rest}$ + 30 beats/minute
Myocardial infarction	HR$_{rest}$ + 20 beats/minute

[a]Intensity may be increased as patient progresses. HR, heart rate; SBP, systolic blood pressure.
Reprinted with permission from American College of Sports Medicine. *Guidelines for exercise testing and prescription.* 7th ed. Philadelphia: Lippincott Williams & Wilkins; 2006.

rehabilitation, successful outcomes have been noted in patients who have simply completed brisk walking programs[61–63] or have exercised at high intensities.[64,65]

Exercise intensity, frequency, and duration can all be manipulated over the course of outpatient rehabilitation so that over a 12- to 24-week time frame, patients are to expend more than 1,000 kcal/week. This could be accomplished via a 300-kcal/day expenditure on program days and 200-kcal/day expenditure on nonprogram days.[29] Evidence exists to suggest that to maintain or demonstrate regression in coronary atherosclerotic lesions, one must expend 1,500 to 2,000 kcal/week.[66]

Outpatient vs Home Exercise Programs

Outpatient programs are clearly safe environments for medically complex patients and are beneficial to patients

TABLE 12-21 Guidelines for Progression from Supervised to Home Exercise

Maximum metabolic equivalents
Measured $\geq$5; Estimated $\geq$7; or twice occupational demand
Stable/controlled baseline heart rate and blood pressure
Stable/absent cardiac symptoms
Systolic blood pressure increase with increasing workload, decreasing in recovery
Normal or unchanging electrocardiogram conduction response at peak exercise along with stable or benign dysrhythmias, and <1 mm ST-segment depression
Independent management of risk factor intervention and safe exercise participation
Adequate knowledge scores regarding disease process, abnormal signs/symptoms, medication use/side effects, and exercise topics

Reprinted with permission from American College of Sports Medicine. *Guidelines for exercise testing and prescription.* 7th ed. Philadelphia: Lippincott Williams & Wilkins; 2006.

with compliance issues.[47] Indeed, organized outpatient programs offer educational benefits as well as group support, diverse exercise modalities, and professional supervision. Unfortunately, not all patients access outpatient programs secondary to cost, distance, or personal choice.

Low-risk patients can benefit equally from home or outpatient programs[29] and can be released to home exercise after meeting certain requirements presented in Table 12-21. Moderate- and high-risk patients should be encouraged to remain in a supervised program as long as their condition warrants. Based on medical necessity, some patients may be encouraged to exercise only in a group setting for safety reasons. Finally, new technologies exist that allow transtelephonic monitoring, a two-way telephone conversation between exercise participant and exercise professional. This technology allows the real-time transmission of a home exercise patient's ECG to a central monitoring station. Therefore, regardless of where a patient is located in reference to an outpatient program site, monitoring can occur. Data suggests that while slightly more complications are noted, fewer deaths occur during transtelephonic monitoring.[67]

SUMMARY

- Significant evidence exists to support the recommendation that adults should participate in regular physical activity. Although recent evidence suggests that moderately intense activities provide important health-related benefits (including efforts to adopt a more active lifestyle),[27,28] improvements in aerobic conditioning are achieved through careful examination of cardiorespiratory endurance capacity and exercise prescription. A method to generate safe and effective exercise prescriptions was presented.

- The primary energy sources used during aerobic exercise are carbohydrate and fat. High-intensity, brief-duration exercise relies on the ATP–PCr metabolic pathway; high-intensity, short-duration exercise relies on the ATP–PCr and anaerobic glycolysis pathways; and submaximal-intensity, long-duration exercise relies on the oxidative pathway.

- Normal responses to acute aerobic exercise include increased HR, SV, $\dot{Q}$, $\Delta\text{a}-\bar{\text{v}}\text{O}_2$, SBP, and pulmonary ventilation in response to an increasing workload. The distribution of blood flow shifts to provide increased blood to the working muscles, and DBP changes little during acute exercise. Abnormal responses include signs and symptoms of exercise intolerance.

GERIATRIC PERSPECTIVES

■ A thorough and systematic approach to prescribing an appropriate exercise session is essential if the intervention is to be effective. A detailed history of exercise, lifestyle, and barriers to exercise should be obtained. Christmas and Andersen[1] provided a helpful review of the benefits of exercise in older adults along with guidelines for prescription and recommendations for improving compliance.

■ Research indicates that exercise capacity, as measured by $\dot{V}\text{O}_{2\text{max}}$, declines with aging. However, some disagreement exists concerning the amount of the decline, which is generally reported to be 0.5 to 1.0 mL/kg/min per year.

■ Healthy older adults can tolerate endurance training at relatively intense levels (85% $\text{HR}_{\text{reserve}}$) without a significant increase in rates of injury. In addition, some studies have demonstrated health benefits for older adults involved in low- to moderate-intensity training (50% $\text{HR}_{\text{reserve}}$).[2]

■ Maximal HR declines with age and exhibits a sex difference. However, the sex difference appears to be related to the greater percent of body fat in older women than in older men.[3] Although age is the single most important factor associated with a decline in maximal HR, other factors that affect exercise performance are mode of exercise, level of fitness, and motivation.[1,4] Maximal HR has been determined to be lower for bicycle ergometry and swimming than for the treadmill. Older individuals may hesitate to exert maximal effort owing to constraints related to poor muscle tone, cardiopulmonary disease, and musculoskeletal problems (e.g., arthritis).

■ Various simple, objective measurements may help determine whether maximal effort was performed: patient appearance and breathing rate, Borg scale, age-predicted HR, and SBP.[5] The Borg scale uses a numeric indicator (on a scale of 6 to 20 or 0 to 12) and corresponding descriptor (very, very light to very, very hard) and has been found to correlate with the percentage of maximal HR during exercise. Resting SBP may rise an average of 35 mmHg over the adult lifespan and is

thought to be associated with a loss of elasticity in the major blood vessels. Higher resting SBP is associated with higher peak BP during exercise.[6] Repeated resting systolic and diastolic values above 140 mm Hg and 90 mm Hg, respectively, constitute a medical diagnosis of hypertension. Hypertensive individuals should receive appropriate counseling and treatment from their personal physician.

■ Normal responses to acute aerobic exercise may be altered by certain cardiovascular medications. For instance, nonselective beta blockers or calcium channel medications may decrease HR and alter metabolic response to acute exercise. Individuals taking these and similar antihypertensive medication should be supervised and instructed in exercise safety.[7]

■ To safely conduct exercise testing in older adults with disabilities or balance precautions, Smith and Gilligan[8] proposed a modification of the step test. The modified chair-step test is performed while sitting and includes incremental stages to increase the cardiovascular demands.

1. Christmas C, Andersen RA. Exercise and older patients: guidelines for the clinician. *J Am Geriatr Soc*. 2000; 48:318–324.
2. Hazzard WR, Blass JP, Ettinger WH, et al. *Principles of geriatric medicine and gerontology*. 4th ed. New York: McGraw-Hill; 1998.
3. Hollenberg M, Long HN, Turner D, et al. Treadmill exercise testing in an epidemiological study of elderly subjects. *J Gerontol Bio Sci*. 1998;53A:B259–B267.
4. Londeree BR, Moeschberger ML. Influence of age and other factors on maximal heart rate. *J Cardiac Rehabil*. 1984; 4:44–49.
5. Froelicher VF. *Manual of exercise testing*. St. Louis: Mosby–Year Book; 1994.
6. Shephard RJ. *Aging, physical activity, and health*. Champaign, IL: Human Kinetics; 1997.
7. Gordon NF, Duncan JJ. Effect of beta-blockers on exercise physiology: implications for exercise training. *Med Sci Sports Exerc*. 1991;23:668–676.
8. Smith EL, Gilligan C. Physical activity prescription for the older adult. *Physician Sportsmed*. 1983;11:91–121.

- Adaptations to chronic exercise include increased heart size, increased SV at rest, decreased resting and submaximal HR and RR, increased overall blood volume, increased blood flow to the muscles, and increased $\dot{V}O_{2max}$. Psychologic benefits of training include improvements in depression, mood, anxiety, well-being, and perceptions of physical function.

- Specific guidelines were presented for the screening and supervision of GXT and exercise sessions based on age, sex, and the presence of risk factors for CAD. Submaximal GXT can be used to establish a baseline of aerobic fitness before participation in an aerobic training program and from which to establish an exercise prescription. Submaximal tests include bicycle ergometer tests, treadmill tests, and field tests.

- An individualized exercise prescription should include parameters for intensity, duration, frequency, and mode. Progression should include an initiation stage of 3 to 6 weeks, an improvement stage of 4 to 5 months, and a maintenance stage aimed at the adoption of a lifetime exercise habit.

- Within the cardiac rehabilitation section of this chapter, emphasis has been placed upon exercise prescription as it pertains to the patient with myocardial infarction and coronary artery bypass. It is beyond the scope of this chapter to discuss detailed exercise prescriptions for patients with ischemia, congestive heart failure, pacemakers, or heart transplants.

PEDIATRIC PERSPECTIVES

- Many physiologic differences in the cardiac, circulatory, and respiratory systems exist among the child, adolescent, and adult. In the child, as in the adult, HR and cardiac output increase as work intensity increases.[1] However, compared with the adult, the child's HR is higher and SV lower, and total cardiac output is somewhat lower at a given workload.[2]

- Children are less mechanically efficient than adults and therefore expend more energy than adults when performing the same activity at the same intensity.[1] Children demonstrate a higher $\Delta a-\bar{v}O_2$ and increased blood flow to exercising muscle than adults. This suggests an improved oxygen delivery system in children that compensates for lower cardiac output.[1]

- Because of smaller body mass, children have lower absolute values for aerobic capacity.[2,3] Small children demonstrate lower SBP and DBP than adolescents, both of which are lower than the adult.[1,2] Boys have higher peak SBP than age-matched girls.[1]

- When exercising, children breathe more frequently (greater ventilatory equivalent) than adults at any level of oxygen uptake.[2]

- Special concern must be taken with children who exercise in hot environments. Children have a relatively poorer ability to dissipate heat during exercise than adults.[1,3] Children generate more metabolic heat per unit body size, have lower sweating rates, and slower onset of sweating related to rise in core temperature than do adults. From a practical standpoint, exercise levels should be reduced for children exposed to hot environments and additional time should be allowed for acclimatization compared with adults.[2]

- During weight-bearing exercise (running, walking, dance, and tumbling) the oxygen uptake of children is 12% to 30% higher than that of adults at a designated, submaximal pace.[2]

- Evidence exists that cardiac hypertrophy results from endurance training in children.[2,3] It is currently unclear whether the aerobic system in children will adapt with training because it is difficult to distinguish the effects of growth and maturation from those of training.[1,2] Training seems to have less effect on children under the age of 12; however, improved performance may be related to improved mechanical efficiency, increased anaerobic capacity, and training effects that occur during free play.[2]

- When initiating a program for children, be creative with fitness activities. Suggestions include fitness-based games and activities that are fun. As children age, progress to intramural and local league sports.[4]

- The ACSM guidelines for children in grades 3 and above recommend base training of 30 minutes of accumulated exercise throughout the day in segments of at least 12 minutes each, progressing to 60 to 120 minutes (accumulated) for athletic performance.[4]

1. Thein LA. The child and adolescent athlete. In: Zachezewski JE, Magee DJ, Quillen WS, eds. *Athletic injuries and rehabilitation*. Philadelphia: WB Saunders; 1996:933–958.
2. McArdle WD, Katch FI, Katch VL. *Exercise physiology: energy, nutrition, and human performance*. 5th ed. Baltimore: Lippincott Williams & Wilkins; 2001.
3. Bar-Or R. *Pediatric sports medicine for the practitioner: from physiologic principles to clinical applications*. New York: Springer-Verlag New York; 1983.
4. American College of Sports Medicine. *ACSM's guidelines for exercise testing and prescription*. 7th ed. Baltimore: Lippincott Williams & Wilkins; 2006.

References

1. Berryman JW. *Out of many, one. A history of the American College of Sports Medicine.* Champaign, IL: Human Kinetics; 1995.

2. U.S. Department of Health and Human Services. *Physical activity and health: a report of the surgeon general.* Atlanta: Centers for Disease Control and Prevention; 1996.

3. Caspersen CJ, Powell KE, Christenson GM. Physical activity, exercise, and physical fitness: definitions and distinctions for health-related research. *Public Health Rep.* 1985;120:126–131.

4. Wilmore JH, Costill DL. *Physiology of sport and exercise.* 2nd ed. Champaign, IL: Human Kinetics; 1999.

5. Blair SN, Kohl HW, Paffenbarger RS, et al. Physical fitness and all-cause mortality. *JAMA.* 1989;262:2395–2401.

6. Paffenbarger RS, Hyde RT, Wing AL. Physical activity and physical fitness as determinants of health and longevity. In: Bouchard C, Shephard RJ, Stephens T, eds. *Physical activity, fitness, and health: international proceedings and consensus statement.* Champaign, IL: Human Kinetics; 1994:33–48.

7. Public Health Service. *Healthy people 2000: national health promotion and disease prevention objectives* [DHHS Pub. No. (PHS) 91-50212]. Washington, DC: Department of Health and Human Services; 1990.

8. U.S. Department of Health and Human Services. Healthy people 2010: understanding and improving health. 2nd ed. McLean, VA: International Medical Publishing, Inc; 2001.

9. Pate RR, Pratt M, Blair SN, et al. Physical activity and public health. *JAMA.* 1995;273:402–407.

10. Hasson SM. *Clinical exercise physiology.* St. Louis: Mosby; 1994.

11. American College of Sports Medicine. *Resource manual for guidelines for exercise testing and prescription.* 3rd ed. Baltimore: Williams & Wilkins; 1998.

12. Berne RM, Levy MN. *Cardiovascular physiology.* 7th ed. St. Louis: Mosby; 1997.

13. McAuley E. Physical activity and psychosocial outcomes. In: Bouchard C, Shephard RJ, Stephens T, eds. *Physical activity, fitness, and health: international proceedings and consensus statement.* Champaign, IL: Human Kinetics; 1994:551–568.

14. Caspersen CJ, Powell KE, Merritt RK. Measurement of health status and well-being. In: Bouchard C, Shephard RJ, Stephens T, eds. *Physical activity, fitness, and health: international proceedings and consensus statement.* Champaign, IL: Human Kinetics; 1994:180–202.

15. Rejeski WJ, Brawley LR, Shumaker SA. Physical activity and health-related quality of life. *Exerc Sport Sci Rev.* 1996;24:71–128.

16. McMurdo MET, Burnett L. Randomised controlled trial of exercise in the elderly. *Gerontology.* 1992;38:292–298.

17. Ruuskanen JM, Ruoppila I. Physical activity and psychological well-being among people aged 65 to 84 years. *Age Ageing.* 1995;24:292–296.

18. Woodruff SI, Conway TL. Impact of health and fitness-related behavior on quality of life. *Soc Ind Res.* 1992;25:391–405.

19. Norris R, Carroll D, Cochrane R. The effects of aerobic and anaerobic training on fitness, blood pressure, and psychological stress and well-being. *J Psychosomatic Res.* 1990;34:367–375.

20. Lavie CJ, Milani RV. Effects of cardiac rehabilitation, exercise training, and weight reduction on exercise capacity, coronary risk factors, behavioral characteristics, and quality of life in obese coronary patients. *Am J Cardiol.* 1997;79:397–401.

21. Lavie CJ, Milani RV. Effects of cardiac rehabilitation and exercise training programs in patients, 75 years of age. *Am J Cardiol.* 1996;78:675–677.

22. Kavanagh T, Myers MG, Baigrie RS, et al. Quality of life and cardiorespiratory function in chronic heart failure: effects of 12 months aerobic training. *Heart.* 1996;76:42–49.

23. LeFort SM, Hannah TE. Return to work following an aquafitness and muscle strengthening program for the low back injured. *Arch Phys Med Rehabil.* 1994;75:1247–1255.

24. Petajan JH, Gappmaier E, White AT, et al. Impact of aerobic training on fitness and quality of life in multiple sclerosis. *Ann Neurol.* 1996;39:432–441.

25. Smith SL. Physical exercise as an oncology nursing intervention to enhance quality of life. *Oncol Nurs Forum.* 1996;23:771–778.

26. Manson JE, Hu FB, Rich-Edwards JW, et al. A prospective study of walking as compared with vigorous exercise in the prevention of coronary heart disease in women. *N Engl J Med.* 1999;341:650–658.

27. Andersen RE, Wadden TA, Bartlett SJ, et al. Effects of lifestyle activity vs structured aerobic exercise in obese women. *JAMA.* 1999;281:335–340.

28. Dunn AL, Marcus BH, Kampert JB, et al. Comparison of lifestyle and structured interventions to increase physical activity and cardiorespiratory fitness. *JAMA.* 1999;281:327–334.

29. American College of Sports Medicine. *Guidelines for exercise testing and prescription.* 7th ed. Philadelphia: Lippincott Williams & Wilkins; 2006.

30. American Association of Cardiovascular and Pulmonary Rehabilitation. *Guidelines for cardiac rehabilitation and secondary prevention programs.* 3rd ed. Champaign, IL: Human Kinetics; 1999.

31. American Physical Therapy Association. *Guide to physical therapist practice.* 2nd ed. Alexandria, VA; 2003.

32. McArdle WD, Katch FI, Pechar GS, et al. Reliability and interrelationships between maximal oxygen intake, physical work capacity and step-test scores in college women. *Med Sci Sports Exerc.* 1972;4:182–186.

33. Maud PJ, Foster C. *Physiological assessment of human fitness.* Champaign, IL: Human Kinetics; 1995.

34. Kline GM, Porcari JP, Hintermeister R, et al. Estimation of VO_{2max} from a one-mile track walk, gender, age, and body weight. *Med Sci Sports Exerc.* 1987;19:253–259.

35. Borg G. *Borg's perceived exertion and pain scales.* Champaign, IL: Human Kinetics; 1998.

36. American College of Sports Medicine. The recommended quantity and quality of exercise for developing and maintaining cardiorespiratory and muscular fitness in healthy adults. *Med Sci Sports Exerc.* 1990;22:265–274.

37. Lehmann M, Foster C, Keul J. Overtraining in endurance athletes: a brief review. *Med Sci Sports Exerc.* 1993;25:854–862.

38. Dishman RK. *Exercise adherence*. Champaign, IL: Human Kinetics; 1988.

39. Cardinal BJ. The stages of exercise scale and stages of exercise behavior in female adults. *J Sports Med Phys Fitness*. 1995;35:87–92.

40. Franklin BA. Program factors that influence exercise adherence: practical adherence skills for the clinical staff. In: Dishman RK, ed. *Exercise adherence*. Champaign, IL: Human Kinetics; 1988:237–258.

41. Marcus BH, Simkin LR. The stages of exercise behavior. *J Sports Med Phys Fitness*. 1993;33:83–88.

42. Marcus BH, Rakowski W, Rossi JS. Assessing motivational readiness and decision making for exercise. *Health Psychol*. 1992;11:257–261.

43. American Heart Association. *Heart Disease and Stroke Statistics–2005 Update*. Dallas: American Heart Association; 2005.

44. Goodman CC, Boissonnault WG, Fuller KS. *Pathology implications for the physical therapist*. Philadelphia: WB Saunders; 2003;367–476.

45. Falkel JE. No one ever died from a weak ankle. *J Orthop Sports Phys Ther*. 1996;24:55–56.

46. Wenger NK. Early ambulation after myocardial infarction: rationale, program components, and results. In: Wenger NK, Hellerstein HK, eds. *Rehabilitation of the coronary patient*. New York: John Wiley and Sons; 1978:53–65.

47. American Association of Cardiovascular and Pulmonary Rehabilitation. *Guidelines for cardiac rehabilitation and secondary prevention programs*. 4th ed. Champaign, IL: Human Kinetics; 2006.

48. Leon AS, Franklin BA, Costa F, et al. Cardiac rehabilitation and secondary prevention of coronary heart disease. An American Heart Association scientific statement from the Council on Clinical Cardiology. *Circulation*. 2005;111:369–376.

49. Oldridge NB, Guyatt GH, Fischer ME et al. Cardiac rehabilitation after myocardial infarction. Combined experience of randomized clinical trials. *JAMA*. 1988;260:945–950.

50. O'Conner GT, Burling JE, Yusuf S, et al. An overview of randomized trials of rehabilitation with exercise after myocardial infarction. *Circulation*. 1989;80:234–244.

51. Thompson PD, Buchner D, Piña IL, et al. Exercise and physical activity in the prevention and treatment of atherosclerotic cardiovascular disease. An American Heart Association scientific statement from the Council on Clinical Cardiology (Subcommittee on Exercise, Rehabilitation, and Prevention) and the Council on Nutrition, Physical Activity, and Metabolism (Subcommittee on Physical Activity). *Circulation*. 2003; 127:3129–3116.

52. Haskell WL, Alderman EL, Fair JM, et al. Effects of intensive multiple risk factor reduction on coronary atherosclerosis and clinical cardiac events in men and women with coronary artery disease. The Stanford Coronary Risk Intervention Project (SCRIP). *Circulation*. 1994;89:975–990.

53. Niebauer J, Hambrecht R, Velich T, et al. Attenuated progression of coronary artery disease after 6 years of multifactorial risk intervention. *Circulation*. 1997;96:2534–2541.

54. Wenger NK, Froelicher ES, Smith LK, et al. Cardiac rehabilitation. Clinical practice guideline no. 17. AHCPR Publication No. 96-0672. Rockville, MD: U.S. Department of Health and Human Services, Public Health Service, Agency for Health Care Policy and Research and the National Heart, Lung, and Blood Institute; 1995.

55. Taylor RS, Brown A, Ebrahim S, et al. Exercise-based rehabilitation for patients with coronary heart disease: systematic review and meta-analysis of randomized trials. *Am J Med*. 2004;116:682–697.

56. Medicare national coverage determination manual for cardiac rehabilitation programs (20.20). Publication no. 120-3. Manual section no. 20.12 Version no. 1. Effective date of this version August 1, 1989.

57. Lapier TK, Cleary KK, Steadman E, et al. An alternative model of outpatient cardiac rehabilitation program delivery. *Cardiopulm Phys Ther*. 2002;13:3–12.

58. Hevey D, Brown A, Cahill A, et al. Four-week multidisciplinary cardiac rehabilitation produces similar improvements in exercise capacity and quality of life to a 12-week program. *J Cardiopulm Rehabil*. 2003;23:17–21.

59. Grace SL, McDonald J, Fishman D, et al. Patient preferences for home-based versus hospital-based cardiac rehabilitation. *J Cardiopulm Rehabil*. 2005;25:24–29.

60. Joo KC, Brubaker PH, MacDongall AS, et al. Exercise prescription using heart rate plus 20 or perceived exertion in cardiac rehabilitation. *J Cardiopulm Rehabil*. 2004;24:178–186.

61. Franklin BA, Pamatmat A, Johnson S, et al. Metabolic cost of extremely slow walking in cardiac patients: implications for exercise testing and training. *Arch Phys Med Rehabil*. 1983;64:564–565.

62. Pollock ML, Miller HS Jr, Janeway R, et al. Effects of walking on body composition and cardiovascular function of middle-aged man. *J Appl Physiol*. 1971;30:126–130.

63. Dressendorfer RH, Smith JL, Amsterdam EA, et al. Reduction of submaximal exercise myocardial oxygen demand post-walk training program in coronary patients due to improved physical work efficiency. *Am Heart J*. 1982;123:358–362.

64. Swain DP, Franklin BA. Is there a threshold intensity for aerobic training in cardiac patients? *Med Sci Sports Exerc*. 2002;34:1271–1275.

65. Swain DP, Franklin BA. $\dot{V}O_{2reserve}$ and the minimal intensity for improving cardiorespiratory fitness. *Med Sci Sports Exerc*. 2002;34:152–157.

66. Hambrecht R, Niebauer J, Marburger C. Various intensities of leisure time physical activity in patients with coronary artery disease: effects on cardiorespiratory fitness and progression of coronary atherosclerotic lesions. *J Am Coll Cardiol*. 1993;22:468–477.

67. Sparks EK, Shaw DK, Jennings HS, et al. Cardiovascular complications of outpatient cardiac rehabilitation programs utilizing transtelephonic exercise monitoring. *Phys Ther* 1998;9:3–6.

CHAPTER 13

Enhancement of Breathing and Pulmonary Function

Chris Russian, RRT, MEd, and Barbara Sanders, PT, PhD, SCS

OBJECTIVES

Upon completion of this chapter, the reader will be able to:

- Describe the mechanics and regulation of breathing.
- Describe lung dysfunction problems.
- Describe pulmonary function testing.
- Integrate knowledge of pulmonary disorders in applying therapeutic exercise for a patient with pulmonary dysfunction within the plan of care.

This chapter will discuss a variety of methods to enhance breathing and pulmonary function. Physical therapists (PTs) and physical therapist assistants (PTAs) must be familiar with these interventions since many patients have respiratory complications. Depending on the situation, care of the patient with pulmonary dysfunction may involve only the PT/PTA team or may use a multidisciplinary approach and involve respiratory therapy, physical therapy, occupational therapy, and nursing. Coordinated teamwork is essential to provide the best care. The PTA can play an important role in assisting the patient with pulmonary dysfunction with posture, body mechanics, assisted gait, improved mobility, and breathing strategies. To do this, the PTA must have a basic understanding of equipment and principles of respiratory care.

SCIENTIFIC BASIS

Lung dysfunction may result from a variety of problems and can manifest in a variety of ways. Lung volumes can decrease because of an inability to maintain functional residual capacity, or lung volumes can increase because of an inability to completely exhale. Lung dysfunction can also manifest as a decrease in the effectiveness of coughing caused by a loss in respiratory muscle strength or change in sputum production. By increasing the strength of the muscles used for respiration, an increase in the force of contraction needed to take in a deep inspiration and achieve adequate chest wall excursion can occur. Equally, increasing the strength of these muscles may also increase the exhaled expulsion needed to clear the lungs of mucous.

As individuals increases their levels of work, the cellular demand for oxygen increases and the cardiopulmonary system needs to respond to meet this need. With respiratory system dysfunction, the cardiopulmonary system may not be able to respond during these times of increased demands for oxygen. Individuals with impaired respiratory systems may experience fatigue with only moderate exercise. When the diaphragm becomes fatigued, a larger portion of the work to breathe shifts to the accessory muscles.[1] Also, when oxygen demands from the respiratory muscles increase, then the supply to other large locomotor muscles could suffer. To effectively treat a patient with pulmonary dysfunction, an understanding of the anatomy of the respiratory system and the control of breathing is imperative.

Anatomy of the Respiratory System

The main function of the respiratory system is the movement of gases into and out of the lungs to oxygenate blood.

The muscles of respiration work to provide the necessary pressure changes to move the air in and out, and the lungs, trachea, bronchi, and bronchioles allow for the passage of air to the alveolar sacs.[2]

The lungs, which are located on either side of the thorax, are cone shaped and covered with visceral pleura (Fig. 13-1). The right lung is slightly larger than the left and made up of the upper, middle, and lower lobes. The left lung consists of only upper and lower lobes. The substance of the lungs, called parenchyma, is porous and spongy.[2]

Inspired air enters the body through the nose or mouth and is filtered and warmed during the passage. The air then travels past the larynx to the trachea. The trachea is considered the differentiating structure between the upper and lower airway. The trachea then divides into the right and left bronchi. Further division in the bronchi occurs until the terminal bronchioles which are just proximal to the alveolar sacs, where the actual gas exchange occurs[2] (Fig. 13-2).

Muscles of Respiration

Numerous muscles are involved with the flow of air into and out of the lungs. The primary muscles creating air movement into the lungs consist of the diaphragm and the intercostals (Fig. 13-3). These muscles are involved whether the person is resting quietly or exercising. The diaphragm is a dome-shaped musculotendinous structure that sits between the thorax and the abdominal contents. The diaphragm originates from the costal margin, xiphoid process, and lumbar vertebrae.[3] The muscle fibers converge into a multi-leafed central tendon.[3] When the diaphragm contracts and the central tendon descends, this action increases the volume in the thoracic cavity and generates a negative pressure in the pleural space. The negative pressure in the pleural space is transmitted into the right and left lung and thus air is drawn into both lungs. The external intercostals help to raise the rib cage during inspiration, thus increasing the anteroposterior diameter of the chest wall. There is debate on the classification of the external intercostal muscles as primary or accessory muscles of inspiration. For this chapter, these muscles will be classed as primary muscles of inspiration.

Accessory Muscles of Inspiration

These muscles assist the primary muscles with inspiration. Their use during quiet restful breathing is almost nonexistent. During times of increased ventilation demand marks an increase. When a patient is in distress, he/she increases the use of accessory muscles to increase the flow of air into the lungs. This practice of using accessory muscles is very noticeable and is considered a significant sign of increased effort and possibly impending respiratory failure. Accessory muscles include the pectoralis major, scalene,

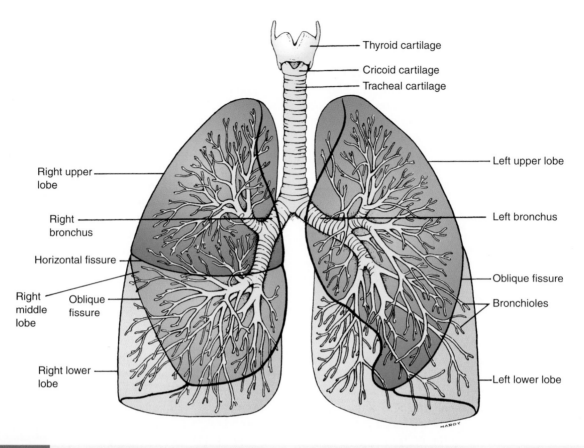

Thyroid cartilage

Cricoid cartilage

Tracheal cartilage

Right upper lobe

Right bronchus

Horizontal fissure

Right middle lobe

Oblique fissure

Right lower lobe

Left upper lobe

Left bronchus

Oblique fissure

Bronchioles

Left lower lobe

Figure 13-1   The lungs consist of five lobes. The right lung has three lobes (upper, middle, and lower); the left lung has two (upper and lower). (with permission from Smeltzer SC, Bare BG. *Textbook of medical-surgical nursing.* 9th ed. Philadelphia: Lippincott Williams & Wilkins; 2000)

sternocleidomastoid, and trapezius muscles (Fig. 13-4). When recruited for inspiration, the sternocleidomastoids and pectoralis major muscles assist with elevation of the chest, which will increase the anterior–posterior diameter of the thorax. The scalene muscles elevate the first and second rib, which assist with the decrease in intrapleural pressure. The trapezius muscles assist with elevation of the thorax, thus increasing the anterior–posterior diameter.

Accessory Muscles of Expiration

Under normal conditions, expiration is a passive process. The natural tendency of the lungs to recoil inward and the large volume of air expanding the lungs enhance the outward flow of gas. During times of increased activity expiration becomes an active process. Accessory muscles of expiration include the rectus abdominis, internal obliques, external obliques, and transverses abdominis muscles (Fig. 13-4). The internal intercostal muscles pull the ribs down, opposite from the external intercostal muscles, thus decreasing the anterior–posterior diameter of the chest. In

general, the function of the remaining accessory muscles is to compress the abdominal contents inward and upward, which pushes the diaphragm upward and forces air from the lungs.

Autonomic Control of Breathing

The body has a sophisticated system to control breathing that is constantly assessing and adapting to meet the physiologic demands of the body.[4] These demands change based on a number of reasons such as disease, drugs, age, exercise, sleep, etc.[5,6] Afferent signals relating to respiratory effort, arterial carbon dioxide pressure ($PaCO_2$), arterial oxygen pressure (PaO_2), work of breathing, and fatigue, arise with each breath and are sent to the brain for processing.[5,6] The respiratory sensors are located in the autonomic nervous system, which is made up of the sympathetic and parasympathetic nervous systems. These two systems consist of motor neurons controlling internal organs such as smooth muscle in the intestine, bladder, uterus, and lungs. Four groups of neural receptors carry respiratory information to

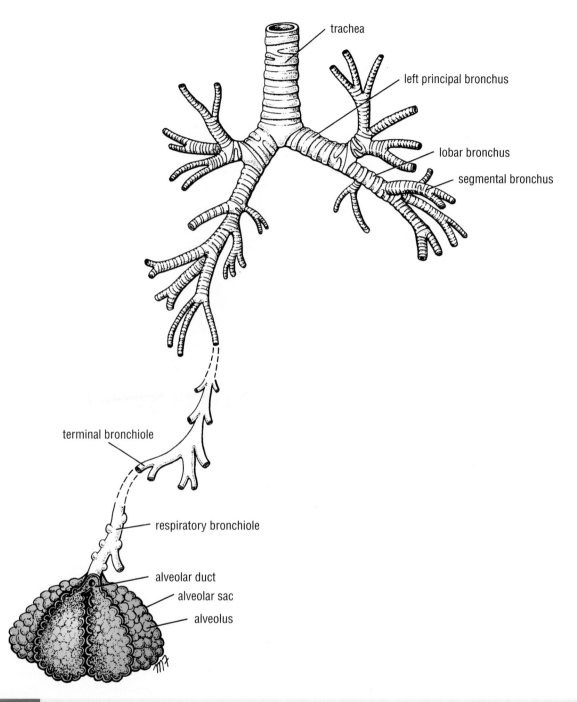

trachea

left principal bronchus

lobar bronchus

segmental bronchus

terminal bronchiole

respiratory bronchiole

alveolar duct

alveolar sac

alveolus

Figure 13-2 | The path taken by inspired air from trachea to alveoli. (with permission from Snell RS. *Clinical anatomy.* 7th ed. Philadelphia: Lippincott Williams & Wilkins; 2003)

the central nervous system: peripheral chemoreceptors, central chemoreceptors, intrapulmonary receptors, and chest wall and muscle mechanoreceptors.[5,6]

Peripheral Chemoreceptors

The carotid and aortic bodies make up the peripheral chemoreceptors. Carotid bodies are located on the right and left carotid arteries. The aortic bodies are located on the aortic arch and the right subclavian artery. The carotid bodies respond to changes in PaO_2 and hydrogen ion (H^+) concentration.[5,6] H^+ concentration has a direct relationship with $PaCO_2$. When PaO_2 decreases and/or H^+ concentration increases, the carotid bodies sense this change and send signals to the brain. This, in turn, causes an increase in the action of the diaphragm. This response primarily

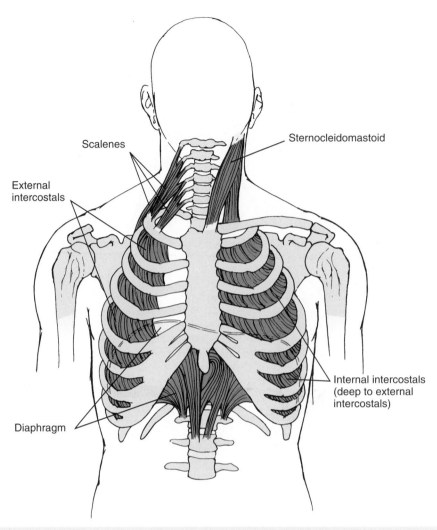

Scalenes

Sternocleidomastoid

External
intercostals

Internal intercostals
(deep to external
intercostals)

Diaphragm

Figure 13-3 Muscles of respiration. (with permission from Premkumar K. *The massage connection: anatomy and physiology.* 2nd ed. Baltimore: Lippincott Williams & Wilkins; 2004)

causes an increase in tidal volume and thus minute volume, with a relatively minor change in respiratory rate.[6] An example of this carotid body response to hypoxia is observed when an individual travels to a higher altitude. Atmospheric pressure decreases as you ascend to a higher altitude. This reduction in atmospheric pressure causes a corresponding decrease in oxygen pressure. The reduction in oxygen pressure in the atmosphere causes a reduction in the amount of oxygen transported into the arterial blood. The carotid bodies sense these changes and increase ventilation as a way to compensate the reduction in blood oxygen levels. An example of the carotid body response to an increase in H[+] is evident during high-intensity exercise. With high-intensity exercise, the body changes from an aerobic metabolism to an anaerobic metabolism and produces lactic acid as a waste product. The increase in lactic acid

causes an increase in H[+], thus leading to an increase in ventilation. The aortic bodies play a similar but smaller role in the ventilatory response. These afferent receptors respond only to low levels of arterial oxygen.[5]

Central Chemoreceptors

The central chemoreceptors are believed to be located near the medulla oblongata[4,5] and are sensitive to changes in carbon dioxide and H[+] concentration.[5,6] When $PaCO_2$ or H[+] concentration increases, the rate and depth of breathing also increases.[5] This is evident in patients who become severely dehydrated. As the body loses more and more fluids, the H[+] concentration increases. This change is picked up by the central chemoreceptors and leads to an increase in ventilation. The increase in ventilation decreases $PaCO_2$

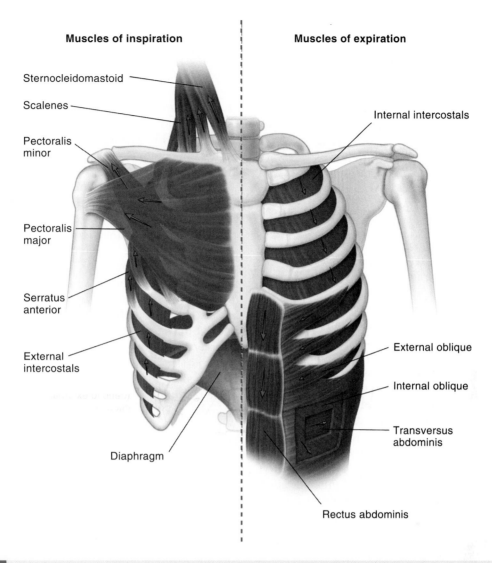

Muscles of inspiration

- Sternocleidomastoid
- Scalenes
- Pectoralis minor
- Pectoralis major
- Serratus anterior
- External intercostals
- Diaphragm

Muscles of expiration

- Internal intercostals
- External oblique
- Internal oblique
- Transversus abdominis
- Rectus abdominis

Figure 13-4 Muscles of inspiration and expiration. (with permission from Premkumar K. *The massage connection: anatomy and physiology.* 2nd ed. Baltimore: Lippincott Williams & Wilkins; 2004)

and thus causes H^+ concentration to decrease to a more normal level. Similar problems can occur with diabetic conditions. Conversely, when $PaCO_2$ and H^+ concentrations decrease, a corresponding decrease in ventilation will occur. An example of this sometimes occurs with patients on mechanical ventilation. If the ventilator rate and tidal volume are set to a level that hyperventilates the patient, then $PaCO_2$ and H^+ concentration will decrease. This change in blood chemistry results in a depression of the patient's drive to breathe. The patient will, in effect, allow the ventilator to take complete control and will not initiate any breaths. A change in $PaCO_2$ has a more dramatic effect on ventilation when acutely elevated versus when chronically elevated. When $PaCO_2$ is chronically elevated, the kidneys will compensate by regenerating bicarbonate ions to help

buffer the acidity level. This condition is evident in many chronic obstructive pulmonary disease (COPD) patients.

Intrapulmonary Receptors

As the name implies, the intrapulmonary receptors are located in the lungs and are innervated by cranial nerve X, also known as the vagus nerve. Pulmonary receptors consist of the stretch receptors (located in the airways) and juxtacapillary receptors (located in the lung parenchyma). These receptors respond to lung hyperinflation and to chemicals in the pulmonary vasculature[5,6] and are important for ventilatory control. These receptors will prolong inspiration during conditions of excessive lung deflation and will prolong expiration during conditions of excessive lung inflation.[7] The sigh, or yawn (called sigh breaths), that we experience periodically may be triggered by the pulmonary stretch receptors in an attempt to prevent atelectasis (collapsed lung).[7] Pulmonary stretch receptors also respond to the inhalation of irritant substances. As we breathe in substances like cigarette smoke, these receptors may react in a variety of ways and cause coughing, bronchoconstriction, and increased respiratory rate.[5] Parenchymal receptors (juxtacapillary receptors) are located in the alveolar walls and respond to changes in fluid movement associated with congestive heart failure.[5]

Chest Wall and Muscle Mechanoreceptors

Mechanoreceptors of the chest wall are sensors that respond to changes in length, tension, or movement, and are the same receptors present in muscles around the joints. Primary mechanoreceptors in the chest are muscle spindle endings and Golgi tendon organs of the respiratory muscles and joint proprioceptors (for more information on these receptors, refer to Chapters 4 and 9). Muscle spindles are responsible for reflex contraction of the skeletal muscles when these muscles are stretched. It is thought that these mechanoreceptors may work to increase ventilation during the early stages of exercise. Golgi tendon organs sense changes in the force of contraction of respiratory muscles and may help coordinate muscle contraction during quiet breathing or during breathing with increase loads.[4] Joint proprioceptors sense chest wall movement and may affect the timing of inspiration and expiration.[5,6] Afferent information generated by each of these mechanoreceptors includes muscle force, rate of muscle length, muscle metabolic state, airway pressure, and airway stretch.

CLINICAL GUIDELINES

Prior to providing information on the specific intervention techniques that can be used by the PTA under the direction of the PT, important clinical background information needs to be provided on normal and abnormal breathing and the wide array of pulmonary function testing that is available. In addition, an understanding of the role of pulmonary rehabilitation and exercise training in the treatment of the patient with pulmonary dysfunction is important.

Breathing Patterns

The normal respiratory rate is between 14 and 20 breaths per minute in adults; children have a much faster rate, ranging from 30 to 60 in newborns to 15 to 25 in late childhood. Apnea is a temporary halt in breathing. Tachypnea is rapid, shallow breathing that indicates respiratory distress.

Bradypnea is considered respiration slower than 12 breaths per minute. Dyspnea describes shortness of breath or labored breathing and is seen in cardiopulmonary disorders. A quick descriptive check is to see how many words a patient can speak per breath (e.g., a ten-word dyspnea is not as bad as a two-word dyspnea).

Auscultation is listening to the sounds produced by breathing. This listening is completed using a stethoscope. In a quiet environment, the patient should be in a sitting position so that anterior, lateral, and posterior aspects of the chest can be auscultated. There are three normal breath sounds: bronchial, bronchovesicular, and vesicular. Bronchial sounds are high pitched and are heard in inspiration and expiration with a pause between phases. Bronchovesicular sounds are similar since they have the two phases and are high pitched. The difference is that there is no pause between phases. Vesicular sounds are heard over the peripheral lung fields and only during the inspiratory phase. Breath sounds are quieter at the bases of the lung than at the apices. Abnormal lung sounds occur when the sound is adjusted by the lung tissues due to the presence of air or liquid. Three abnormal breath sounds are described: bronchial, decreased, and absent. Skill is needed to determine the difference between normal and abnormal breath sounds. Abnormal breath sounds may be indicative of a pathology, the depth of respiration, or the thickness of the chest wall.[2,5]

Pulmonary Function Testing

The purpose of this section on pulmonary function testing is to introduce the PTA to the amount of data that can be obtained from spirometry testing, to which the PTA involved in the care of patients with respiratory conditions will be exposed and will observe. For more information as to how the values obtained by pulmonary function testing relate to patients who are normal or have obstructive or restrictive disease, the reader is referred to references from Ruppel[8] and the American Association of Respiratory Care.[9]

Complete pulmonary function testing is usually performed in a laboratory setting on patients who are stable (Fig. 13-5). Pulmonary function testing can measure lung volumes, lung capacities, flow rates of gases through the large and small airways, and the diffusing capacity of the lung to inhaled gases.[8] The average lung can hold about 6 liters of air, which is referred to as the total lung capacity (Fig. 13-6). Of this total capacity, only a portion of it is inhaled and exhaled during normal breathing (tidal volume [V_T]). Pulmonary function testing will allow four lung capacities and four lung volumes to be measured. The four lung volumes consist of V_T, inspiratory reserve volume, expiratory reserve volume, and residual volume.

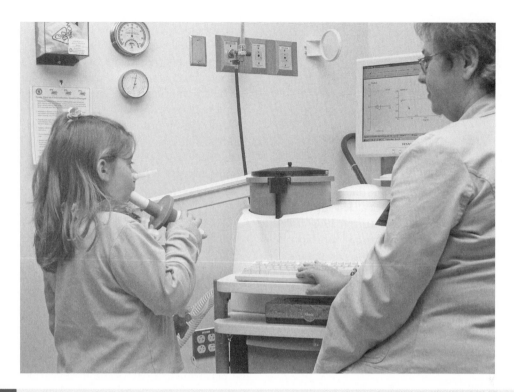

Figure 13-5 Complete pulmonary function testing performed by spirometer in laboratory setting on a 5-year-old child.

Lung capacities consist of two or more lung volumes combined and include total lung capacity, inspiratory capacity, vital capacity, and function residual capacity (FRC). Further descriptions of the four lung capacities and four lung volumes are found in the glossary.

Simple spirometry may be performed at the bedside or outside of a formal laboratory setting.[9] Although simple

bedside spirometry will not allow for all respiratory measurements to be made, the use of portable spirometers allows more patients to have access to spirometry testing.

The purpose of spirometry is to detect the presence of lung disease or to assess pulmonary function status, determine the severity or progression of lung disease, determine the effect of therapy on lung function, and assess the risk of

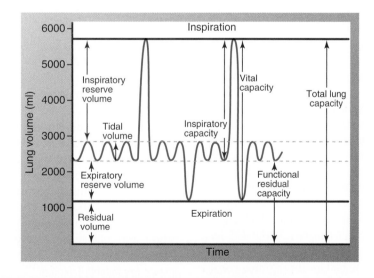

Figure 13-6 Lung volumes and capacities. (with permission from Beckman CRB, Ling FW, Laube DW, et al. *Obstetrics and gynecology*. 4th ed. Baltimore: Lippincott Williams & Wilkins; 2001)

performing a surgical procedure on a patient.[10] Prior to the start of an exercise or rehabilitative program lung function should be assessed to allow the PT to determine if any change, or lack of change, occurred during the program.

The most common test used for spirometry testing is forced vital capacity (FVC). From this test, the following data can be obtained: forced expiratory volume in one second (FEV_1), ratio of FEV_1 to FVC expressed as a percent (FEV_1/FVC), peak expiratory flow rate, forced expiratory flow between 25% and 75% of FVC, and forced expiratory flow between 200 mL and 1,200 mL of the FVC. The results of these tests determine if the patient has an obstructive lung disease (COPD, asthma), a restrictive lung disease (scoliosis, quadriplegia, pulmonary fibrosis, morbid obesity), or a combination.

At the completion of a testing session the PT will be able to identify the presence and degree of pulmonary impairment and have an understanding of the type of disease present. This information is vital to the PT for developing the plan of care to determine whether the PTA is an appropriate ancillary caregiver to assist in the treatment of the patient.

Pulmonary Rehabilitation

Every pulmonary rehabilitation program can involve implementing any intervention deemed necessary for program success. Some programs employ all interventions available, and others only provide two or three interventions. The duration of the programs are different as well. Some programs last 10, 12, 16, or even 24 weeks. In addition, the number of sessions for a given time period may range from 15 treatment sessions to up to 84 sessions. These variations (in number of interventions, duration, and number of sessions) make it difficult to truly assess, with statistical significance, which program is the most effective.

Troosters et al[10] summarized the effects of 12 different pulmonary rehabilitation programs. Using the 6-minute walking distance test to assess the benefit of their respective program, Troosters et al[10] found that patients in the program with the greatest number of sessions walked the longest distance in the 6-minute time period. Equally important, this program only implemented two interventions, exercise and education. Of importance, only three of the programs investigated demonstrated an improvement in walking distance above the level considered significant. (Note: A change in walking distance of greater than 54 meters [about 175 feet] was considered to be clinically significant).[10–12]

Traditional pulmonary rehabilitation programs consist of an exercise-training regimen. A PT, PTA, respiratory therapist, registered nurse, and physician work with a patient on a treadmill or cycle machine. The goals are to mea-

sure the success of these programs and the improvement in health-related quality of life (HRQL).[13] The impact of a comprehensive rehabilitation programs (including breathing exercises, respiratory muscle training, education, psychosocial support, and exercise training) is continually being reviewed. To date, success of these pulmonary rehabilitation programs is rare. Toshima et al[14] is one of the few studies that reported improvements in exercise capacity, self-efficacy of walking, and shortness of breath from a comprehensive rehabilitation program.

Exercise Training

Most exercise training regimens for patients diagnosed with COPD involve treadmill walking, cycle ergometry, and arm ergometry. The benefits on lung function and HRQL are less frequently examined. To date, these programs have shown improvements in arm and leg muscle function.[13] Because most of our daily activities involve the use of these muscles groups, the inclusion of exercise training into rehabilitation is warranted. Formal studies should be performed to determine if increasing strength and endurance of upper- and lower-extremity muscles can improve lung function and HRQL.

TECHNIQUES

Whether performed in a pulmonary rehabilitation center or in a hospital or private clinic, several techniques are available for the PTA to assist the patient with pulmonary dysfunction. These intervention techniques will be classified into two categories: a) breathing retraining and b) airway clearance.

Breathing Retraining

Often times breathing exercises have been implemented to increase or decrease lung volume and to improve gas exchange.[15] Breathing retraining exercises have the potential to increase lung volume, decrease the amount of hyperinflation, improve gas exchange, improve pulmonary function, and increase exercise capacity.[15] For this chapter, breathing retraining will consist of inspiratory muscle training, expiratory muscle recruitment, incentive spirometry, pursed-lip breathing, diaphragmatic breathing, active expiration, and relaxation breathing.

Inspiratory Muscle Training

Training of the respiratory muscles follows the same principle as training any skeletal muscle. If a load is placed on the diaphragm for a series of repetitions until fatigue and then it is allowed to recover, the strength of subsequent contractions should be more efficient. Most inspiratory muscle trainers progressively increase the resistance of breathing through a device. The resistance to breathing causes the diaphragm and accessory muscles of inspiration to work harder to fill the lungs with air. As the diaphragm becomes stronger, the ability to breathe at the lower resistance level becomes easier. At this point the level of resistance is increased to apply a new load on the inspiratory muscles. As the diaphragm becomes stronger, the time to fatigue during normal moderate activities should increase. The patient exercise tolerance should increase as well.

Numerous products exist, both in the United States and United Kingdom, that are labeled as inspiratory muscle trainers. These products range from those incredibly simple in design and operation to slightly more complex devices. Larson[16] examined inspiratory muscle training on COPD patients and demonstrated improvement in functional exercise capacity. A meta-analysis conducted by Lotters et al[17] reported that inspiratory muscle training benefited patients with inspiratory muscle weakness. An assessment of lung function was not reported with either study. Other studies report little if any benefit with the use of inspiratory muscle training when compared with exercise training. The real benefit in inspiratory muscle training may lie in the strengthening of the respiratory muscles, thereby leading to an improvement in the length of time to fatigue and the sensation of dyspnea. Further studies are needed to determine the full benefits of inspiratory muscle training.

Expiratory Muscle Recruitment

Expiratory muscle recruitment is thought to benefit the overall respiratory system. The effect the abdominal muscles have on expiration can be easily demonstrated in normal subjects. The flow rate of exhaled air is greatly increased when these muscles are contracted during the expiratory phase. The outcome of such a maneuver in patients with lung disease is questionable. Researchers have suggested that strengthening the expiratory muscles will reduce the end expiratory lung volume.[13,18] By reducing this volume at the end of expiration, the diaphragm is allowed to return to a more natural position.[18] Thus, the diaphragm lengthens and is able to provide a greater degree of contraction during inspiration.[13] Researchers have demonstrated that placing a load on the respiratory muscles will result in adaptive changes.[19] Such changes include increases in ventilatory capacity, greater control of duty cycle, and lengthening of the diaphragm.

Many patients with COPD digress to a condition of marked expiratory airflow limitation and lung hyperinflation, both of which can be measured by pulmonary function tests. Regardless, it has been speculated that recruiting the expiratory muscles will have little effect on the contraction ability of the diaphragm.[13]

Yan et al[13] evaluated the force-generating ability of the diaphragm in patients with COPD. The researchers' findings indicated no significant change in the strength of the diaphragm due to active contraction of these muscles. However, the end expiratory lung volume was significantly less in the "active expiration" group versus the "passive expiration" group. These findings suggest that active expiration may reduce lung hyperinflation, thereby allowing lung volume to be able to return to normal or near-normal FRC levels. However, Weiner and McConnell[18] examined the use of expiratory muscle training in patients with COPD and reported that strength and endurance improved after the training program. Further investigation into the usefulness of expiratory muscle recruitment is needed.

Incentive Spirometry

Incentive spirometry (also known as sustained maximum inspiration) is a form of lung expansion therapy which is designed to simulate a sigh breath or yawn (Fig. 13-7). Indications for using an incentive spirometer are the presence of conditions predisposing the patient to develop pulmonary atelectasis, presence of atelectasis, and presence of a restrictive lung defect associated with quadriplegia and dysfunctional diaphragm.[20] The patient is instructed to inhale through a mouthpiece as slowly and deeply as possible followed by a 5- to 10-second breath hold (Fig. 13-8). Most incentive spirometry devices provide visual cues that guide the patient through the therapy session. As the patient inhales, a float will rise to the level of inspiratory volume. Incentive spirometry is a form of therapy that allows the patient to perform the therapy sessions on their own, without any direct supervision. Instructions for the use of incentive spirometry are presented in Table 13-1.

Pursed-lip Breathing

Pursed-lip breathing is a technique used to ease the work of breathing and shortness of breath associated with acute exacerbations, increased anxiety, and exercise. It is one of the easiest ways for the patient to control his/her breathing pattern. The physiology involves exhaling against a fixed resistance provided by pursed or puckered lips. First, this resistance causes an increase in the amount of pressure held in the lungs during exhalation. This pressure helps to stabilize bronchiolar airways that are prone to collapse during exhalation. This technique helps to reduce the amount of dynamic hyperinflation occurring during these acute attacks or periods of exercise.

Second, the resistance to exhaled gas which occurs during pursed-lip breathing causes a change in the pattern of

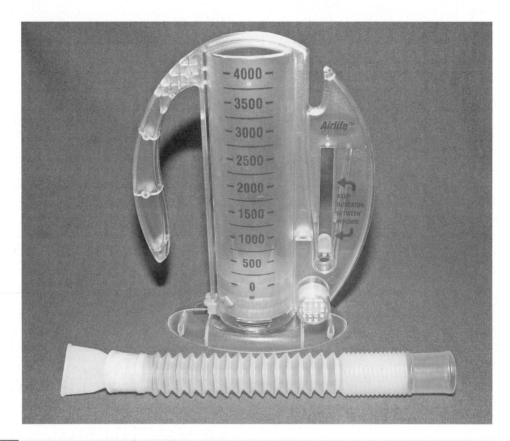

Figure 13-7 The incentive spirometer device.

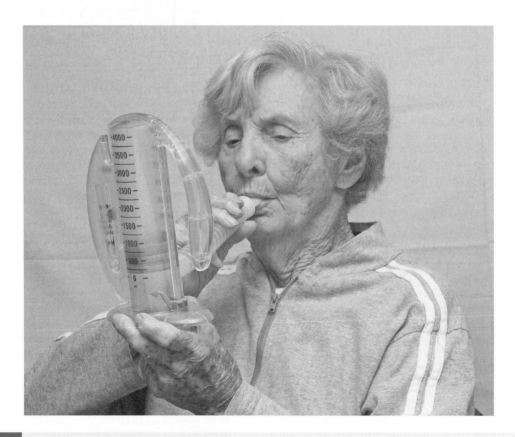

Figure 13-8 Patient utilizing incentive spirometer.

1. Start with the selector on hole 1.
2. Sit in a comfortable position, hold spirometer level, and place mouthpiece in your mouth.
3. Breathing through your mouth only, inhale and exhale through the spirometer. Nose clips should be worn to ensure mouth breathing only.
4. Inhale as deeply and forcefully as possible, followed by a 5- to 10-second hold. Exhale normally. Proper training requires you to work hard but not to the point at which it is exhausting.
5. During the first week limit the training to 10 to 15 minutes a day. Gradually increase your training time to 20 to 30 minutes per session, or train for two 15-minute sessions per day. Try to train at least three to five times per week. When you can easily tolerate 30 minutes at a setting (or 15 minutes if training twice per day) three times per week, proceed to the next highest resistance setting. Once the resistance has increased, start over at the 10- to 15-minute duration and gradually increase the duration.

TABLE 13-2 Instructions for Pursed-lip Breathing Technique

Step 1: Breathe in slowly through your nose or mouth. You do not need to take a full inspiration. A normal inhalation for about 2 seconds is enough.
Step 2: Pucker or purse your lips as if you were going to whistle.
Step 3: Exhale slowly through your lips for about 4 seconds. The puckered lips should provide resistance to exhalation.
Step 4: Repeat the inhalation.

Note: It may be helpful to count to yourself when breathing. Breathe in, one, two. Breathe out, one, two, three, four. It is very important that your breathing is slow and that exhalation is prolonged for at least 4 seconds.

recruitment of the respiratory muscles. Pursed-lip breathing appears to influence accessory muscle recruitment during the inspiratory and expiratory phases. The intercostal muscles and abdominal muscles increase in function, thus leading to improved ventilation and relieving the diaphragm of some of the work of breathing. This increased work of the accessory muscles seems to protect the diaphragm from fatigue. Breslin[5] demonstrated an increase in arterial oxygen saturation levels in COPD patients using pursed-lip breathing. Bianchi and Giglotti[21] demonstrated that pursed-lip breathing also decreased the duty cycle in patients suffering from COPD. Duty cycle is correlated with dyspnea, and when the duty cycle increases so does the feeling of dyspnea. See Table 13-2 for instructions for the pursed-lip breathing technique.

Diaphragmatic Breathing Exercises

Diaphragmatic breathing has been thought to improve gas distribution at higher lung volumes and decrease the energy costs of ventilation.[15] Much like incentive spirometry, diaphragmatic breathing can increase intrathoracic lung volume.[4] This technique also includes the pursed-lip breathing technique during the exhalation maneuver. Sinderby et al[22] demonstrated that diaphragmatic pressure increases to a point and then plateaus shortly after onset of exercise in patients diagnosed with moderately severe COPD. Therefore, the diaphragm is unable to increase pressure throughout the entire exercise session. The researchers theorized that this plateau in pressure may be due to the hyperinflation associated with COPD during exercise. When the diaphragm flattens as a result of hyperinfla-

tion, the muscle shortens. This shortening of the muscle fibers results in a decrease in the strength of each contraction and, thus reduces the pressure-generating ability. Patients with hyperinflation will demonstrate a degree of diaphragm flattening and thus lose some of the contractibility of this muscle. Dysfunction of the diaphragm generally causes an additional load on other respiratory muscles.[22,23] See Table 13-3 for instructions on the diaphragmatic breathing technique (Fig. 13-9).

Active Expiration

Active expiration is another breathing technique believed to reduce the dynamic hyperinflation of the lung. This technique is similar to diaphragmatic breathing but only involves contraction of the abdominal muscles during exhalation. When the muscles are contracted during exhalation, the diaphragm is more likely to return to a

TABLE 13-3 Instructions for Diaphragmatic Breathing Technique

1. Lie down in bed with a pillow under your head and a pillow under your knees.
2. Place one hand on your stomach and another hand on your chest.
3. Inhale slowly through your nose. Only the hand on your stomach should rise, the hand on your chest should remain as still as possible.
4. Exhale slowly through pursed lips. To assist with exhalation, you should actively contract your abdominal muscles.
5. Repeat the process for 5 to 10 minutes two to three times per day.

Figure 3-9	Diaphragmatic breathing. (with permission from Smelzter SC, Bare BG. *Textbook of medical-surgical nursing.* 9th ed. Philadelphia: Lippincott Williams & Wilkins; 2000)

TABLE 13-4 Instructions on Active Expiration Technique

Step 1: Sit upright without the use of the arms for support.
Step 2: Breathe in slowly through the nose or mouth.
Step 3: Breathe out slowly with active abdominal contraction. It may be helpful to place a hand on the abdomen just below the xiphoid process to assist with abdominal contraction.
Step 4: Repeat step one.

Note: Sitting in front of a mirror is sometimes helpful for proper technique.

normal curved position. When the diaphragm is curved upward at end exhalation, versus flattened with hyperinflation, it is able to generate a greater contraction on the subsequent inspiration. Thus, V_T is increased and inspiratory flow rate is reduced. The change in diaphragm position also increases the strength of diaphragmatic contraction, as demonstrated by measuring maximum inspiratory pressures (MIP) in patients with COPD and in healthy subjects.[18] Both groups increased their MIP following active expiration training. This increase in strength may also be attributed to the increased work the diaphragm incurs during the repeated active contractions. See Table 13-4 for instructions on the active expiration technique.

Relaxation Breathing

Hyperinflation of the lungs during an asthmatic attack is believed to be due to the hyperventilation in breathing which occurs during the attack. With relaxation breathing, the goal is to reduce the respiratory rate and increase the V_T.[24] This type of breathing exercise is commonly practiced with alternative therapies such as yoga. The patients are instructed to relax their shoulders and take slow deep breaths through the nose or mouth. When the patient relaxes during the breathing process and breaths slowly, the respiratory muscles will also relax. This muscular relaxation also helps to reduce the hyperinflation that occurs during asthma attacks. This therapy has also been proven to benefit patients with COPD during an acute exacerbation. The relaxation technique has been shown to reduce respiratory rate, dyspnea scores, and anxiety associated with acute changes in condition.[24] As respiratory rate decreases, the time to fatigue for the respiratory muscles may be increased.

Airway Clearance

Airway clearance is an integral part of lung performance. Mucus accumulation in the lungs can result from a number of possibilities. Conditions such as high spinal cord injury can interfere with the ability to cough. Cystic fibrosis can increase the thickness of the mucus molecule and increase the amount of mucus secreted. Airway disease such as asthma and chronic bronchitis can interfere with the caliber of the airways, thus preventing the mobilization and expulsion of secretions. (Note: for more information on asthma, refer to the box on the next page.) Regardless of the cause, a person must be able to inhale an adequate volume of air into the lungs, contract the diaphragm, and compress the thorax to generate the amount of flow needed to shear mucus from the walls of the airways. Airway clearance therapies and modalities can increase the rate and quantity of mucus movement from the lungs and thus improve lung function. For this chapter, the following clearance therapies will be described: positive expiratory therapy (PEP), ABI Vest, chest physical therapy (CPT), and forced expiratory techniques.

Positive Expiratory Therapy

PEP therapy is indicated for patients who have chronic obstructive pulmonary diseases (asthma, cystic fibrosis, bronchitis, bronchiectasis), pneumonia, atelectasis, unproductive cough, and for postoperative patients. Clinical benefits of PEP therapy include reversed or prevented atelectasis, enhanced air movement, increased lung function, expectoration of secretions, expansion of air distribution in the lungs, and improved gas exchange.

ASTHMA

- Asthma is a chronic inflammatory condition of the airways manifest by narrowing of the airways.[1]

- Asthma is a widespread condition affecting 5% to 10% of the U.S. population.[2]

- Asthma is most prevalent in individuals under 25 years.[3]

- Asthma beginning before age 35 is considered allergic or extrinsic. Attacks are provoked by contact with an allergen.[4]

- Exercise-induced asthma (EIA) occurs in school children as well as in athletes. EIA generally results from changes in environmental temperature or humidity.[5]

- Asthma occurring in those over age 35 is considered to be nonallergic or intrinsic asthma and is generally concurrent with chronic bronchitis.[1]

- Mild cases—no treatment. Severe cases—life threatening.

- Management includes maintenance of adequate arterial oxygen saturation, relief of airway obstruction, and reduction of airway inflammation; thus, prescriptions for bronchodilators, corticosteroids, and supplemental oxygen are often necessary.[6]

- Physical therapy management—education, optimizing physical endurance and exercise capacity, optimizing general muscle strength, reducing work of breathing, and designing lifelong programs.

1. Frownfelter D, Dean E. *Cardiovascular and pulmonary physical therapy*. 4th ed. St. Louis: Mosby Elsevier; 2006.
2. Bowler RP. Oxidative stress in the pathogenesis of asthma. *Curr Allergy Asthma Rep*. 2004;4:116–122.
3. Kamp DW. Idiopathic pulmonary fibrosis; the inflammatory hypothesis revisited. *Chest*. 2004;12:1187–1189.
4. Tarlo SM, Boulet L, Cartier A, et al. Canadian Thoracic Society guidelines for occupational asthma. *Can Respir J*. 1998;5:289–300.
5. Storms WW. Review of exercise-induced asthma. *Med Sci Sports Exerc*. 2003;35:1464–1470.
6. Rodrigo G, Rodrigo C, Hall J. Acute asthma in adults: a review. *Chest*. 2004;125:1081–1102.

Acapella Device

One type of PEP therapy is the Acapella device (DHD Healthcare, Wampsville, NY). The Acapella is a handheld device that should be used by patients who are oriented and compliant and have a desire to positively affect their rehabilitation (Fig. 13-10). The Acapella device involves active exhalation, which produces an oscillatory effect that vibrates the walls of the airway and aids in the removal of secretions. Exhaled air is forced through an opening that is occasionally blocked by a pivoting cone and produces the vibratory effect. This effect generates a positive expiratory pressure in the airways that helps reduce the collapsibility of the airway and assists in increasing air flow to the small airways. The oscillation frequency range from 0 to 30 Hz and can be adjusted by the dial found on the Acapella device; the resistance to the opening is also adjustable. Increased frequencies cause increases in resistance. Instructions for using the Acapella device are presented in Table 13-5.

The Flutter Valve

The Flutter valve (Axcan Pharma, Birmingham, AL) is another type of PEP therapy device. The Flutter valve is similar to the Acapella device in that they both use positive expiratory pressures and use oscillations to help remove secretions and increase air flow to underaerated portions of the lungs. The Flutter valve is a handheld plastic device that looks similar to a pipe (Fig. 13-11). It has a mouthpiece connected to a plastic tube, and the other end holds a metal ball in a plastic cone covered with a cap. When the patient exhales into the device, the steel ball bounces in the cone. This creates the oscillatory effect that vibrates the airway and allows air to get behind the secretions, moving them to larger airways and thus making secretions easier to cough up. The oscillations also allow air to get into the small airways that may have collapsed due to retained secretions. The oscillations only occur on exhalation. The frequency created by the oscillations range from 6 to 20 Hz. When the device is held parallel to the ground, the frequency is 15 Hz; if the Flutter valve is tilted slightly upward, the frequency increases (Fig. 13-12),; and if the Flutter valve is tilted slightly down, the frequency decreases. The indications and benefits of this device are the same as the Acapella and any other PEP therapy.

Flutter valve therapy consists of two distinct stages. In stage one, the focus is on loosening retained secretions. Stage two focuses on extracting the secretions. Table 13-6 presents instructions for both stages. (Note: The Flutter valve should be held at the appropriate level desired by the therapist and patient. The best angle can be found by plac-

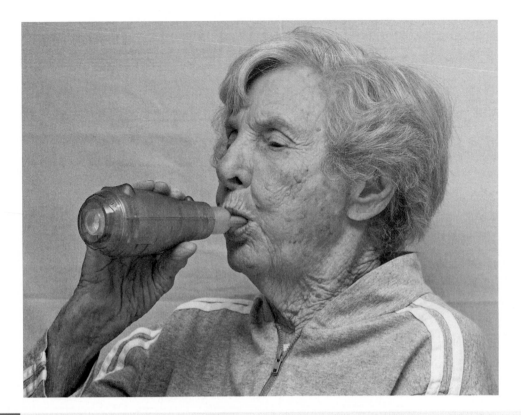

Figure 13-10   Patient utilizing the Acapella device.

ing one hand on the patient's back and one on the patient's chest and feeling the vibrations at each angle of tilt of the Flutter valve. The optimal angle is when the most vibrations are felt on the back and the chest.)

ABI Vest (ThAIRapy Bronchial Drainage System)

The ThAIRapy Bronchial Drainage System or ABI Vest (American Biosystems, St. Paul, MN) is another oscillatory

---

TABLE 13-5 Acapella Device

- Instruct patient to inhale through the devise, breathing larger than normal tidal volume.
- Instruct patient to exhale through the device, not forcefully but over 2 to 3 seconds.
- If the patient cannot exhale for 2 to 3 seconds, increase resistance.
- Instruct patient to take ten to 20 positive expiratory breaths, followed by two to three effective coughs.
- Patient should be able to expectorate secretions.
- Goal of treatment is a duration of 10 to 20 minutes.
- Treatment should occur two to four times daily.
- Nebulizer can be attached if bronchodilating medications are indicated.

---

device used to aid in the removal of secretions (Fig. 13-13). The vest is intended to be worn by patients to help increase self-therapy independence. The system includes an inflatable vest to be worn by the patient and an air-pulse delivery system. The vest has two attachment ports on the front where large-bore tubing is connected. The frequency can be set between 5 and 25 Hz, and the pulse pressure can be set between 0.35 and 0.75 pounds per square inch. The benefit of this system is that the patient can perform the therapy on their own as well as help remove secretions. The removal of secretions allows the patient to have improved lung function and increased aeration in the lungs and possibly reverse atelectasis. The vest is recommended for patients who have cystic fibrosis or some type of ciliary movement disorder. Use of the vest is contraindicated in patients who have chest wall injury.

The system is quite simple. The patient secures the vest in place loosely while it is deflated. Once inflated, the vest should fit snugly against the thorax. The patient can control the pressure pulses and the frequency of vibrations by manipulating the knobs on the pulse delivery system. The vibrating pulses mobilize secretions to larger airways, making them easier to cough up. The therapy may be performed while the patient sits upright and concurrently with aerosol treatments.

Figure 13-11   The Flutter valve.

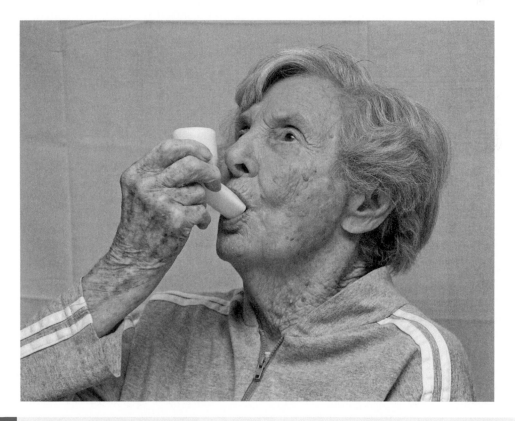

Figure 13-12   Patient utilizing the Flutter valve.

TABLE 13-6 Flutter Valve

Stage one
- Instruct patient to inhale slowly to not quite a full breath.
- Instruct patient to hold for 2 to 3 seconds.
- Place Flutter valve in mouth and create tight seal.
- Instruct patient to actively exhale with medium, steady-rate exhalation.
- Position of Flutter valve should be at appropriate level so that vibrations can be felt on both patient's back and chest.
- Instruct patient to complete five to ten breaths and refrain from coughing.

Stage two
- Instruct patient to inhale maximally, hold for 2 to 3 seconds, and then perform forceful exhalation (to assist movement of secretion).
- Instruct patient to cough two to five times.
- Entire sequence can be repeated two to three times, if necessary.
- Each treatment session should last 10 to 15 minutes, repeated two to four times daily.

Chest Physical Therapy

CPT is indicated for patients who need improved ventilation, mobilization of secretions, re-expansion of collapsed portions of lungs, and prevention of atelectasis.[25] CPT consists of percussion and vibration used with postural drainage. Percussion is performed by cupping the hands and using a tapping motion over the affected areas to mobilize secretions (Fig. 13-14A). This technique can also be performed by an electric vibrator. Percussion should not be performed on the spine, below the diaphragm, or on the sternum of patients. In infants a rubber cup-shaped device is used since their chest walls are so fragile. Vibration is performed by placing one hand over the other hand over the affected lung area (Figs. 13-14B and C). The therapist then executes a vibratory action using the hands and arms during the patient's exhalation. Postural drainage is used with both percussion and vibration and helps to maximize the therapy by positioning the patient to drain specific affected lobes. See Table 13-7 for instructions on postural drainage positions with some of the positions illustrated in Figure 13-15.

Forced Expiratory Technique

Any maneuver that involves a less than full cough effort in an attempt to dislodge mucus from the walls of the airways can be classed as a directed cough. For many patients with spinal cord dysfunction, muscle dysfunction, airway instability, or pain associated with coughing, a full explosive cough effort is not possible. The forced expiratory techniques (controlled cough, huff cough) involve a series of coughs from a mid to low lung volume. With huff coughing, the airways are less likely to experience the collapse that typically occurs with a full explosive cough.[26] The patient is instructed to take a slow deep inspiration followed by a rapid huff exhalation. This process may be repeated several times in a row until mucus production occurs.

Figure 13-13 Patient with cystic fibrosis wearing ABI Vest while concurrently undergoing aerosol treatment.

| Figure 13-14 | Percussion and vibration. **A.** Proper hand positioning for percussion. **B.** Proper technique for vibration. **C.** Proper hand position for vibration. (with permission from Nettina SM. *The Lippincott manual of nursing practice*. 7th ed. Philadelphia: Lippincott Williams & Wilkins; 2001) |

TABLE 13-7 Postural Drainage Positions

The proper position for postural drainage for the each lobe is as follows:
- Upper lobes, apical segments: patient sits upright, and percussion is performed above the clavicle and next to the neck.
- Upper lobes, anterior segments: patient lays flat in supine position; percussion is done below the clavicle.
- Right upper lobe, posterior segment: patient lays on his/her left side and leans 45 degrees forward; percussion is done on the scapula next to the spine.
- Left upper lobe, apical–posterior segment: patient sits in semi-Fowler's position or with the head of the bed elevated to 30 degrees, laying on the right side, rotated 45 degrees to the front; percussion is performed on the scapula next to the spine.
- Right middle lobe, lateral and medial segments: patient lays in Trendelenburg position on the left side leaning 45 degrees to the back; percussion is done two hands below the clavicle.
- Left upper lobe, superior and inferior lingula segments: patient lays in Trendelenburg position on the right side, leaning 45 degrees back; percussion is done two hands below the clavicle.
- Right and left lower lobes, superior segments: patient lays flat in prone position, and percussion is performed below the scapula.
- Right and left lower lobes, posterior basal segments: patient lays in Trendelenburg prone position; percussion is performed two hands below the scapula.
- Right lower lobe, anterior basal and medial basal segments: patient lays in Trendelenburg supine position, and percussion is performed two hands below clavicle.
- Left lower lobe, anterior–medial basal segment: patient lays in Trendelenburg supine position with percussion done two hands below the clavicle.
- Right lower lobe, lateral basal segment: patient lays on left side in Trendelenburg position, rotated 45 degrees to the front; percussion is done two hands below the scapula and to the side.
- Left lower lobe, lateral basal segment: patient lays on right side in Trendelenburg position, rotated 45 degrees to the front; percussion is done two hands below the scapula and to the side.

Upper lobes
apical segments

Upper lobes
posterior segments

Left lingula

Right
middle lobe

Lower lobes
posterior segments

Right lower lobe
lateral segment

Lower lobes
anterior segments

Figure 13-15 Position for postural drainage. (with permission from Nettina SM. *The Lippincott manual of nursing practice.* 7th ed. Philadelphia: Lippincott Williams & Wilkins; 2001)

CASE STUDY

PATIENT INFORMATION

An 18-year-old man diagnosed with cystic fibrosis at 1 year presented to the outpatient clinic for routine spirometry and chest radiography. His vital signs were as follows: heart rate, 89 beats/min; respiratory rate, 15 breaths/min; oxygen saturation level, 93% while breathing room air; blood pressure, 130/85; breath sounds were diminished; air movement bilaterally with expiratory wheezes on the right side greater than the left side. Patient stated that he had been a little short of breath while doing routine activities and had shortened his exercise routine recently due to dyspnea. The radiologist reported that the chest x-ray revealed a patchy density in the right upper and middle lobes consistent with possible pneumonia and also noted that the patient had a flattened diaphragm consistent with hyperinflated lungs.

The pulmonary function testing data showed the following: $FEV_1/FVC = 65\%$ of predicted; $FEV_1 = 70\%$ of predicted. The patient stated that he had been coughing up more mucus than he normally does in the past few days. His current regimen of therapy was bronchodilator treatments as needed, postural drainage and percussion therapy two times per day, inhaled steroids twice per day, and treadmill brisk walking for 10 minutes in the morning (down from 20 minutes in the morning). The patient was on a high-energy and high-fat diet due to his condition.

LINKS TO
GUIDE TO PHYSICAL THERAPIST PRACTICE

The patient's diagnosis was consistent with pattern 6C of the *Guide to Physical Therapist Practice*[27] "impaired ventilation, respiration/gas exchange, and aerobic capacity/endurance associated with airway/clearance dysfunction." Included in this diagnostic group is "cystic fibrosis, pneumocytosis, pneumonia, bronchitis, asthma, pleurisy and other respiratory related diseases" and direct intervention involves "breathing strategies, positioning activities, and conditioning exercises."

INTERVENTION

The initial intervention was directed at increasing airway clearance and encouraging deep breathing, with instructions for pursed-lip breathing and use of a bronchodilator. The PT instructed the PTA to perform the following treatment and report the patient's response to the treatment at a posttreatment review session:

1. Perform postural drainage and percussion with emphasis on education of patient for correct positioning (Figs. 13-14 and 13-15).
2. Review with patient correct use of Flutter device for positive expiratory pressure for airway stability and vibration of secretion mobilization (Fig. 13-12 and Table 13-6).
3. Review deep breathing techniques and diaphragmatic breathing during rest (Fig. 13-9).
4. Instruct patient in pursed-lip breathing technique for use during periods of distress (Table 13-2).
5. Instruct patient to maintain home program of percussion and postural drainage but increase to three times per day, use of the inhaler, and treadmill walking at 10 minutes per session.

PROGRESSION

One Week After Initial Treatment

At the time of re-examination by the PT the patient presented with improved breath sounds and less congestion and reported feeling better. The PT directed the PTA to review the current home program with the patient, monitor him on the treadmill walking for 12 to 15 minutes, and instruct him in exercise progression for the treadmill.

Two Weeks After Initial Examination

After 2 weeks of intervention the PT's examination indicated normal breath sounds, no reports of dyspnea, and increased endurance during activities of daily living. The PT instructed the PTA to review the home program, set the patient up with a final appointment and schedule a repeat pulmonary function test.

OUTCOMES

Three weeks after initial intervention the patient was re-evaluated by the PT and cleared for continued home management of his lung disease.

SUMMARY—AN EFFECTIVE PT–PTA TEAM

This case study demonstrates an effective relationship between the PT and PTA. The PT trusts the PTA in management of the appropriate techniques for the patient's improvement. The PTA must be knowledgeable of treatment techniques for breathing/lung sounds, exertion assessments or scales, airway clearance, breathing management, and aerobic conditioning. Good communication between the PT and PTA necessitates documentation and reporting of patient response to treatment including any unexpected responses. The working relationship between this team provided the patient with quality care and a successful outcome of intervention.

▼ ▼ ▼ GERIATRIC PERSPECTIVES ▼ ▼ ▼

- Age-related changes in the respiratory system do affect the efficiency of breathing. However, aging is a heterogenic process in that individuals age at varied rates and therefore will exhibit different levels of change. Age-related changes[1,2] include:
  - Structural changes in lung tissue
  - Changes in volume of air moved through the lungs
  - Diminished or altered exchange of gases—oxygen and carbon dioxide
  - Altered inspiration and expiration mechanics

- The lung of the older adult has an increase in the physiologic dead space as a result of a decrease in lung elasticity or compliance. The volume of air remaining in the lung following a maximal expiration is increased, which ultimately affects the total capacity of the lung to exchange air.[1,3]

- Inspiratory reserve volume and expiratory reserve volume remain fairly constant with aging, while the residual capacity increases. The overall result is a decrease in the forced vital capacity.[4] Functionally, the change in FVC means that the older adult has less inspiratory and expiratory reserve to support the added demands of activity and exercise.

- Exercise studies with elderly subjects have demonstrated that cardiovascular factors (heart rate, for example) rarely limit exercise performance; rather, the older individual is constrained by pulmonary factors like depth of rate of breathing or threshold for maximal oxygen uptake ($\dot{V}O_{2max}$).[5] Stathokostas et al[6] reported that over a 10-year period in a sample of 62 healthy, ambulatory, independent men and women $\dot{V}O_{2max}$ declined 14% in the men and 7% in the women.

- Important age-related changes impacting respiratory function are related to decreases in the elastic recoil and increases in chest wall stiffness. The changes are associated with age-related postural changes, stiffening of intercostal cartilage, as well as rib and vertebral joint arthritis.[1] A decrease in diaphragmatic strength, although not in diaphragmatic mass, also occurs with aging, but it is not known if the strength loss is related to the structural changes.

- Expiratory and inspiratory muscle strength changes in the fifth decade have been implicated in a decreased ability to produce a forceful cough to effectively clear secretions.[7,8]

1. Spirduso WW, Francis KL, MacRae PG. *Physical dimensions of aging*. 2nd ed. Champaign, IL: Human Kinetics; 2004.
2. Kauffman TL. *Geriatric rehabilitation manual*. New York: Churchill Livingstone; 1999.
3. Hazzard WR, Blass JP, Halter JB, et al. *Principles of geriatric medicine and gerontology*. 5th ed. New York: McGraw-Hill; 2003.
4. Pride NB. Ageing and changes in lung mechanics. *Eur Respir J*. 2005;26:563–565.
5. Paterson DH, Cunningham DA, Koval JJ, et al. Aerobic fitness in a population of independently living men and women aged 55–86 years. *Med Sci Sports Exerc*. 1999;31:1813–1820.
6. Stathokostas L, Jacob-Johnson S, Petrella RJ, et al. Longitudinal changes in aerobic power in older men and women. *J Appl Physiol*. 2004;97:781–789.
7. Kim J, Sapienza CM. Implications of expiratory muscle strength training for rehabilitation of the elderly: tutorial. *J Rehabil Res Dev*. 2005;42:211–224.
8. Shaker R, Ren J, Bardan E, et al. Pharyngoglottal closure reflex: characterization in healthy young, elderly and dysphagic patients with predeglutitive aspiration. *Gerontology*. 2003;49:12–20.

SUMMARY

- Matching the best option for breathing enhancement with the appropriate patient is very important. Some therapies that might not work for some patients might work extremely well for others.

- Every therapy session should be tailored to fit the individual. Compliance with the therapy is another important issue. When patients miss therapy, the results will also be missed. Stressing that adhering to the assigned schedule will produce the maximum amount of benefits and lung improvement is very important.

- Equally important is the proper technique with the therapy. If the device is used improperly or the instructions are ignored, then the gains will not be evident.

- This chapter did not introduce every therapeutic option available to enhance pulmonary function. A myriad of devices and breathing techniques exist and may be of benefit to patients. The reason for inclusion of the information in this chapter was based on available research. The devices and breathing tech-

PEDIATRIC PERSPECTIVES

- A misconception exists that respiratory and chronic pulmonary diseases are primarily adult issues.[1]

- Children with asthma miss 10.1 million more days of school than their peers without asthma.[2]

- Children with a central nervous system disorder such as cerebral palsy are at high risk for pulmonary/respiratory problems.[3]

- A child's airway size and poor mechanical advantage predisposes him/her to increased likelihood of, and generally, more severe respiratory illness than adults.[1]

- The child has a higher metabolic rate than the adult, requiring increased consumption of oxygen, increased heat loss, and increased water loss secondary to a faster respiratory rate.

- Three general categories of interventions are common in children: a) removal of secretions, b) breathing exercises and retraining, and c) physical reconditioning. Depending on the area of the country in which the PTA practices, respiratory therapists may be doing more of the removal of secretions with overlap occurring between respiratory therapy and physical therapy relative to breathing exercises and retraining, and physical therapy being responsible for physical reconditioning.

- Breathing exercises may incorporate "child-friendly" games and activities such as blowing a feather across the table, blowing to keep a feather up in the air, blowing bubbles, blowing a pinwheel, etc.

- The most commonly known childhood diseases with pulmonary complications are cystic fibrosis and asthma.

- Studies performing aerobic conditioning activities in children with asthma reported improved aerobic capacity and increased general health.[4,5]

- Results are mixed with aerobic conditioning in children with cystic fibrosis, depending on the severity of the disease and if the child has concurrent infection.[6,7]

- Oxygen saturation in children with cystic fibrosis who require hospitalization should be monitored during aerobic activity with the use of a pulse oximeter. Readings should be done every 15 minutes for patients whose baseline saturation is 93% to 96% and more frequently if below 93%. If the oxygen saturation drops below 90% and does not return with a short rest (2 to 3 minutes), supplemental oxygen should be given until the saturation returns to 93%.[8]

- Improved upper-body strength, aerobic capacity, and independence in activities of daily living have been reported in adolescents with cystic fibrosis who underwent a combination of strengthening and aerobic exercises.[7,9]

1. Tecklin JS. Pulmonary disorders in infants and children and their physical therapy management. In: Tecklin JS, ed. *Pediatric physical therapy.* Philadelphia: Lippincott Williams & Wilkins; 1999.

2. Taylor WP, Newacheck PW. Impact of childhood asthma on health. *Pediatrics.* 1992;90:657–662.

3. Carlson SJ, Ramsey C. Assistive technology. In: Campbell SK, ed. *Physical therapy for children.* Philadelphia: WB Saunders Co; 1995.

4. Counil FP, Varray A, Matecki S, et al. Training of aerobic and anaerobic fitness in children with asthma. *J Pediatr.* 2003;142:179–184.

5. Matsumoto I, Araki H, Tsuda K, et al. Effects of swimming training on aerobic capacity and exercise induced bronchoconstriction in children with bronchial asthma. *Thorax.* 1999;54:196–201.

6. Orenstein DM, Franklin BA, Doershuk CF, et al. Exercise conditioning and cardiorespiratory fitness in cystic fibrosis. *Chest.* 1981;80:392–398.

7. Orenstein DM, Hovell MF, Mulvihill M, et al. Strength versus aerobic training in children with cystic fibrosis: a randomized controlled trial. *Chest.* 2004;126:1204–1214.

8. Arkansas Children's Hospital. *Cystic fibrosis clinical pathway.* Little Rock, AR: Arkansas Children's Hospital; 2006.

9. de Jong W, Grevink RG, Roorda RJ, et al. Effect of a home exercise training program in patients with cystic fibrosis. *Chest.* 1994;105:463–468.

niques presented have been shown to be successful with patients.

- If the patient reports a reduction in dyspnea or an improvement in walking distance or activities of daily living, then the therapeutic regimen produced a positive outcome.

References

1. Scherer TA. Respiratory muscle endurance training in chronic obstructive pulmonary disease: impact on exercise capacity, dyspnea, and quality of life. *Am J Respir Crit Care Med.* 2000;162:1709–1714.

2. Wolfson MR, Shaffer TH. Respiratory physiology: structure, function, and integrative responses to intervention with special emphasis on the ventilatory pump. In: Irwin S, Tecklin T, eds. *Cardiopulmonary physical therapy: a guide to practice.* 4th ed. St. Louis: Mosby; 2004;39–81.

3. Man WD. Postprandial effects on twitch transdiaphragmatic pressure. *Eur Respir J.* 2002;20:577–580.

4. Gubaidullin RR, Butrov AV. Relationship between transdiaphragmatic pressure and oxygen consumption in patients with intestinal obstruction. *Crit Care.* 2002;6:6.

5. Breslin H. The pattern of respiratory muscle recruitment during pursed-lip breathing. *Chest.* 1992;101:75–78.

6. Cherniack NS, Pack AI. Control of ventilation. In: Fishman AP, ed. *Fishman's pulmonary diseases and disorders.* 3rd ed. New York: McGraw-Hill; 1998.

7. Caruana-Montaldo B, Gleeson K, Zwillich CW. The control of breathing in clinical practice. *Chest.* 2000;117:205–225.

8. Ruppel GE. *Manual of pulmonary function testing.* 6th ed. St. Louis: Mosby; 1994.

9. American Association for Respiratory Care. Clinical practice guidelines: spirometry. *Respir Care.* 1996;41:629–636.

10. Troosters T. Pulmonary rehabilitation in chronic obstructive pulmonary disease. *Am J Respir Crit Care Med.* 2005;172:19–38.

11. Decramer M. Treatment of chronic respiratory failure: lung volume reduction surgery versus rehabilitation. *Eur Respir J Suppl.* 2003;22:47s–57s.

12. Solway S, Brooks D, Lacasse Y, et al. A qualitative systematic overview of the measurement properties of functional walk tests used in the cardiorespiratory domain. *Chest.* 2001;119:256–270.

13. Yan S, Sinderby C, Bielen P, et al. Expiratory muscle pressure and breathing mechanics in chronic obstructive pulmonary disease. *Eur Respir J.* 2000;16:684–690.

14. Toshima MC, Kaplan RM, Ries AL. Experimental evaluation of rehabilitation in chronic obstructive pulmonary disease: short-term effects on exercise endurance and health status. *Health Psychol.* 1990;9:237–252.

15. Levenson CR. Breathing exercises. In: Zadai C, ed. *Pulmonary management in physical therapy.* New York: Churchill Livingstone; 1992.

16. Larson JL. Inspiratory muscle training with a pressure threshold breathing device in patients with chronic obstructive pulmonary disease. *Am Rev Respir Dis.* 1988;138:689–696.

17. Lotters F, van Tol B, Kwakkel G, et al. Effects of controlled inspiratory muscle training in patients with COPD: Aa meta-analysis. *Eur Respir J.* 2002;20:570–576.

18. Weiner P, McConnell A. Respiratory muscle training in chronic obstructive pulmonary disease: inspiratory, expiratory, or both? *Curr Opin Pulm Med.* 2005;11:140–144.

19. Sheel WA. Respiratory muscle training in healthy individuals: physiological rationale and implications for exercise performance. *Sports Med.* 2002;32:567–581.

20. American Association for Respiratory Care. Clinical practice guideline. Incentive spirometry. *Respir Care.* 1991;36:1402–1405.

21. Bianchi R. Gigliotti F. Chest wall kinematics and breathlessness during pursed-lip breathing in patients with COPD. *Chest.* 2004;125:459–465.

22. Sinderby C, Spahija J, Beck J, et al. Diaphragm activation during exercise in chronic obstructive pulmonary disease. *Am J Respir Crit Care Med.* 2001;163:1637–1641.

23. Babcock MA. Effects of respiratory muscle unloading on exercise-induced diaphragm fatigue. *J Appl Physiol.* 2001;93:201–206.

24. Gosselink R. Controlled breathing and dyspnea in patients with chronic obstructive pulmonary disease (COPD). *J Rehabil Res Dev.* 2003;40:25–34.

25. Frownfelter D, Dean E. *Cardiovascular and pulmonary physical therapy.* 4th ed. St. Louis: Mosby Elsevier; 2006:326–328.

26. Fink JB. Positive pressure techniques for airway clearance. *Respir Care.* 2002;47:786–796.

27. American Physical Therapy Association. *Guide to physical therapist practice.* 2nd ed. Alexandria, VA; 2003.

Functional Progression is Therapeutic Exercise

Functional Progression for the Spine

Ginny Keely, PT, MS, OCS, FAAOMPT

OBJECTIVES

Upon completion of this chapter, the reader will be able to:

- Identify the dynamic and inert structures responsible for postural equilibrium.

- Identify appropriate goals for a spinal stabilization program based on principles of position, progression, and functional loss.

- Apply to clinical practice appropriate postural correction techniques and maintenance methods within the established plan of care.

- Apply to clinical practice proper observation skills and education techniques concerning body mechanics within the established plan of care.

- Apply appropriate spinal stabilization techniques using proper initiation and profession principles with and without therapeutic equipment within the established plan of care.

Treating the spine can be an ominous task for the novice physical therapist (PT) and physical therapist assistant (PTA). The spine, with its intricacies, might intimidate one who is looking for a black and white picture that dictates specific intervention. It has been estimated that 5.6% of the U.S. population, or approximately 10 million people, have back pain at any one point in time.[1] It is therefore important for all practitioners to gain a reasonable arsenal of intervention skills aimed at getting the client back to work or play. This chapter gives the PTA a framework in which to treat individuals with spinal injuries, with the intended outcome of returning the client to premorbid level of function.

SCIENTIFIC BASIS

Biomechanical Considerations

Although the spine is actually just a series of joints, the intimate relationships among the joints give the spine a variety of special qualities. The anterior–posterior curves enable the spine to sustain compressive loads ten times greater than if the column were straight.[2] The hydraulic nature of the discs permits controlled movement while forces are transferred vertically to the trabecular system of the adjacent vertebral bodies.[2] The synovial facet joints guide motion in multiple planes, permitting the human body to move freely in three dimensions. Together, the vertebral bodies, discs, facet joints, supportive ligaments, and muscles coalesce to create an extremely dynamic structural system.[2]

Posture

To function in a world with strong gravitational forces, the body has adapted by integrating delicate architectural and dynamic supportive designs, allowing for relatively effortless upright positioning. This design, however, is combated by 21st century lifestyle. Most people, regardless of age, have lived a life full of sitting, flexed postures, and restricted activity and movement. Good posture "is a state of musculoskeletal balance that protects the supporting structures of the body against injury or progressive deformity."[3] This musculoskeletal balance is important at rest and with the dynamic activity of the body in motion.

To achieve balance, one must consider both the dynamic and inert structures responsible for postural equilibrium. Muscles provide dynamic counterforces to moments of extension and flexion caused by gravitational torque at joints, and they require an intact nervous system to provide sensorimotor feedback.[4] The inert osseous and ligamentous structures provide passive tension at joints and support for weight bearing in the upright posture. At equilibrium, the line of gravity falls near or through the axes of rotation of the joints, and compression forces are optimally distributed over weight-bearing surfaces.[5] Gravitational forces are then balanced by counter torque generated either by inert structures or by minimal muscle activity.[5] When the center of mass moves, the line of gravity falls a distance away from the joint axes, often approaching the limits of the base of support. A need exists for increased counter torque to balance gravitational forces and maintain upright posture.[5]

When considering spinal alignment and the interplay of inert and dynamic structures, the PTA should note the influence of the lower biomechanical chain. Structural or functional faults may contribute to a less than optimal foundation on which the spine must function. Structural alignment issues include limb length difference and bony alignment of the femur, and functional problems include postural and muscle imbalances about the hip, knee, or foot.

Structural Malalignment

Limb length differences may lead to spinal asymmetry by effectively lowering the pelvis on one side and elevating the other. For example, if a patient has a short left extremity, the pelvis will drop on the left, carrying the spine with it. Hence, the spine will be leaning to the left. As the individual seeks optical righting, a compensatory curve of the lumbar spine may occur back to the right. If an overcorrection is achieved, yet another compensatory curve back to the left may be noted in the thoracic spine. This positioning asymmetry leads to unnatural forces through the spine. The concave side of the curve has increased facet weight bearing and narrowing of the intervertebral foramen, and the hydraulic disc is at risk for injury on the convex side. In addition, the muscles on the convex side tend to lengthen and become weaker, whereas the muscles on the concave side tend to shorten.

Femoral structure may also influence spinal mechanics. If a patient has coxa vara, the pelvis tends to be brought into a position of anterior tilt, or anterior inclination. The opposite is true with coxa valga, in which the pelvis tends toward a posterior tilt, or posterior inclination. If the pelvis is positioned in an anterior tilt, the lumbar spine is brought into a greater lordosis. An accentuated anterior tilt increases forces on the posterior elements of the spine, such as the facet joints, putting these structures at risk for injury. Conversely, if the pelvis is tilted posteriorly, the lumbar spine may lose normal lordosis. This position of relative kyphosis may put the anterior structures at risk for injury, especially the disc. With the loss of lordosis, the annular structure of the disc is stressed posteriorly and may lead to annular incompetence and possibly an inability for the annulus to adequately control the nucleus.[6,7]

Knee posture may also affect stress in the spine. A genu valgum, or "knock-kneed," posture tends to guide the pelvis into either an anterior or a posterior tilt because of compensatory femoral rotation. With faulty knee alignment in the frontal plane, the hip tends to compensate in the transverse plane with either a medial or lateral rotation. The pelvis then responds with sagittal plane compensation, leading to excessive anterior or posterior tilt. Again, these postures direct forces through the spine in an anterior or posterior manner, as discussed previously. Owing to effects on pelvic position, genu recurvatum (knee hyperextension) may also promote a shearing compensation in the upper lumbar spine. The spine transitions from an excessive lordosis caused by an excessive anterior pelvic tilt and adopts a position of flexion (kyphosis) to bring the body into anterior–posterior balance.[6]

Functional (Muscle) Imbalance

Functional imbalance is a dysfunction in the musculoskeletal system, potentially leading to a less than optimal spinal foundation. The musculoskeletal system can be likened to a balanced system of guy wires or springs attached to a structural foundation (Fig. 14-1). The overall length of the supportive guy wires affects the balance of the structural foundation. In addition, the extensibility, or quality of overall length of the supportive guy wire, affects the balance within the system.

Janda and Jull[8] suggested that the pelvic crossed syndrome may affect the balance of the muscles surrounding the joints of the lower extremity. For example, if the pelvis is in a position of anterior tilt, the muscular system may develop compensatory qualities. The hip flexors, placed in a relaxed position, may shorten along with the lumbar extensors. Conversely, the gluteals and abdominals are in a lengthened position, subjecting them to stretch weakness. Given that it weakens the passive components of the muscles, chronic stretch may neurologically inhibit the active components, making the muscle less stiff.[9,10] Similarly, the chronically shortened muscles may lose passive elasticity and be actively facilitated toward a higher state of contractility, becoming increasingly stiff.[9,10] Because of these factors, it is a difficult task to overcome the postural tendency promoted by the crossed pelvic syndrome.[8]

Balance of the musculature around the pelvis is important for postural reasons and because the iliopsoas, tensor fascia lata, quadriceps, hamstrings, gluteus maximus, hip rotators, abductors, and adductors play a crucial role in the ability of the pelvis to appropriately transmit ground reaction forces.[4] Table 14-1 lists the primary muscles involved in postural assessment.

Figure 14-1 Springs demonstrate a mechanical model of lumbopelvic stability.

TABLE 14-1 Postural Muscles Prone to Loss of Flexibility or Weakness

Muscles Prone to Tightness	Muscles Prone to Weakness
Erector spinae	Rectus abdominus
Quadratus lumborum	Serratus anterior
Iliopsoas	Gluteus maximus, medius, and minimus
Tensor fascia lata	
Piriformis	Lower trapezius
Rectus femoris	Vastus medialis and lateralis
Hamstrings	Short cervical flexors
Gastrocsoleus	Extensors of upper limb
Pectoralis major	Tibialis anterior
Upper trapezius	
Levator scapula	
Sternocleidomastoid	
Scalenes	

Adapted from Janda V, Jull G. Muscles and motor control. In: Twomey LT, Taylor JT, eds. *Physical therapy of the low back. Clinics in physical therapy series.* 3rd ed. New York: Churchill Livingstone; 2000:253–278.

Body Mechanics

Proper body mechanics are considered crucial both for control of symptoms and for prevention of future episodes of back pain. However, no one definition of proper body mechanics is accepted, which can lead to confusion in patient management. Floyd and Silver[11] advocated full posterior pelvic tilt with lumbar flexion for lifting, which employs the neurologic protective mechanism of extensor muscle relaxation in the full end of range position. This end-range relaxation suggests that a posterior pelvic tilt may protect the spinal musculature from injury.

McGill[12] supported the idea of extreme anterior pelvic tilt to protect the spine during lifting, but this may compromise the posterior structures that are not designed for such weight-bearing capabilities. McGill countered with the idea of pelvic and lumbar "neutral" for lifting and for most functional tasks. As described later, this neutral position varies among individuals.

The appropriate (proper) body mechanics can greatly influence the musculoskeletal environment in which functional tasks are performed, leading to improper stresses in the spine.[12] Consider the potential effect of shortened or stiff hamstring muscles. When a task such as squatting is performed, short or stiff hamstrings limit the ability of the pelvis to maintain its relatively neutral alignment because of the effect of the muscles at their attachments on the ischial tuberosities. As the hamstrings become taught throughout hip flexion, the muscles eventually pull on the ischial tuberosities, causing the pelvis to tilt posteriorly. A similar phenomenon occurs in the upper extremity with

overhead reaching. A stiff or short latissimus dorsi muscle (extending from the posterior aspect of the pelvis to the intertubercular groove of the humerus) can limit the ability of the humerus to move upward, causing the pelvis to tilt anteriorly to allow for a greater range of overhead reach.

As noted earlier, the body functions most efficiently when in a state of postural equilibrium. When the center of mass moves, the line of gravity falls away from joint axes, often toward the perimeter of the base of support. In this situation, the muscles act to balance gravitational forces and maintain postural balance.[13] If a joint remains in a locked (or close-packed) position, the gravitational forces are attenuated and the inert support structures are at risk.[5] Therefore, the basic idea of proper body mechanics is the safe maintenance of a loose-packed joint position while external gravitational forces are imposed, often near the limits of the base of support and while external loads are supported. To achieve this balance, the client needs both the knowledge of safe joint position and the necessary muscular strength to maintain musculoskeletal balance.

Spinal Stabilization

The idea of spinal stabilization evolved because of the belief that to recover and maintain health, patients with low back pain must exercise.[14] Such functional exercise techniques emphasize movement re-education and apply a combination of principles derived from neurodevelopmental techniques, proprioceptive neuromuscular facilitation (PNF), and basic body mechanics. The goal of this type of training is to improve the patient's physical condition and symptoms and to facilitate efficient movement.[14,15]

The basic philosophy behind stabilization training is that spinal pain is a movement or postural disorder that has resulted in or perpetuated spinal dysfunction.[14] The actual pathoanatomy of spinal pain is poorly understood. Multiple potential pain generators exist in spinal pain syndromes, and often the anatomic structure at fault does not matter.[4] The crucial matter is to determine the activities and postures in which the patient is unable to tolerate stresses. The concept of stability of the spine actually considers a combination of the osseoligamentous system, muscle system, and neural control system.[16] The PT should avoid getting caught up in the guessing game of pathoanatomic diagnosis and focus on improvement of function and, hence, stability. Therefore, the basis of functional stabilization training is to provide the patient with movement awareness, knowledge of safe postures, and functional strength and coordination that promote management of spinal dysfunction. Freedom of movement while maintaining a stable foundation is the goal. Table 14-2 presents the expectations and goals that should be considered when developing an individualized stabilization program.[15]

TABLE 14-2 Expectation and Goals of a Spinal
           Stabilization Program

Patients complain less and become more functional with
   exercise intervention.
The neurologic influences of muscles and joints are
   inseparable; thus, the physical therapist assistant must
   be concerned with the neuromotor system and not treat
   muscles and joints in isolation.
Regardless of anatomic involvement or stage of recovery, all
   patients with low back pain can engage in a training
   program.
Patients are trained to improve physical capacity; to
   facilitate more functional movement; and to prevent,
   control, or eliminate symptoms.
Training should include increasing flexibility, strength,
   endurance, and coordination.

Reprinted with permission from Biondi, B. Lumbar functional stabilization program. In: Goldstein TS, ed. *Functional rehabilitation in orthopedics*. Gaithersburg, MD: Aspen; 1995:133–142.

Many PTs use exercise in the treatment of low back problems. However, the type of exercise and the emphasis in training are not standardized. What is known from research investigations is that exercise programs facilitate management of spinal symptoms.[17–23] O'Sullivan et al[24] demonstrated a significant decrease in pain and disability immediately, 3 months, 6 months, and 30 months after initiation of an exercise intervention. In a retrospective study, Saal and Saal[21] found that a high percentage of patients with objective radiculopathy had successful outcomes with stabilization training, even when surgery had previously been recommended. Nelson et al[20] demonstrated that a large number of patients for whom surgery was recommended had successful outcomes in the short term by performing aggressive strengthening exercises. Thus, although it has been shown that exercise is beneficial, a variety of training programs have been used.

The exercise format for stabilization emphasizes both strength and endurance, as well as addressing proprioception. If a client is aware of the safe-functioning neutral position of the spine, then the ability to maintain safe posture is the key. This ability has a basic strength requirement; however, because postural muscles must have endurance, the strengthening exercises should progress toward endurance.[12,25] Consider the evidence that shows that patients with back pain have selective wasting of the type 1 (slow-oxidative) muscle fibers.[26] The loss of type 1 fibers renders the muscles less equipped for endurance activities.[4] This information provides further incentive to address endurance as much as strength.

Therefore, the PT needs to identify the muscles on which to focus when initiating any type of therapeutic exercise regime. Research suggests that the core stabilizers are not the larger, external muscles—such as the rectus abdominus and external oblique muscles—but rather the inner, deep muscles, such as the lumbar multifidus (segmentally), the transversus abdominus, and (to some extent) the internal oblique muscles. The multifidus muscles are important for reducing shear forces in the lumbar spine,[21,22] and recent evidence supports the ability of the lumbar extensor muscles, even at low levels of activity, to increase lumbar posteroanterior stiffness.[12,27,28]

Through ultrasonographic imaging, Hides et al[29] identified selective ipsilateral multifidus wasting at the level of spinal injury. Although they identified selective wasting of type 2 (fast-twitch) fibers, they also found an internal structural change of the type 1 fibers, described as "moth eaten" in appearance.[30] This selective wasting of muscle appears to have long-lasting implications for recovery.[30] Again, emphasis in training of the type 1 fibers is warranted. The multifidus atrophy develops acutely and continues for at least 10 weeks, even when pain-free status has been achieved, with or without exercise intervention.[31] However, in the experimental group who received exercise therapy, multifidus size was restored. On follow-up, individuals in the exercise group had a significantly lower recurrence rate of pain than those in the control group.[16]

Indahl et al[32] demonstrated in porcine experiments that although the multifidus muscles increased in electrical activity when subjected to annular stimulation, they underwent reflex inhibition when saline was injected into the associated facet joint, demonstrating a complex pattern of neurologically mediated events. It has been postulated that the loss of muscle size of the multifidus after injury is not related to the presence of electrical activity. In fact, it may be possible that because of high electrical activity, the muscle undergoes wasting as a result of the increased metabolic demands.[29]

The transversus abdominus muscle has been confirmed as a primary stabilizer of the lumbar spine. In fact, support by the transversus abdominus is considered to be the most important of the abdominal muscles. Its action seems to be independent of the other abdominal muscles and is most closely tied to the function of the diaphragm and pelvic floor muscles and intimately relates to the thoracolumbar fascia. The transversus abdominus, with some contribution from the internal oblique muscle, assists in increased intra-abdominal pressure. Its normal action, along with the action of deep fibers of the lumbar multifidus muscles, may function to form a deep internal corset. This pattern of motor control is disrupted in patients with low back pain.[16]

Given that stabilization, as an exercise intervention, is meant to both condition the muscles and address motor programming, the obvious question is whether motor programs can really be changed. One concept to emphasize is that stabilization training in general works the core stabilizers in their natural fashion—not as prime movers but as primary stabilizers. The limbs are providing the resistance, and the core muscles respond to the postural challenge. In healthy individuals, the stabilizers act in a feed-forward manner; the trunk muscles precede the limb muscles in order of motor recruitment.[33] In other words, the trunk muscles "turn on" in preparation for the limb movement. Conversely, in the patient population, the firing of the abdominal muscles is delayed, often occurring after the limb movement.[34]

Recent findings support the idea that skill training can indeed change the motor-firing pattern of abdominal muscle activity in response to limb movement.[16,35] In addition, some researchers have demonstrated that it is possible to alter movement patterns and muscle recruitment patterns by training individuals in spinal stabilization techniques.[36,37]

Finally, in addition to working the core stabilizers, conditioning of the major postural muscles is encouraged. These muscles include the gluteals, erector spinae, latissimus dorsi, and lower-extremity muscles. The PT should include upper-extremity exercises as an adjunct because spinal stresses increase as upper-extremity loads are maneuvered.

CLINICAL GUIDELINES

Posture

Addressing posture is probably the single most important aspect of treating spinal injuries. By examining an individual's posture using the vertical compression test, the implications of postural faults are easily demonstrated.[38] During the test, forces of gravity in the vertical plane are exaggerated and stress points are manifested. The patient usually is able to feel the gravitational stresses, and postural correction then becomes a powerful tool.

To examine the ability of an individual to attenuate loads through the body in relaxed stance, provide a smooth, direct downward pressure through the trunk, accentuating gravitational load. This action essentially provides the PT with a visual representation of the potential effects of increased gravitational load on a patient in the standing position. The results of the test can be used to project the possible shearing forces exerted on the body when an upright position must be maintained for an extended period of time (Fig. 14-2).

After postural correction, employ the vertical compression test again. A firm resistance to gravity that is balanced through the load-bearing joints will diffuse the forces, enabling the client to feel the difference in an immediate and applicable way. Regardless of diagnosis, the patient must be educated regarding posture if any noticeable postural inefficiencies are present, as most individuals demonstrate.

Body Mechanics

Although body mechanics are dynamic while posture appears static, each is truly an extension of the other. When the body moves through space, gravitational forces impart moments of force that vary in direction and intensity. The body must constantly adapt to these forces, but the uninformed individual is not aware of potentially efficient and safe positions in which to best handle the external forces. Therefore, it is imperative to observe the client in functional movements, scrutinizing the mechanics of the movement to identify inefficient and potentially unsafe maneuvers.

Functional testing need not be complicated. Simple observation of normal activities can be quite valuable. This examination can begin as soon as the client stands from the seated position. Notice the position of the body over the legs. Observe whether the individual uses momentum or pushes from the upper extremities to attain the standing position. Is the pelvis in an extreme position as it moves forward over the lower extremities? Is there unnecessary internal rotation torque of the femurs, with accompanying pronation of the subtalar or midtarsal joints? Is the thoracic spine in a compromised position of end-range kyphosis during the movement to standing? Any of these compensatory movements indicates decreased ability to withstand the forces of gravity for that particular maneuver. Look for similar compensatory behaviors in all functional tests, including partial squatting, unilateral balance, lifting an item from the floor, reaching forward or overhead, pushing or pulling, and the prone leg lift for multifidus stability.

Frequently body mechanics are compromised by the patient's lack of understanding of safe functional performance and by a physical limitation that makes proper performance impossible. Recall the example of stiff hamstrings and the influence on squatting. Loss of mobility in the hamstrings will limit the ability of the pelvis to maintain neutral alignment because the hamstrings may mechanically influence the pelvis into a posterior tilt. The PTA should watch for such compensations and seek to address the physical as well as the functional limitations.

Spinal Stabilization

If the goal is to improve the protective stabilizing ability of the spinal muscles, it is imperative that the exercise load not overtax the muscles. If the muscles are fatigued, this may create compensation and potential inhibition of the targeted muscles. Initially, the spinal stabilization program begins with the learning of an isolated contraction of the targeted muscle, which enhances the client's proprioceptive abilities needed for the progression of exercise. Light resistance

Figure 14-2   The vertical compression test.

PURPOSE: Examine vertical loading responses throughout the system.

POSITION: Client standing relaxed. Physical therapist (PT) on stool behind.

PROCEDURE: PT applies gravitational overpressure directly down through client's shoulders.

with isolated contraction follows, with gradual progression to functional and weight-bearing activities. Although limb movement alone imposes the initial challenge to the muscle, resistance to the limbs follows as the client progresses. In the early phases, it is important for the client to perform slow movements because the proximal stabilizing muscles may weaken or become inhibited when exposed to ballistic limb movement.[39]

Stabilization exercise is encouraged for young adults and for all ages. Adolescents have been successfully treated with these techniques, and it is well established that exercise in the aging population has numerous health benefits.[40] Remember to monitor risk factors in older adults when teaching them an exercise program.

Neutral Position

The neutral position, also called the "functional range of motion," is the position in which the spine is asymptomatic or least symptomatic and corresponds to the optimal position within which the spine functions most efficiently.[14] This position, or range of motion (ROM), varies among individuals and pathologies. Exercising at the end of ROM in either direction is not recommended.[12]

When given the opportunity to identify the least painful position, most people will indicate a relatively neutral position. This position is roughly achieved when the spine is resting and the patient is in the hook-lying position. When the hips are flexed to approximately 60 degrees, as naturally occurs in hook-lying, the lumbar spine tends to adopt a position that is closest to the mid-range. Therefore, the hook-lying position is a good one for initiating the patient's discovery of the neutral position.

The client's least painful position may be one of relative flexion of the lumbar spine, corresponding to a posterior pelvic tilt (called a flexion bias).[15] Some clients are most comfortable toward the extension ROM of the lumbar spine, with an anteriorly tilted pelvis, which indicates an extension bias.[15] Although these biases may change as the pathology changes, the PTA should always be aware of a patient's bias when designing an exercise prescription.

Training Progression

The PT should consider the following basic principles when beginning a training progression: (a) monitor the effects of weight bearing, (b) use stable before unstable postures, (c) use simple motions before combined movements, and (d) integrate gross motions before isolated, fine motor patterns. The patient's tolerance to weight bearing or load bearing should be kept in mind when prescribing exercise because some movements inherently involve more gravitational forces than others. An exercise in supine naturally decreases the gravitational stresses, whereas a loaded upright activity could exacerbate a condition in a patient with load sensitivities. The supine position also naturally provides more external stability than does the quadruped, kneeling, or upright position. Simple movements should be mastered before progressing to motions that require stability in diagonal planes, which challenge the body in three planes of motion. Lastly, the patient should be competent in mass body movements before the PTA superimposes isolated movements. For example, the action of rising from the seated position is less challenging than rising from the seated position and simultaneously reaching for the phone.

To teach stabilization concepts to a client, begin by helping the client produce and explore lumbopelvic movement in the sagittal plane (anterior–posterior direction), which is best done in the supine position. Then ask the client to identify the position in which symptoms are reduced or absent. This position constitutes the neutral position. If the client is asymptomatic within a range of movement, then he or she is free to move within the neutral ROM rather than maintain a strict neutral position. After the client accomplishes muscle control to maintain the neutral position (or ROM), teach the client to perform simple movements, gradually progressing to advanced, functional actions.

Individuals progress at different rates. The easiest way to help the client maintain the neutral ROM is to assist him or her with the use of external support, referred to as passive prepositioning. For example, the neutral position for a patient with a flexion bias is to be adequately supported in a supine position with the hips and knees in the 90/90 position, which encourages lumbar flexion. In contrast, the neutral position for a patient with an extension bias may be achieved with passive support to the spine in extension. The PTA may place a towel roll under the lumbar spine for support or simply ask the patient to allow the lower extremities to lie flat, which tilts the pelvis anteriorly and extends the lumbar spine. Exercising in this supported position assists the patient in maintaining a safe position for the spine.

Active prepositioning refers to the next level of stabilization in which the client uses muscular contraction to maintain a safe, stable posture for exercise. After exploring lumbopelvic motion and identifying the neutral position, the patient actively contracts the deep stabilizers to maintain the neutral position. When the patient can achieve adequate active contraction, the PTA can begin to focus on challenging the stabilizing musculature. The patient should begin with slow, controlled limb movement, while the PTA looks for any sign of subtle compensation. One common error is for the patient and PTA to get stuck in this phase of active cocontraction in preparation for movement. When time does not permit the PTA to help the patient move to a more advanced phase of intervention, the patient's concept of stabilization is of rigid holding to protect the spine. It is important that the patient does not move while the spine is locked in isometric holding but rather progresses to the next phase, dynamic stabilization.

In the dynamic stabilization phase, the muscles (via proprioceptive properties) protect the spine from unwanted motions. Muscles are not precontracted to protect the spine from undesired movement, but the muscles are on call, so to speak, and are recruited as needed to control spinal movements within the safe range. This phase also requires that the individual has the ability to freely transition from use of agonist and antagonist stabilizing musculature.

Functional Loss Characteristics

Of particular importance in the development of a stabilization program are the patient's functional loss characteristics: position sensitivity, weight-bearing sensitivity, stasis sensitivity, and pressure sensitivity. Although they may be found in isolation or may occur in combination, they will be discussed individually.[12,15]

Position Sensitivity

The patient who is position sensitive is usually the easiest to treat. Such a patient can easily identify the position of comfort when searching for the neutral position and when given the tools to manage the spine in or about that position, can learn to satisfactorily control symptoms. In addition to stabilization training, these individuals need to have a good understanding of which postures in daily living tend to place them in precarious positions. For example, patients with a flexion bias should be taught to avoid the relaxed standing posture because it creates an anterior pelvic tilt and lumbar extension.

Weight-bearing Sensitivity

A common finding, weight-bearing sensitivity is manifest quickly in an examination. A person who is weight-bearing sensitive frequently employs load-reducing maneuvers. For example, if the PTA notices that the patient is slouched in a chair with the buttocks forward and the trunk leaning back on the upper thoracic spine, the patient may be seeking the most supine position available at the moment. It is tempting to interpret this behavior as poor posture, but the position may be used as a load-reducing maneuver. Individuals with weight-bearing sensitivity will do anything possible to decrease the influences of gravity. In the examination room, such patients tend to lean on the upper extremities for support, often shifting position to vary the weight distribution.

To progress to an exercise program for patients with this functional loss characteristic, the PT needs to be creative in developing exercises that keep the spine unloaded or that actually provide distraction through exercise. Examples include the basic principles of unloading via nonweight-bearing positions. Another consideration is the use of traction harness supports for both gravity-eliminated and antigravity positions. Eventual progression might include upright unweighting exercises, such as pull-ups and dips, while paying attention to basic stabilization principles.

Stasis Sensitivity

Stasis sensitivity is commonly found in individuals with hypermobile or unstable conditions. This sensitivity is evidenced by the tendency for the patient to prefer moving to staying still and to feel worse in any sustained posture. The position, unless close to anatomic neutral, is irrelevant; if the posture is sustained, pain occurs. Nights are often difficult because the body remains still during sleep. The patient may need to get up in the night and walk around to decrease symptoms. Treatment considerations for these patients should include adherence to a relatively anatomic neutral posture, with controlled flexion/extension movement permitted during functional activities. Aerobic exercise, because of its oscillatory effects, often helps reduce symptoms. However, the emphasis should be on control of spinal movement during activity.

Pressure Sensitivity

Patients with pressure sensitivity on the posterior aspect of the spine will need modifications to any supine exercise and will best tolerate any activity in which there is no external pressure applied to the spinous processes or sacrum. For supine positioning, place two mats side by side with a slight gap to suspend the pressure-sensitive areas between the supportive surfaces.

Examination by the Physical Therapist

A thorough examination by the PT is always an important aspect of stabilization training and exercise prescription. As indicated, muscle imbalances may limit appropriate performance of certain exercises, and these imbalances must be dealt with before advancing the program. Compensatory movements during exercise may indicate a physiologic condition that warrants further investigation. The PT should always pay close attention to pain response and to compensatory movements that may occur with activity. Pain during safe exercise is often different from the symptoms for which the patient sought treatment. Often the muscle action will trigger different but benign symptoms related to muscle activity and not to pathology. The PTA should be alert to these symptoms to communicate the patient's status to the PT.

When the PT is embarking on a stability program for a patient with a hypermobile segment, it is important to have some objective measures regarding the stabilizing function of the multifidus muscles. The recommended testing procedure for segmental multifidus testing is shown in Figure 14-3. The lumbar spine is flexed up to the level of the involved segment; an attempted lateral displacement of the femurs will be poorly resisted in the presence of weak multifidi. This pressure should be light.

The multifidi primarily function as contralateral rotators; however, because the forces are applied through the pelvis, the side on which the pressure is applied is the side providing the resistance. In other words, if the pressure is applied to the femur on the left side (with the force directed toward the right), the left multifidus is being tested (Fig. 14-3). Because the multifidus muscles are inhibited at the level of spinal injury,[29] it is helpful to track the function of the multifidus using this testing procedure.

An alternate method of multifidus testing is a screening procedure recommended by Richardson et al.[16] This test relies on palpation and comparison of the contractions on each side. With the patient in the prone position, the PT palpates adjacent to the spinous process and tells the patient, "gently swell out your muscles under my fingers without moving your spine or pelvis." The PT assesses the ability of the muscles to perform this action. This technique can also be used as a training tool for isolated multifidus contraction.[16]

Another objective measurement that helps document recovery is the assessment of weight-bearing symmetry. Using two scales side by side, observe the load distribution on examination and on re-examination. As the spine gains stability, weight distribution should be increasingly symmetric, providing that no other biomechanical factors are interfering with the balance of load.

Figure 14-3 Segmental multifidus muscle testing.

PURPOSE: Examine core stability of the segmental lumbar muscles.

POSITION: Client lying supine. Physical therapist (PT) palpating intersegmentally to flex the lower trunk up, isolating to the desired level.

PROCEDURE: PT gives gentle, gradual lateral pressure to distal femurs, creating a rotational force through the lumbar spine. PT compares side to side and segments above and below, observing for weakness, as demonstrated by lack of resistance to the rotational force.

Summary: Spinal Stabilization

Movement with stability is the ultimate goal of stabilization training. The client should develop freedom of movement, without rigid spinal-holding patterns, and should function more efficiently during all activities. This improved movement is accomplished through enhanced proprioceptive abilities, strength, postural endurance, and balanced, efficient motor programming.

TECHNIQUES

Posture

Making changes in posture is often difficult and frustrating for both the client and the PTA. It seems that even if the client's posture can be corrected, he or she drifts back into the old dysfunctional position as soon as appropriate pos-

ture is no longer the focus of concentration. Therefore, in addition to educating the patient on posture in a proprioceptive manner, adjuncts should be used to help reinforce proper posture throughout the day. The objective is to offer some useful postural correction and education techniques and then to suggest adjuncts to assist the patient in maintaining the postural changes.

The use of the vertical compression test, as indicated earlier, is recommended for initial examination and after postural correction to evaluate the patient's static alignment (Fig. 14-2). After correction procedures, the vertical compression test checks the correction both for examination purposes and to illustrate the difference to the patient. Often the patient will feel off balance and must be convinced of the benefits of the change. Usually, a mirror or photograph will help demonstrate the value of the correction.

To correct faulty posture, the use of verbal and physical cues is recommended. Begin from the foundation and move superiorly. Use of a plumb line helps when the client is initially learning to look for postural deviations.[5] If the knees are locked into hyperextension, ask the patient to soften them. If the pelvis is anteriorly tilted, provide manual cues while asking the client to tuck the tail under. For example, to encourage inferior movement of the sacrum, the PTA places a finger of one hand on the sacrum and taps or presses lightly in an inferior direction while a finger or the hand is placed on the midline of the abdomen inferior to the umbilicus and skin-drags the anterior abdomen in a superior direction. If the pelvis is posteriorly tilted, the PTA can reverse the same manual cues and ask the client to tip the pelvis forward as though it were a bucket and he or she were trying to pour water out of the front of it.

For a patient with a rounded, forward shoulder posture, addressing the upper trunk will alter the faulty posture inferiorly. Place a finger on the upper sternum, and tap it gently, asking the patient to breathe while lifting the sternum up and forward slightly and then to exhale without allowing the chest to drop (Fig. 14-4). Besides offering the cervical spine relief from the often-associated forward head posture, this technique has the added benefit of promoting abdominal breathing.

Although a temporary solution, simple taping is a powerful tool for postural education. Both in the lumbar and thoracic spine, posterior taping offers a primitive but effective form of biofeedback. The tape pulls when the patient moves into a flexed posture. To tape the lumbar spine, begin in the standing or prone position. Ask the patient to produce and explore lumbopelvic movement, coming to rest in the neutral position. Then apply (a) horizontal anchor strips at the thoracolumbar junction and the sacrum, (b) diagonal strips to form an X across the low back (Fig. 14-5), (c) a few longitudinal strips from anchor to anchor, and (d) a couple of horizontal closing strips. Thoracic taping can be applied in a similar manner, emphasizing the direction of desired support. Athletic tape usually works well for these techniques but usually quickly loosens. Fortunately, taping does not take long to make an impact. As soon as the client sits in the car, the learning is intensified. Other more adhesive types of tape are available, and they may be used to maintain postural feedback over a longer period of time. However, the PT must be aware of any potential skin allergies that may preclude leaving the tape on for more than a few hours.

Additional methods for promoting maintenance of corrected posture include techniques that periodically remind the client to self-correct. Setting a watch to beep every 30 minutes or so is an easy method. Clients who work at a computer may use an alarm program that sounds every 30 minutes; besides serving as a reminder of postural correction, it may encourage the client to stand up and perform 1 minute of stretching exercises.

Body Mechanics

Before moving on to techniques of body mechanics education, the importance of the lower extremities must be discussed. One of the most frustrating aspects of training body mechanics is the fact that lower-extremity strength can be the limiting factor in one's ability to move efficiently and safely through daily activities. The most basic of body mechanics education is the use of proper lifting techniques. When lifting from the floor, the individual must achieve a position that is close to the floor, which requires strong lower extremities that can safely lower and raise the body. Therefore, lower-extremity strength is as fundamental to spinal care as is spinal strength.

By following a few basic ergonomic principles, workers can protect themselves on the job (Table 14-3). Patient education in these basic concepts will provide guidance for a lifetime of active prevention of workplace injury or exacerbation of symptoms.

When possible, videotape the client performing on the job or videotape simulated job or sports activities. Review the tape in slow motion, looking for subtle movement faults of which the patient may be unaware. When dealing with a work or sports environment, it is important for the PTA to understand the necessary activities. The PT and/or PTA can seek out educational videos on the sport or job or can obtain the assistance of a reputable teaching professional, work manager, or coach to gain knowledge in basic techniques. This information, combined with professional knowledge on biomechanics and rehabilitation, provides a wealth of intervention potential for the client in question and for future clients.

Obstacle course training is a powerful way to assist the patient in problem solving while focusing on maintaining a functional, neutral posture. Varying the environment in which an individual is performing a task is known to improve overall learning. Therefore, setting up a simple obstacle course in the clinic is an inexpensive and valuable tool for effective training and can provide objective measures in the form of time to completion. Examples of tasks that can be used are pushing a weighted cart, pulling a vacuum cleaner, lifting cuff weights from the floor to an overhead shelf, placing a child seat into the back of a car, bending over to scrub the bathtub, leaning over the sink to simulate brushing the teeth, moving wet clothes from a washer to dryer, and sitting in an office chair and reaching to answer the phone or use the computer.

Spinal Stabilization

Initiation of Training

Before an exercise routine is started, the tissue should be prepared and the PT should try to optimize the healing en-

| Figure 14-4 | Technique for correcting faulty posture. |

PURPOSE: To correct a rounded, forward-shoulder posture.

POSITION: Client standing. Physical therapist assistant (PTA) standing to side.

PROCEDURE: PTA places a finger on client's upper sternum and taps it gently, asking client to breathe while lifting the sternum up and forward slightly and then to exhale without allowing chest to drop.

| Figure 14-5 | Lumbar spine taping to provide feedback. |

PURPOSE: To provide primitive postural feedback.

POSITION: Client standing in neutral lumbopelvic position.

PROCEDURE: Physical therapist assistant applies horizontal anchor strips at the thoracolumbar junction and sacrum, diagonal strips in an X across the low back, a few longitudinal strips from anchor to anchor, and a couple of horizontal closing strips.

TABLE 14-3 Summary of Basic Ergonomic Principles

Keep frequently used materials close to avoid reaching.
Position work at elbow height for sitting and standing.
Place heavier objects lower and lighter objects higher.
Keep loads close to the body
Push loads instead of pulling whenever possible.
Maintain neutral posture.
Eliminate excessive repetition.
Minimize fatigue by avoiding static loads and grips, taking breaks, and rotating stressful jobs.
Use adjustable workstations and chairs; change postures frequently.
Provide clearance and access so that proper movements are possible.
Create a comfortable environment with adequate lighting and temperature.
Eliminate vibration.

vironment.[4] For the patient with lumbar pathology, the exercise preparation technique of choice is aerobic activity. In fact, aerobic exercise itself has been shown to have positive effects on low back pain.[41] This activity may be performed in numerous postures, and the PT should consider the patient's specific characteristics and positional bias when choosing an aerobic modality. Giving consideration to the client's specific concerns, the PT may recommend walking, bicycling, using a ski machine, or supine bicycling. Occasionally the client is not ready for aerobic exercise; in this case therapeutic modalities may be used to prepare the tissue for intervention.

The aerobic activity in the initial phases of stabilization training should be specifically for warmup purposes and should not be overly aggressive. Fast, or ballistic, movements of the extremities can be detrimental to the training of the core stabilizers and should be reserved for those individuals who have demonstrated proper stabilization techniques in early-phase activities.

The individual's flexibility and mobility must be considered so that all stabilization exercises are safe and appropriate. Simply stated, specific flexibility or mobility limitations may interfere with the physical performance of an activity. For example, if the hip is unable to flex beyond 100 degrees before recruiting the pelvis into a posterior tilt, any exercise requiring more than 100 degrees of hip flexion is unsafe. Watch for compensation that may originate from such a physical limitation. The PT should use other therapeutic interventions to correct the limitation to allow for progression of the stabilization program.

The PT begins stabilization training by providing the patient a relatively easy position in which to produce and explore lumbopelvic motion (this is usually the hook-

lying position). One good method is for the PT to ask the patient to envision the face of a clock on his or her abdomen, with 12:00 at the belly button and 6:00 at the pubic bone. The PT then asks the patient to alternately tilt the pelvis so that 12:00 rocks toward the floor and then 6:00 rocks toward the floor. The PTA then instructs the patient to move back and forth from the 12:00 to 6:00 positions gently, slowly, and with awareness ten times each direction. The patient then identifies the point within that range that is most comfortable. Because this point is the most comfortable spot, training is focused on teaching the patient how to stay near that point during daily life. As noted, this position is referred to as the neutral or functional position of the spine and should be emphasized and maintained for all movements performed during spinal stabilization activities.

When progressing a patient to a new exercise, the PTA should always ensure proprioceptive accuracy before embarking. Again, the initial phase of stabilization training should include isolated stabilizing muscle contractions (passive preconditioning), followed by challenge to the stabilizing musculature via limb movement (active preconditioning), with eventual progression to functional activities for neuromotor retraining (dynamic stabilization). Each new exercise should be initiated with the patient exploring the lumbopelvic motion, safely and accurately identifying the neutral position. Remember that the neutral position may change as the pathology changes; therefore, the patient should re-explore each movement with each new activity. The pelvic rocking has the added benefit of providing input to the type 2 mechanoreceptors[42] and thus reducing pain.

As the patient demonstrates awareness of the neutral or functional position, the PTA begins to train the isolated transversus abdominus contraction. The PTA asks the client to place a finger or two just medial to the anterior–superior iliac spine (ASIS) and lightly press into the tissue. Then the patient is told to draw the abdominal muscles inward and upward, without altering the spinal position, and to feel a simultaneous tensing in the pelvic floor muscles. An alternate position for transversus contraction is in quadruped next to a mirror.[16] As the transversus contraction is achieved, the abdomen draws upward, narrowing the waist. With either technique, the idea is to isolate contraction and avoid overexertion, which tends to recruit all of the abdominal muscles.

A great tool for assisting the patient in awareness of abdominal contraction is a biofeedback instrument. Simple, single-channel electromyographic devices can give the patient auditory and visual feedback regarding electrical activity in the targeted muscles. If choosing this adjunct, the PTA should remember to document the parameters during each session in which the device is used to obtain additional objective information. Usually, if needed at all, electromyography will be necessary for only a few visits. Recommended placement for electrodes is just inferior and medial to the ASIS.[43]

Phase I: Basic

If the patient understands the concepts of selective muscle contraction and the neutral spine position, the next aspect of training is to challenge the muscle's ability to maintain postural control while subject to perturbation. This challenge is accomplished via subtle movement of the upper and lower extremities. Again, emphasize slow, controlled movement with awareness. Parameters used during phase I are presented in Table 14-4.

The main thing to remember during phase I is that protocols are not used; instead, the PTA is encouraged to use his or her imagination to best facilitate the patient's learning. The usual approach is to follow a developmental sequence path, beginning with supine exercises (including bridging) and progressing to prone, quadruped, kneeling, and standing exercises. This framework may be adapted to specific patient situations, and some postures may need to be avoided according to patient tolerance and abilities. For example, if a patient has particularly tight rectus femoris muscles but the positional bias for intervention is flexion, the bridging posture may be too difficult, owing to the anatomic limitations. These important data are obtained from physical examination and through careful observation of the patient while he or she is performing the exercises.

In addition, it must be emphasized that the neutral (functional) position of the spine should be maintained during all activities. If the patient performs an activity and the neutral position cannot be maintained, pain will occur, which indicates that the program is being progressed too aggressively.

Supine Activities

Supine exercises typically begin with simple, supported, upper-extremity movement. This movement may be performed bilaterally for balanced abdominal recruitment or unilaterally for asymmetric recruitment that challenges the spine in the transverse plane (rotation). The patient should be asked to lift the arms overhead first without abdominal contraction because the lumbar spine will usually extend slightly and the patient will become aware that movement of the upper extremities can influence the spine (Fig. 14-6).

To progress from upper-extremity movement, ask the client to attempt to lift one lower extremity slightly and then lower it before attempting to lift the other. The tendency is for the patient to get a rotational shift in the pelvis and lumbar spine during the transition from one side to the other. If this rotation occurs, the PTA should emphasize that maintaining a level pelvis during the transition will promote depth in the contraction of the core stabilizers (Fig. 14-7).

One method used to facilitate deep stabilizer recruitment is to ask the patient to imagine that gum is stuck on the bottom of one shoe. As the patient tries to lift the foot, he or she imagines the gum pulling strongly back down. After the foot has been lifted just a few inches, the patient imagines that the foot is being pulled back down and should permit the foot to slowly return to the support surface. Supine exercises can be progressed by having the patient lift one leg and the contralateral arm simultaneously. This activity is sometimes referred to as the dying bug exercise (Fig. 14-8).

Another technique to facilitate deep stabilizer recruitment is manual resistance. The PTA applies gentle resistance to the limbs, either supported or unsupported, to facilitate irradiation of contraction from the stronger muscles to the targeted, deeper muscles.[44]

The initial stabilization experience for the patient is more of a learning session than an exercise session. The PTA should remember this when providing directions for the home exercise program. The patient should be instructed to take time to practice the movements instead of being told to do specific sets of repetitions. The patient should also be advised to practice in a quiet environment that is conducive to concentration. This initial training is probably the most important aspect to the overall success of the stabilization program. If the patient becomes sloppy with movements early on, neither pain reduction nor improvement in functional performance will occur.

To increase the challenge to the stabilizing muscles in supine, exercises can be advanced so that the limbs are no longer providing support. Advancement of exercise should include the addition of ankle and hand weights or exercise tubing for further challenge. As the patient improves in the ability to maintain a stable trunk with these exercises, both the duration and the speed of the activity should be increased.

Exercising supine can include bridging activities, which can be challenging, especially when progressing to single lower-extremity support. Bridging exercises chal-

---

TABLE 14-4 Phase I (Basic) Stabilization Training

Goals

Improve proprioceptive awareness.
Increase strength, flexibility, and coordination.
Become proficient in basic body mechanics.
Promote independence in exercise.
Decrease symptoms.

Exercises

Short lever arms.
Minimal, if any, weights.
Stable, supported postures.

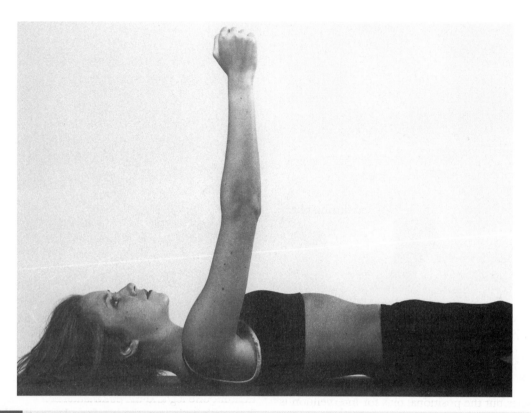

Figure 14-6 Unilateral upper-extremity lift in supine.

PURPOSE: Facilitate proprioceptive awareness of abdominal contractions associated with upper-extremity movement.
POSITION: Client lying supine in neutral lumbopelvic position.
PROCEDURE: Client lifts one arm overhead, noting forces that occur in lumbar spine. Client counteracts forces with abdominal contraction, maintaining a still lumbopelvic spine.

Figure 14-7 Unilateral lower-extremity lift in supine.

PURPOSE: Facilitate proprioceptive awareness of abdominal contractions associated with lower-extremity movement.
POSITION: Client lying supine in neutral lumbopelvic position.
PROCEDURE: Client lifts one limb slightly and then lowers it while counteracting forces with abdominal contraction and maintaining a still lumbopelvic spine.

Figure 14-8   Dying bug exercise in supine.

PURPOSE: Facilitate proprioceptive awareness of spinal stress with limb movement and strengthen abdominal stabilizers.
POSITION: Client lying supine in neutral lumbopelvic position.
PROCEDURE: Client raises right arm and left leg and then left arm and right leg (similar to a supine running motion).
NOTE: Emphasis should be placed on control before speed. Resistance is optional. Neutral position of spine should be maintained.

lenge the core stabilizers and require strong gluteal contraction. All motions should be performed slowly at first, with speed increasing as the patient's abilities increase. As with all exercises, it is possible to add weights, tubing, or manual resistance to increase the level of difficulty (Figs. 14-9 and 14-10). When the patient has experience in firing the core stabilizers, sit-ups can be added (Figs. 14-11 and 14-12).

Prone Activities

Prone exercises are excellent for strengthening the lumbar extensors and gluteal muscles, and they provide a direct challenge to the anterior stabilizing muscles to hold the pelvis from posterior tilting. The PTA should watch for sequence of contraction, emphasizing the stabilizing muscle contraction before any gluteal activity. If gluteals are recruited first, prevention of extension moment through the low back is impossible. If the patient has a flexion bias or has difficulty with prone positioning, use of pillows for abdominal support is recommended. Again, to progress the

exercises, use upper- and lower-extremity lifts to challenge the core stabilizers (Figs. 14-13 and 14-14).

Quadruped exercises offer less external support than supine and prone exercises (Figs. 14-15 and 14-16). Therefore, these activities are usually started after the more supported postures. The patient's hands should be placed directly below the shoulders and the knees below the hips. Ask the patient to grip a towel or hand weight if he or she has difficulty with the wrist extension position in quadruped. Care should be given to the thoracic spine, making sure that the scapulae are stable and that thoracic kyphosis is relatively neutral. The tendency is for the thoracic spine to arch into flexion. Patients often attempt to lift the leg high during lower-extremity extension, resulting in lumbar extension. Keeping the foot low along the support surface will usually eliminate lumbar extension and may improve contraction of the stabilizing multifidus. Another common error is excessive lateral weight shift toward the supporting lower extremity. To reduce this tendency, the PTA can position the patient next to a wall, effectively blocking a weight shift.

Figure 14-9   Bridge position.

PURPOSE: Facilitate proprioception and isolate stabilizing muscles and hip extensors.
POSITION: Client hook-lying.
PROCEDURE: Client elevates hips while maintaining lumbopelvic neutral position.
NOTE: Client raises hips only as high as proper form can be maintained. Resistance is optional.

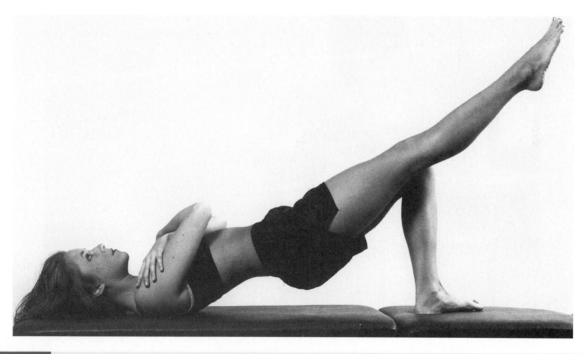

Figure 14-10   Unilateral lower-extremity lift in bridge position.

PURPOSE: Progress the bridging exercise to emphasize rotational stability and balance.
POSITION: Client lying in bridge position in lumbopelvic neutral position.
PROCEDURE: Client extends one leg while maintaining neutral pelvis.
NOTE: Requires solid contraction of the gluteals. Resistance is optional.

Figure 14-11 Partial sit-up.

PURPOSE: Strengthen abdominal stabilizers.
POSITION: Client lying supine in hook-lying position with arms folded across chest.
PROCEDURE: Client lifts shoulders from the support surface.

Figure 14-12 Abdominal muscle strengthening.

PURPOSE: Strengthen abdominal musculature.
POSITION: Client lying supine on incline bench with knees flexed and feet firmly on floor; hands clasped in front of body.
PROCEDURE: Client gradually lifts head and trunk off bench until spine is flexed.

Figure 14-13 Unilateral hip extension in prone.

PURPOSE: Facilitate proprioception while attempting limb movement in a new position.

POSITION: Client lying prone with arms overhead or by side.

PROCEDURE: Client barely lifts leg, focusing on gluteal contraction and avoiding lumbar rotation.

NOTE: Physical therapist assistant may palpate anterior–superior iliac spine to observe for excessive anterior pelvic tilting or rotation through pelvis. Resistance is optional.

Kneeling and Standing Activities

To continue the developmental progression, the client is advanced to kneeling, a position of less stability and potentially greater challenge than the quadruped position. Simple alternate shoulder flexion, with or without weights, can be a great exercise to begin functional stabilization of the spine (Figs. 14-17 and 14-18).

Although it is a more challenging position for stability, standing should be addressed early. As soon as the client understands the neutral position, the PTA should begin to teach basic body mechanics. Include supine to sit, sit to stand, forward bending, and basic lifting as soon as possible. Lunges while maintaining the neutral position of the spine are excellent. Such activities can be used as a part of a home exercise program. The PTA should continue to refine functional activities as the patient is progressed to more advanced training.

Phase II: Advanced

Table 14-5 summarizes the goals and exercises of phase II, the advanced program. In addition to adding weights and

Figure 14-14 Bilateral upper- and lower-extremity lift in prone.

PURPOSE: Provide endurance strengthening of stabilizing muscles of trunk while facilitating proprioceptive awareness.

POSITION: Client lying prone in Superman position.

PROCEDURE: Client barely lifts all four extremities off support surface.

NOTE: May be performed with static holds or limbs can be moved in various patterns. Resistance is optional.

Figure 14-15   Unilateral lower-extremity lift in quadruped.

PURPOSE: Facilitate proprioception while attempting limb movement in a new position.

POSITION: Client kneeling in quadruped, with hands directly beneath shoulders and knees directly below the hips.

PROCEDURE: Client produces and explores lumbopelvic motion and locks in neutral position. Client extends one hip so foot just clears support surface (to avoid unnecessary lumbar extension).

NOTE: Resistance is optional.

Figure 14-16   Opposite upper- and lower-extremity lift in quadruped.

PURPOSE: Provide endurance and strengthening of stabilizing muscles of trunk while facilitating proprioceptive awareness.

POSITION: Client kneeling in quadruped with hands directly beneath shoulders and knees directly below hips.

PROCEDURE: Client starts in neutral position, extends one hip, and flexes opposite shoulder while maintaining neutral cervical positioning.

NOTE: Resistance is optional.

Figure 14-17 Kneeling upper-extremity lift.

PURPOSE: Facilitate proprioception while attempting limb movement in a new position. Strengthens shoulder girdle and trunk-stabilizing muscles.
POSITION: Client kneeling tall in neutral lumbopelvic position.
PROCEDURE: Client lifts one arm overhead, only as high as possible without losing form. Client alternates arms.
NOTE: Resistance is optional.

increasing the lever arm for any of the aforementioned exercises, training a patient for return to dynamic activity requires dynamic exercises. Use of unstable surfaces is recommended to add challenge and reality to the dynamic spinal stabilization training program. An unstable surface can range from a foam floor mat to single-leg support on a foam roll. PTAs can also use wall pulleys, ankle platforms, balance boards, slider boards (Figs. 14-19 to 14-28), and the therapeutic ball.

Any one exercise may be performed for 2 to 5 minutes to address true learning and endurance. Although thousands

of repetitions are required to create a new habit, learning retention can be promoted by varying the environment of an activity and changing the order in which activities are performed.[39] Therefore, it is recommended that activities be rotated in and out of an exercise routine. Feedback to the patient should be monitored. Initial training requires quite a bit of immediate verbal and manual cuing, but the PTA's assistance should quickly diminish so that the patient concentrates on providing self-feedback. The PTA should then provide feedback after the patient completes a particular bout of activity.[45]

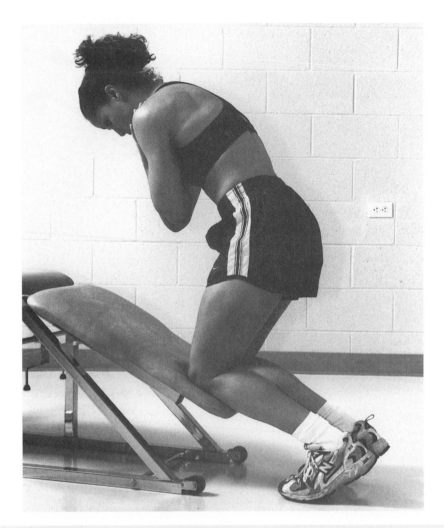

Figure 14-18   Back muscle strengthening in kneeling.

PURPOSE: Strengthen back extensor musculature.

POSITION: Client kneeling on incline bench, toes on floor. Hips and spine in flexed position. Hands hold shoulders.

PROCEDURE: Client extends spine to neutral position, lifting body from bench.

TABLE 14-5 Phase II (Advanced) Stabilization Training

Goals

Train for endurance.
Focus on specific coordination training.
Achieve controlled and safe functioning in combined axes.

Exercises

Longer lever arms.
Less stable surfaces.
Transitional and functional movement patterns and postures.
Move around combined axes.
Increased speed, repetition, and weights for functional
  endurance training.

The use of a patient journal or flow sheet is recommended to track and encourage compliance. The more the patient feels responsibility for the rehabilitation plan, the more successful the outcome. Again, the goal is for the patient to learn new motor skills; lots of practice is necessary for new movement patterns to become second nature.

Special Consideration: Therapeutic Ball

Among the wide variety of activities and props that can be used to add challenge to a dynamic spinal stabilization program, the therapeutic ball has become popular. Thus, this section reviews a spinal stabilization program that uses the therapeutic ball to treat individuals with spinal

Figure 14-19 Upper-extremity exercise in supine with weights (proprioceptive neuromuscular facilitation pattern).

PURPOSE: Strengthen stabilizing musculature in stable, functional pattern.
POSITION: Client hook-lying in neutral lumbopelvic position.
PROCEDURE: Client performs upper-extremity diagonal patterns against resistance. Client maintains neutral spine position.

Figure 14-20 Upper-extremity exercise in quadruped with weights (proprioceptive neuromuscular facilitation pattern).

PURPOSE: Strengthen stabilizing musculature in stable, functional pattern.
POSITION: Client kneeling in quadruped in neutral lumbopelvic position.
PROCEDURE: Client performs upper-extremity diagonal patterns against resistance. Client maintains neutral spine position.

Figure 14-21   Side bending.

PURPOSE: Strengthens abdominal muscles, back muscles, and hip abductors.

POSITION: Client lying on side on adjustable bench with trunk in 15-degree decline; hands can be placed on shoulders **(A)** or behind head **(B;** increases difficulty). To make exercise easier, lower extremities can be secured at ankles. Roll at trunk determines axis of movement. Spine is bent to left side.

PROCEDURE: Client actively bends to right side.

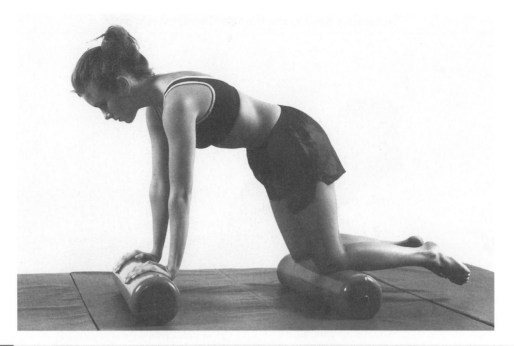

Figure 14-22   Use of foam roller in quadruped.

PURPOSE: Challenge trunk stability on unstable surfaces.
POSITION: Client kneeling in quadruped with hands and knees on foam rollers.
PROCEDURE: Client maintains lumbopelvic control.
NOTE: To increase the muscular and proprioceptive challenge, client flexes arms or extends hips and knees.

Figure 14-23   Use of balance board in prone.

PURPOSE: Challenge trunk stability on unstable surfaces.
POSITION: Client lying in push-up position in neutral lumbopelvic position with hands on balance board.
PROCEDURE: Client shifts weight side to side, front to back, or in diagonals or may perform push-up activity. Client maintains neutral spine position.

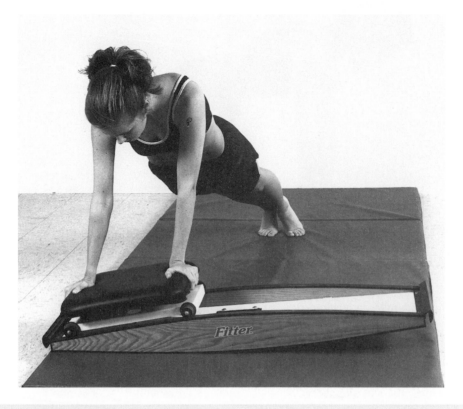

Figure 14-24   Use of sliding board in prone.

PURPOSE: Challenge trunk stability on unstable surfaces.
POSITION: Client lying in push-up position in neutral lumbopelvic position with hands on sliding board.
PROCEDURE: Client shifts weight side to side or performs push-up activity. Client maintains neutral spine position.

dysfunction. Such a program promotes activity patterns that use appropriate muscles working in a coordinated fashion; the goal is returning the individual to pain-free movement.

As for other techniques of spinal stabilization, two points must be emphasized. First, it is important that the therapeutic ball activities do not cause or increase spinal pain. Second, the PTA must carefully monitor the quality of the patient's movement to ensure that the neutral position is maintained during all activities. Finding and maintaining the neutral (functional) position of the spine

enables the patient to perform the exercises without pain and allows the patient to move the arms and legs with less fatigue.

Therapeutic ball exercises can be performed in the supine and prone positions. From the supine position, bridging (and modifications of bridging) are emphasized (Figs. 14-29 and 14-30). Prone exercises include activities in which the upper extremity, lower extremity, and both extremities can be used to challenge the muscles required to stabilize the spine in the neutral position (Figs. 14-31 to 14-35).

A

B

Figure 14-25 Trunk rotation with wall pulleys.

PURPOSE: Actively increase extension, side bending, and rotation of spine while strengthening spinal extensor and rotator musculature.

POSITION: Client sitting with hips and knees flexed to 90 degrees, feet firmly on floor. Spine flexed, side bent left and rotated left, allowing client to grasp pulley handle with both hands. Placement of roll determines axis of rotation **(A)**.

PROCEDURE: Client turns head and cervical spine to right and extends trunk while rotating to right; arms raised overhead **(B)**.

Figure 14-26   Trunk rotation with wall pulleys.

PURPOSE: Actively increase flexion, side bending, and rotation of spine while strengthening abdominal musculature.

POSITION: Client sitting with hips and knees flexed to 90 degrees, feet firmly on floor. Spine extended and rotated left, allowing client to grasp pulley handle with both hands **(A)**.

PROCEDURE: Client actively turns head and cervical spine right; then flexes, side bends, and rotates spine right as pulley handle is pulled toward floor **(B)**.

Figure 14-27 Advanced sit-up.

PURPOSE: Strengthen abdominal stabilizers.

POSITION: Client lying supine with legs extended and arms folded across chest.

PROCEDURE: At the same time the client lifts shoulders from support surface (as in partial sit up), the client lifts the extended legs to 60 to 70 degrees hip flexion.

Figure 14-28 Abdominal muscle strengthening.

PURPOSE: Strengthen abdominal musculature.

POSITION: Client lying supine on incline bench with hips and knees held in extended position.

PROCEDURE: Client lifts pelvis and bilateral lower extremities off bench.

Figure 14-29   Use of therapeutic ball in bridging.

PURPOSE: Challenge stabilizing musculature on unstable surface and in a position that requires endurance and strength of gluteals.

POSITION: Client lying supine with head, neck, and upper thoracic spine supported on therapeutic ball.

PROCEDURE: Client elevates hips to maintain upper thoracic position on ball. Client elevates hips while maintaining lumbopelvic neutral position.

NOTE: Client raises hips only as form can be maintained.

Figure 14-30   Unilateral lower-extremity lift on therapeutic ball in bridge position.

PURPOSE: Challenge stabilizing musculature on unstable surface and in a position that requires endurance and strength of gluteals.

POSITION: Client lying in bridge position in lumbopelvic neutral with hips elevated.

PROCEDURE: Client lifts one foot off support surface while maintaining lumbopelvic neutral and solidly contracting gluteals **(A)**.

NOTE: To increase difficulty, client extends one leg while maintaining lumbopelvic neutral **(B)**.

Figure 14-31   Upper- and lower-extremity lift over therapeutic ball.

PURPOSE: Challenge spinal stability, emphasizing spinal extensor muscles.

POSITION: Client lying in prone over therapeutic ball with body horizontal or shoulders higher than hips. Client in neutral lumbopelvic and cervical spine position.

PROCEDURE: Client lifts arms, legs, or opposite arm and leg.

NOTE: Resistance is optional. More hip flexion encourages lumbar flexion; more hip extension encourages lumbar extension.

Figure 14-32   Bilateral lower-extremity lift over therapeutic ball.

PURPOSE: Challenge spinal stability, emphasizing spinal extensor muscles.

POSITION: Client lying in push-up position with therapeutic ball under hips. Client in neutral lumbopelvic and cervical spine position.

PROCEDURE: Client maintains neutral spine position.

NOTE: Clinician may provide manual resistance at trunk or legs to increase challenge.

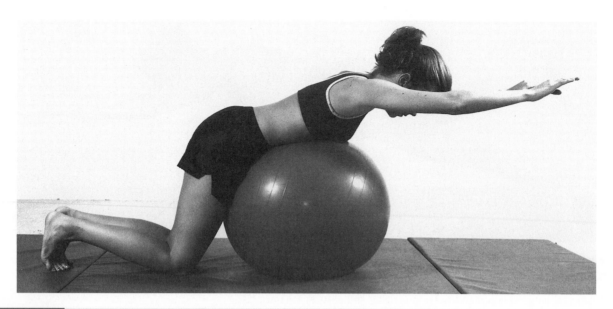

Figure 14-33 Scapular retraction with knees flexed on therapeutic ball.

PURPOSE: Strengthen upper back and shoulder girdle muscles.

POSITION: Client kneeling in quadruped with therapeutic ball under hips and knees on floor.

PROCEDURE: Client flexes shoulders overhead in Superman position and holds position.

NOTE: *To decrease challenge, client holds hands behind back.* To increase challenge, client performs upper-extremity movements (swimming, reciprocal flexion/extension). Resistance is optional.

Figure 14-34 Scapular retraction with knees extended on therapeutic ball.

PURPOSE: Strengthen upper back and shoulder girdle muscles.

POSITION: Client kneeling in quadruped with therapeutic ball under hips and knees on floor.

PROCEDURE: Client extends hips and knees, keeping ball under hips. Client flexes shoulders overhead in Superman position and holds position.

NOTE: To increase challenge, client performs upper-extremity movements (swimming, reciprocal flexion/extension). Resistance is optional.

Figure 14-35 Gluteal-abdominal hold with therapeutic ball.

PURPOSE: Strengthen upper back and shoulder girdle muscles.

POSITION: Client in quadruped with therapeutic ball under shin or ankles (depending on desired level of challenge).

PROCEDURE: Client holds position or shifts weight bearing forward and backward and side to side. Client maintains neutral spine position.

CASE STUDY 1

PATIENT INFORMATION

A 22-year-old female college student presented to the clinic with the diagnosis of L4-L5 disc injury. She reported right low back and right lower-extremity pain with a duration of 2 weeks. The patient described the pain as dull and achy, with numbness in the right calf. She rated her pain as 3/10, with the worst being 5/10. The patient believed her pain was the result of an increase in frequency and duration of sitting over the previous 4 months. Her medical history was significant for microscopic discectomy at L5-S1 4 years earlier. She reported that her calf numbness had been present since the surgery. Her symptoms were worse with sitting, bending, and hamstring stretching and better with distraction. The patient's goals were to lift weights, jog, and swing a golf club without pain.

Examination by the PT revealed positive neural tension signs in the right lower extremity and decrease in both active and passive segmental stability at L4-L5. Repeated movement testing revealed centralization with standing extension and peripheralization with standing flexion. The use of a vertical compression test caused an increase in pain (4/10); performance of the test after a postural correction did not change the pain response. The piriformis and gluteus medius muscles on the right demonstrated moderate soft tissue restriction. The right Achilles reflex was absent, and decreased sensation was present in the distribution of S1. The patient reported that these findings were related to the previous injury and surgery. She had decreased flexibility of the hamstrings bilaterally, and a positive straight-leg-raising (SLR) test at 50 degrees on the right. Lower abdominals and L4-L5 multifidus stability tests demonstrated 3+/5 strength. Findings indicated sciatic nerve inflammation and annular incompetency at the level of L4-L5.

LINKS TO
GUIDE TO PHYSICAL THERAPIST PRACTICE

Pattern 4F of the *Guide to Physical Therapist Practice*[3] relates to the diagnosis of this patient. This pattern is described as "impaired joint mobility, motor function, muscle performance, range of motion, or reflex integrity secondary to spinal disorders." Included in the patient diagnostic group of this pattern are nerve root disorders. Anticipated goals include an increase in the "ability to perform physical tasks," using verbal instruction, demonstration, and modeling for teaching, and an increase in the ability to "perform physical tasks related to work and leisure activities," using aerobic endurance activities, balance and coordination training, posture awareness training, strengthening, and stretching.

INTERVENTION

Initial goals of intervention were to educate the patient on the neutral spine and appropriate body mechanics and improve neural tension signs. The PT discussed the initial goals with the PTA and instructed the PTA to treat the patient as follows:

1. Pain-free stretching of the hamstrings (Fig. 4-7) and piriformis.
2. Instruct the patient on proprioceptive neutral posture in the unloaded supine position.
3. Instruct on proper body mechanics of supine to sit and straight-back bending (as bending forward to brush teeth).

PROGRESSION

One Week After Initial Examination

Examination by the PT 1 week after the initial examination indicated that the patient was able to control her leg symptoms with an extension-biased posture. Her SLR had improved to 75 degrees bilaterally, and a faint Achilles reflex was present on the right. The vertical compression test resulted in pain rated as 2/10; performance of the test after postural correction resulted in no pain. Abdominal and multifidus strength were graded as 4/5.

Given this improvement, the goals of intervention were revised by the PT to address active segmental stability. The PT discussed the patient's progress and revised goals with the PTA. The PT asked the PTA to perform the following intervention:

1. Use of lumbar taping for biofeedback for extension-biased posturing (Fig. 14-5).
2. Stretches: hamstrings, piriformis.
3. Initiation of supine and prone active prepositioning stabilization activities (Figs. 14-6, 14-7, and 14-13).

Two Weeks after Initial Examination

After 2 weeks of intervention, upon re-examination by the PT, the patient presented with normal abdominal and multifidus strength, a negative vertical compression test, a negative SLR test, and positive neural tension signs. She continued to avoid sitting because it aggravated the symptoms. The goals of intervention were advanced by the PT to improve neural tension signs and increase sitting tolerance. The PT discussed the patient's progress with the PTA and revised the patient's goals. The PT reviewed the following intervention with the PTA. Communication between the PT and the PTA indicated that there was a proper level of understanding of the additional interventions. The PTA, following the revised plan of care, instructed the patient on the following:

1. Treadmill walking focused on maintaining stability of lumbopelvic spine (Fig. 12-8).
2. Continued stretching.
3. Increase stabilization activities: supine activities using resistance for upper (Fig. 14-19) and lower extremities; dying bug exercise (Fig. 14-8).

Three Weeks after Initial Examination

After 3 weeks of intervention, upon re-examination by the PT, the patient presented with negative neural signs. She continued to avoid sitting because it aggravated the symptoms. The goals of intervention were to improve sitting tolerance and begin dynamic stabilization activities. The PT discussed the re-examination with the PTA and asked the PTA to instruct the patient on the intervention consisting of the following:

1. Treadmill jogging focused on maintaining stability of lumbopelvic spine.
2. Continued stretching.
3. Increase stabilization activities: upright lunge (Fig. 8-10) and push/pull weighted cart.

Four Weeks after Initial Examination

Examination by the PT at the 4-week follow-up indicted that the patient presented with normal objective findings. The goals of intervention were to progress dynamic stabilization activities, including running 2 miles without onset of lower-extremity pain, and to initiate a gym weightlifting program. Upon discussing the examination findings and intervention with the PT, the PTA instructed the patient on the following:

1. Recumbent bicycling focused on maintaining stability of lumbopelvic spine and continued treadmill work: combined total up to 60 minutes (Fig. 12-4).
2. Increase stabilization activities: resisted baseball swing using elastic band and throwing a ball.
3. Gym weightlifting program: leg press, hamstring curls, lunges, pull-ups, dips, and PNF with elastic band (Fig. 7-20).

OUTCOMES

After 5 weeks of intervention, upon re-examination by the PT, the patient was able to control her leg and back symptoms and had resumed prior activities. She had met all goals and was discharged by the PT to a home stabilization program to be completed three times per week. All exercises were to be performed to fatigue, and a gym program was to be completed two or three times per week.

SUMMARY—AN EFFECTIVE PT-PTA TEAM

This case study demonstrates an effective and trusting working relationship between the PT and PTA. Since the plan of care is to only see the patient once a week, it is necessary for the PT to re-examine the patient at each return visit to assess change in status and progress the patient's program. The PT is then able to discuss and effectively communicate the findings with the PTA and request that the PTA instruct the patient on the progression of the intervention. It is imperative that the PT is comfortable with the skills and level of understanding of the PTA. The intervention requested by the PT requires advanced training by the PTA; therefore, good communication and a trusting working relationship is a must. In this scenario the PT is able to examine other patients while the PTA is instructing this patient on the intervention; however, the PT remains available if problems or questions occur, providing a safe and effective environment.

CASE STUDY 2

PATIENT INFORMATION

The patient was a 33-year-old carpenter complaining of low back pain radiating into the left buttock. The patient reported that three to four times per day he felt numbness and tingling in the back of his left leg. Ten days ago he was working under a house in a crawl space with a 5-foot ceiling. At one point he had difficulty standing fully erect and walked home in a stooped posture. The next day the pain in his back and buttock was worse, and he was unable to stand fully erect and has been unable to work since.

Examination by the PT indicated a patient who walked in with a flexed posture and sat slumped. A diagram of the patient's pain pattern showed that the patient indicated pain across the low back and into the left buttock. The patient had no complaints of sensation changes at the time of initial examination. When asked to perform flexion in standing, the patient indicated pain across the low back and left buttock. When repeating the flexion, the patient reported the pain increased in his buttock and moved into his thigh. The patient reported the same occurrence when lying supine and bringing the knees to the chest and repeating this movement. Extension in the standing position caused pain in the low back and buttock. Repeating this activity caused increased pain in the low back but alleviated the buttock pain. The same results occurred with performing extension in prone (prone press-up) and repeating the movement. Results of a neurologic screening (which included testing of sensation, reflexes, and muscle strength) were negative.

The examination revealed flexion activities causing an increase in distal symptoms and extension activities decreasing the distal symptoms. Based on the examination and evaluation, the PT diagnosed the patient as having a posterolateral disc protrusion.

LINK TO
GUIDE TO PHYSICAL THERAPIST PRACTICE

Utilizing the *Guide to Physical Therapist Practice*, this patient fell in musculoskeletal practice pattern 4F: "impaired joint mobility, motor function, muscle performance, range of motion, or reflex integrity secondary to spinal disorder." Anticipated goals for this patient include "ability to perform physical tasks" is improved and "performance levels in employment activities" are improved.[3]

INTERVENTION

Goals set by the PT were to reduce the disc protrusion. The patient was educated as to the cause of the problem and to avoid any activities involving trunk flexion. The patient was provided a lumbar roll and instructed in proper sitting posture with the assistance of the roll. The patient was instructed in the proper procedure for performing a prone press-up (Fig. 4-29) and instructed to perform five press-ups every waking hour. The patient was warned that the home exercise program may result in an increase in low back pain and pain across the shoulders as the press-up was not an activity to which the patient was accustomed. The PT introduced the patient to the PTA, and the patient was set up to receive treatment by the PT three times per week for 2 weeks, at which time the patient was scheduled with the PT for re-evaluation and progression of the plan of care. The PTA was instructed to monitor the patient's appropriate performance of the prone press-ups, to progress the patient's home exercise program over the 2 weeks from hourly press-ups to press-ups three times per day, and to inform the PT if the patient's distal symptoms increased.

PROGRESSION

One Week After Initial Examination

During the first week after the initial examination by the PT the PTA worked with the patient in the performance of appropriate press-ups. Upon return for the first return visit, the patient was walking more erect. He reported that his low back pain had increased, he had a slight increase in muscle pain in the posterior shoulders and triceps, and the pain in the buttock was more intermittent. The PTA assured the patient that these changes were positive. The pain in the low back was due to his lack of flexibility, the pain in the shoulders was due to using muscles he was not used to using, and the fact that the buttock pain was more intermittent and not as frequent was a sign of improvement. In observing the patient performing the prone press-up, the PTA corrected the fact that the patient was not allowing his paraspinal muscles in the lumber spine to completely relax at the point that the patient fully extended his arms. The PTA then observed the patient performing the press-up correctly ten times. The PTA instructed the patient to perform the prone press-up five times every 2 hours.

Upon return at the second visit during the first week after the initial examination, the patient reported that the low back pain had decreased and he had not had buttock pain for an entire day. The PTA observed the press-up, which the patient performed correctly ten times. The PTA reviewed the precautions to any flexion activity and the proper use of the lumbar roll when sitting. The PTA instructed the patient to perform the press-up five times every 3 hours.

Upon return at the third visit during the first week after the initial examination, the patient reported that he had no pain in the buttock or low back. The PTA instructed the patient to perform the prone press-ups ten times three times per day. In addition, the PTA made an appointment for the patient to see the PT, thereby moving up that PT appointment 1 week because the patient had made significant improvement, had reduced the posterior disc protrusion, and needed to have his plan of care progressed by the PT.

Two Weeks After Initial Examination

Examination by the PT indicated that the patient had made significant progress and was pain free with the activities he was allowed to do (flexion was not allowed). The PT changed the plan of care to recover function. The PT instructed the PTA to see the patient two times per week for 1 week to begin a series of exercises to recover function—progressing from knees to chest activities to flexion in standing. Exercise sessions were to always end with the prone press-up. Then the PTA was to see the patient one time per week for 2 weeks, at which point the patient would see the PT for re-evaluation. The PTA was to inform the PT if the patient's pain returned. The PTA instructed the patient in the following home exercise program and to return in 3 days:

1. Double knee to chest (Fig. 4-32B): ten times three times per day.
2. Prone press-up: ten times three times per day. (Press-ups should always be performed after the knees to chest.)

Upon return to the clinic 3 days later, the patient reported no problems with the exercise program and no change in status. The PTA progressed his exercise program to the following:

1. Standing, bend over and touch the toes: ten times three times per day.
2. Rotation in sitting (Fig. 4-31): ten times to the right and left three times per day.
3. Prone press-up: ten times three times per day. (Press-ups should always be performed as the last activity.)

Three Weeks After Initial Examination

The patient returned and reported no problems. The PTA progressed his exercise program to the following:

1. Standing, bend over, touch the toes, and pick up a 2-pound object: ten times three times per day.
2. Rotation in sitting: ten times to the right and left three times per day.
3. Prone press-up: ten times three times per day. (Press-ups should always be performed as the last activity.)

Four Weeks After Initial Examination

Examination by the PT indicated that the patient was pain free with all activities. The PT discontinued the flexion and rotation activities from the home exercise program and instructed the patient on the importance of continuing the prone press-up exercises. In addition, the patient was instructed to use the press-up if the pain returned. The PT added unilateral hip extension in prone (Fig. 14-13) and bridging exercises (Figs. 14-9 and 14-10) to the home exercise program to increase the strength of the core musculature. The PT also instructed the patient as to how to slowly begin to return to work.

OUTCOMES

Four weeks after the initial examination the patient had no back pain and no pain radiating into the buttock. The patient was now ready to slowly return to work, realizing that he should attempt to avoid prolonged trunk flexion activities. If his job required trunk flexion, the patient was instructed to interrupt this flexed posture frequently by placing his hands on his hips and extending five to ten times.

SUMMARY—AN EFFECTIVE PT–PTA TEAM

This case study demonstrates components of an effective working relationship of the PT and PTA. The PT set the original plan of care for the PTA to take at least 2 weeks to reduce the posterior disc protrusion. However, the PTA realized that the patient was improving quickly and would not need the full 2 weeks. The PTA correctly notified the PT that the patient was pain free after only 1 week of treatment by the PTA, and the PT progressed the patient's plan of care.

SUMMARY

- Intervention for the individual with low back pain can be challenging. If a painful problem is caused or perpetuated by a movement disorder, the PTA needs to focus on correcting the faulty movement pattern. A thorough examination will assist the PT in choosing appropriate intervention strategies that can facilitate more efficient, comfortable function. The PT and PTA should remember to:
  - Observe the patient in functional tasks.
- Examine how the patient is responding to gravitational forces.
- Evaluate the lower biomechanical chain for deficits that may lead to increased spinal stresses.
- Educate the patient in static posture before progressing to dynamic activities.
- Emphasize proprioceptive awareness before progressing the patient to higher-level exercises.
- Train the patient in supported positions before progressing to more challenging, unsupported conditions.

▼ ▼ ▼   GERIATRIC PERSPECTIVES   ▼ ▼ ▼

■ The ability to maintain an erect posture during static and dynamic movement requires a complex coordination of systems: central nervous, motor, somatosensory, and biomechanical. In healthy old age, the ability to maintain an upright posture and alignment remains intact. The classic flexed posture depicted by the media is largely the result of a combination of age-related changes and neurologic and musculoskeletal disorders.[1]

■ Spinal flexibility does change with aging and may decrease as much as 50% compared with younger adults.[2] Spinal flexibility is an essential component of typical movement and therefore may affect biomechanical performance of functional tasks.[3] With advancing age, altered neuromuscular control, decreased muscle strength, and degenerative joint changes will result in a tendency to stand with slightly flexed hips and knees, rounded shoulders, forward head, increased kyphosis, and decreased lumbar lordosis. These postural changes affect flexibility in extension and axial rotation and may limit the ability to take a deep breath.[4]

■ Postural re-education, flexibility, and spinal stabilization exercises may result in tremendous functional gains for most older adults. In sedentary older adults, the trunk flexors are more prone to weakness and

tightness whereas trunk extensors are more prone to stretch weakness. Iliopsoas, tensor fascia lata, and hip adductor muscles are usually tight as well. Caution should be exercised when designing programs for spinal stabilization for older adults, especially if using prone positioning and a balance board. Overall health, strength, and presence of comorbid conditions (e.g., osteoporosis) should be examined closely.

■ Activities using the therapeutic ball may be problematic and may require adaptations for safety. Use of a foam roll or square of foam on the floor may be a better choice. To further improve safety, the training may take place within parallel bars or within reach of a stabilizing surface or person.

1. Pathy MSJ. Neurologic signs of old age. In: Tallis RC, Fillit HM, Brocklehurst JC, eds. *Brocklehurst's textbook of geriatric medicine and gerontology*. 5th ed. London: Churchill Livingstone; 1998.
2. Schenkman M, Shipp KM, Chandler JM, et al. Relationships between mobility of axial structures and physical performance. *Phys Ther*. 1996;76:276–285.
3. Bergstrom G, Anainsson A, Bjelle A, et al. Functional consequences of joint impairment. *Scand J Rehabil Med*. 1985;17:183–190.
4. Goldstein TS. *Geriatric orthopaedics*. Gaithersburg, MD: Aspen; 1999.

- Use tactile and verbal cues to facilitate the desired movements and muscle contractions.

- Notice that the neutral position varies among individuals and may change as the pathology changes.

- Focus on the core stabilizers: the multifidus, transversus abdominus, and internal obliques.

- Include the whole body in the training regimen.

- Exercise postural muscles with endurance-training principles.

- Monitor the patient's responses to weight bearing, movement, and static postures; modify exercises as needed.

- Watch for subtle compensatory movements during training.

- Incorporate functional tasks in training, either mimicking an activity in the clinic or conducting treatment sessions in the actual environment in question.

- Include flexibility, strength, endurance, functional movement re-education, and coordination in the complete training package.

- The PTA should understand that the ultimate goal is to facilitate function. Thus, the PTA should help the patient focus on active participation in the recovery process because this form of intervention is geared toward reduction of symptoms and prevention of reinjury. It is not a quick fix but a lifelong learning process.

- The current level of quality research in this area gives the PT and PTA scientific evidence to support a program of developing motor control and muscle function for rehabilitation of low back injuries. In this process, the client should develop freedom of movement, without rigid spinal holding patterns. Efficiency in functional movements should be enhanced through improved proprioceptive abilities, strength, postural endurance, and balanced and efficient motor programming.

PEDIATRIC PERSPECTIVES

▲ ▲ ▲   ▲ ▲ ▲

- Age affects posture and movement throughout the lifespan. Children are not expected to conform to adult standards for posture and movement, primarily because the developing child has much greater flexibility and mobility than the adult.[1] The child is developing muscular, vestibular, visual, and other systems during growth and maturation. Children, therefore, cannot be expected to have the same motor programs as adults.

- The literature fails to describe the exact sequence of postural response development in children. Variations in descriptions are likely due to children using multiple postural control strategies as their sensory and motor systems develop.[2] Very young children commonly have immature and unsteady control of posture and gait. Postural abilities needed to control balance and lower-extremity musculature are not attained until 5 or 6 years.[3] By 7 to 10 years children demonstrate similar eyes-closed postural sway to adults.[2]

- Most postural deviations in the growing child are developmental and related to age. Such deviations usually improve without treatment as a part of neuromuscular development. Examples include protruding abdomen posture, varus/valgus lower-extremity alignment, and flat feet.[1] A young child is not likely to have habitual postural faults and could be harmed by corrective measures that are not needed. Rather, development and maturation will correct most minor childhood postural faults. Postural faults may develop in response to intense childhood participation in some sports such as gymnastics, swimming, and dance. Severe postural deviations should be treated regardless of age.[1]

- Scheuermann's kyphosis can occur in the adolescent,[4] which can mistakenly be attributed to poor posture; caution is required. Radiologic studies confirm this diagnosis.

- In infants, the posterior (extensor) muscle group of the trunk develops first, making an imbalance between trunk extensors and flexors. The abdominals are relatively much stronger in adults than in children.[1] Therefore, although trunk stabilization exercises are appropriate for all age groups, young children may have difficulty with mastery of stabilization exercises owing to incomplete strength development of the abdominals.

1. Kendall FP, McCreary EK, Provance PG. *Muscles: testing and function.* 4th ed. Baltimore: Lippincott Williams & Wilkins; 1993.
2. Campbell SK. *Pediatric physical therapy.* Philadelphia: WB Saunders; 1995.
3. Breniere Y, Bril B. Development of postural control of gravity forces in children during the first 5 years of walking. *Exp Brain Res.* 1998;121:255–262.
4. Salter RB. *Textbook of disorders and injuries of the musculoskeletal system.* 3rd ed. Baltimore: Lippincott Williams & Wilkins; 1999.

References

1. Loney PL, Stratford PW. The prevalence of low back pain in adults: a methodological review of the literature. *Phys Ther.* 1999;79:384–396.
2. Kapandji IA. *The physiology of the joints.* Vol. 3 Edinburgh: Churchill Livingstone; 1982.
3. American Physical Therapy Association. *Guide to physical therapist practice.* 2nd ed. Alexandria, VA; 2003.
4. Porterfield J, DeRosa C. *Mechanical low back pain: perspectives in functional anatomy.* 2nd ed. Philadelphia: WB Saunders; 1998.
5. Kendall FP, McCreary EK, Provance PG, et al. *Muscles: testing and function with posture and pain.* 5th ed. Baltimore: Lippincott Williams & Wilkins; 2005.
6. Riegger-Krug C, Keysor JJ. Skeletal malalignments of lower quarter: correlated and compensatory motions and postures. *J Orthop Sports Phys Ther.* 1996;23:164–170.
7. Levine D, Whittle MW. The effects of pelvic movement on lumbar lordosis in the standing position. *J Orthop Sports Phys Ther.* 1996;24:130–135.
8. Janda V, Jull G. Muscles and motor control. In: Twomey LT, Taylor JT, eds. Physical therapy of the low back. Clinics in physical therapy series. 3rd ed. New York: Churchill Livingstone; 2000:253–278.
9. Cholewicki J, McGill SM. Mechanical stability of the in vivo lumbar spine: implications for injury and low back pain. *Clin Biomech.* 1996;11:1–15.
10. Johansson H, Sjolander P, Sojka P. A sensory role for the cruciate ligaments. *Clin Orthop Relat Res.* 1991;268:161–178.
11. Floyd WF, Silver PHS. The function of the erector spinae muscles in certain movements and postures in man. *J Physiol.* 1955;129:184–190.
12. McGill SM. Low back exercises: evidence for improving exercise regimes. *Phys Ther.* 1998;78:754–765.
13. Norkin CC, Levangie PK. *Joint structure and function: a comprehensive analysis.* 3rd ed. Philadelphia: FA Davis Co; 2000.
14. Morgan D. Concepts in functional training and postural stabilization for the low back injured. *Top Acute Care Trauma Rehabil.* 1988;2:8–17.

15. Biondi B. Lumbar functional stabilization program. In: Goldstein TS, ed. *Functional rehabilitation in orthopedics.* Gaithersburg, MD: Aspen; 1995:133–142.

16. Richardson C, Jull G, Hodges P, et al. *Therapeutic exercise for spinal segmental stabilization in low back pain.* London: Churchill Livingstone; 1999.

17. DiFabio RP. Efficacy of comprehensive rehabilitation programs and back school for patients with low back pain: a meta-analysis. *Phys Ther.* 1995;75:865–878.

18. Frost H, Klaber J, Moffett JA, et al. Randomized controlled trial for evaluation of a fitness program for patients with chronic low back pain. *BMJ.* 1995;310:151–154.

19. Frost H, Lamb SE, Klaber J, et al. A fitness program for patients with chronic low back pain: 2-year follow-up of a randomized controlled trial. *Pain.* 1998;75:273–279.

20. Nelson BW, Carpenter DM, Dreisinger TE, et al. Can spinal surgery be prevented by aggressive strengthening exercises? A prospective study of cervical and lumbar patients. *Arch Phys Med Rehabil.* 1999;80:20–25.

21. Saal JA, Saal JS. Nonoperative treatment of herniated lumbar intervertebral disc with radiculopathy. *Spine.* 1989;14:431–437.

22. Saal JA. Dynamic muscular stabilization in the nonoperative treatment of lumbar pain syndromes. *Orthop Rev.* 1990;19:691–700.

23. Weber D, Woodall WR. Spondylogenic disorders in gymnasts. *J Orthop Sports Phys Ther.* 1991;14:6–13.

24. O'Sullivan PB, Twomey LT, Allison GT. Evaluation of specific stabilizing exercise in the treatment of chronic low back pain with radiologic diagnosis of spondylolysis or spondylolisthesis. *Spine.* 1997;22:2959–2967.

25. Lee HWM. Progressive muscles synergy and synchronization in movement patterns: an approach to the treatment of dynamic lumbar instability. *J Man Manipulative Ther.* 1994;2:133–142.

26. Mannion AF, Weber BR, Dvorak J, et al. Fiber type characteristics of the lumbar paraspinal muscles in normal healthy subjects and in patients with low back pain. *J Orthop Res.* 1997;15:881–887.

27. Cholewicki J, Panjabi MN, Khachatryan A. Stabilizing function of trunk flexor-extensor muscles around a neutral spine posture. *Spine.* 1997;22:2207–2212.

28. Shirley D, Lee M, Ellis E. The relationship between submaximal activity of the lumbar extensor muscles and lumbar posteroanterior stiffness. *Phys Ther.* 1999;79:278–285.

29. Hides JA, Stokes MJ, Saide M, et al. Evidence of lumbar multifidus muscle wasting ipsilateral to symptoms in patients with acute/subacute low back pain. *Spine.* 1994;19:165–172.

30. Rantanen J, Hurme M, Falck B, et al. The lumbar multifidus muscle five years after surgery for a lumbar intervertebral disc herniation. *Spine.* 1993;18:568–574.

31. Hides JA, Richardson CA, Jull GA. Multifidus muscle recovery is not automatic after resolution of acute, first-episode low back pain. *Spine.* 1996;21:2763–2769.

32. Indahl A, Kaigle AM, Reikeras O, et al. Interaction between the porcine lumbar intervertebral disc, zygapophyseal joints, and paraspinal muscles. *Spine.* 1997;22:2834–2840.

33. Hodges PW, Richardson CA. Contraction of the abdominal muscles associated with movement of the lower limb. *Phys Ther.* 1997;77:132–142.

34. Hodges PW, Richardson CA. Inefficient muscular stabilization of the lumbar spine associated with low back pain: a motor control evaluation of transversus abdominus. *Spine.* 1996;21:2640–2650.

35. O'Sullivan PB, Twomey LT, Allison GT, et al. Specific stabilizing exercise in the treatment of chronic low back pain with a clinical and radiological diagnosis of lumbar segmental instability. Paper presented at the 10th biennial conference of the Manipulative Physiotherapists Association of Australia, St. Kilda, Melbourne, 1997. (Cited in Richardson C, Jull G, Hodges P, et al. *Therapeutic exercise for spinal segmental stabilization in low back pain.* London: Churchill Livingstone; 1999.)

36. Elia DS, Bohannon RW, Cameron D, et al. Dynamic pelvic stabilization during hip flexion: a comparison study. *J Orthop Sports Phys Ther.* 1996;24:30–36.

37. O'Sullivan PB, Twomey LT, Allison GT. Altered abdominal muscle recruitment in patients with chronic back pain following a specific exercise intervention. *J Orthop Sports Phys Ther.* 1998;27:114–124.

38. Saliba VL, Johnson GS. Lumbar protective mechanism. Functional orthopedics I. Course outline. San Antonio, TX: The Institute of Physical Art; 1999.

39. Umphred DA. *Neurological rehabilitation.* 4th ed. St. Louis: Mosby; 2001.

40. Menard D, Stanish WD. The aging athlete. *Am J Sports Med.* 1991;17:187–196.

41. Nutter P. Aerobic exercise in the treatment and prevention of low back pain. *Occup Med.* 1988;3:137–145.

42. Wyke BD. Neurological aspects of low back pain. In: Jayson MIV, ed. *The lumbar spine and back pain.* London: Sector; 1976:189–256.

43. Barnett J, Zaharoff A. Surface EMJ in dynamic lumbar stabilization training. Unpublished manuscript, 2000.

44. Voss DE, Ionta MK, Myers BJ. *Proprioceptive neuromuscular facilitation: patterns and techniques.* 3rd ed. Philadelphia: Harper & Row; 1985.

45. Frank JS, Earl M. Coordination of posture and movement. *Phys Ther.* 1990;70:855–863.

Functional Progression
for the Extremities

Steven R. Tippett, PT, PhD, SCS, ATC, Michael L. Voight, PT, DHSC, OCS, SCS, ATC, and
Kevin E. Wilk, PT, DPT

OBJECTIVES

Upon completion of this chapter, the reader will be able to:

- Define the specific adaptations to imposed demands (SAID) principle appropriately as it relates to a functional progression program.

- Identify both physical and psychologic patient benefits of a functional progression program.

- Apply appropriate techniques including aerobic sequences, sprint sequences, jump–hop sequences, and cutting sequences for a lower-extremity functional progression rehabilitation program within the established plan of care.

- Identify appropriate clinical guidelines for upper-extremity functional progression concerning criterion-based intervention and its related phases.

- Identify the classification system for the effect of pain on athletic performance within a functional progression program.

Rehabilitating injured individuals so they can resume preinjury activity levels is both a science and an art. Intervention to regain preinjury function must begin promptly after injury and proceed until the patient is once again performing at the highest possible level. Therapeutic measures must be incorporated that sufficiently prepare the healing tissue for the inherent demands of a given activity, and just as important, these interventions must take place at the appropriate time during the healing process. A rehabilitation program that does not adequately address the function of the injured tissue will result in inadequate physiologic loading, minimizing the readiness of the tissue to return to activity. Therapeutic intervention too late or too early in the rehabilitation program may predispose the patient to reinjury.

Functional progression is a planned sequence of activities designed to progressively stress the injured patient in a controlled environment to return the patient to as high a level of activity (competition) as possible without reinjury.[1] Functional progression depends on the specific work and leisure activities in which the individual participates or wants to participate. Based on the demands imposed, the physical therapist (PT) must design a rehabilitation program that stimulates and replicates functional activities tailored to the patient's goals. If the program does not result in the unrestricted return to participation in work and leisure activities, it cannot be considered complete or successful.

The PT routinely establishes treatment goals, which are addressed during the formal rehabilitation program. The goals are directed at pain, swelling, loss of muscle strength, and loss of joint range of motion (ROM). Simply satisfying these clinical goals does not ensure that the patient is ready to return to work or athletic competition. Reducing pain and swelling and increasing strength and ROM must be accompanied by specific activities that are interjected in the treatment program in a safe and timely manner.[2] After satisfying the clinical goals and before being released from the formal treatment program, the patient must be challenged in specific activities to help ensure his or her readiness for work or competition. This challenge is when the functional progression program comes into play. The physical therapist assistant (PTA) can play an integral part in this functional progression program.

To reach the ultimate goal, the patient is advanced along a continuum of functional skills, trying more advanced activities as each set of exercises is mastered. The PT and PTA must carefully monitor the patient's tolerance to the new, more aggressive exercises to ensure a safe return to work or leisure activities.

SCIENTIFIC BASIS

Whether the treatment is conservative or surgical, intervention plays a vital role in achieving a successful outcome.

TABLE 15-1 Six Principles of a Reliable Functional Progression Program

Successful treatment is based on a team approach: the physician, patient, physical therapist, and physical therapist assistant work together toward a common goal.
The effects of immobilization must be minimized; early motion and strengthening are preferred whenever possible.
Healing tissue should never be overstressed.
The patient must fulfill specific objective criteria before progressing to the next rehabilitative stage.
The rehabilitation program must be based on sound, current clinical, and scientific research.
The rehabilitation program must be individualized to the patient's specific work- and leisure-related activities.

The process must be sequential and progressive in nature, with the ultimate goal of a rapid return to pain free function. A reliable functional progression program is based on six basic principles, presented in Table 15-1.

The patient's goal is usually to return to participating in unrestricted, symptom-free competitive or recreational activity. Patients with upper-extremity dysfunction generally want to participate in a wide range of pain-free activities including working overhead, painting, combing one's hair, and throwing a ball. Patients with lower-extremity impairment want to be able to run, cut, and jump with no pain or discomfort. The rehabilitative program must be designed to progress the patient to the ultimate level of desired function. The functional approach to treatment suggests that patients with extremity dysfunction must exhibit dynamic joint stability before any functional sport-type movement can be safely and effectively initiated. For example, because the function of the rotator cuff and biceps brachii is to stabilize the humeral head within the glenoid, rehabilitation of these muscles must be emphasized early in the rehabilitative program to enable dynamic motion to occur at the glenohumeral joint without complications.

In addition, the concept of proximal stability for distal mobility must be addressed. For example, for overhead sport movements to occur without complications, proximal stability should be accomplished via the scapulothoracic joint, thereby enabling the arm to move effectively through space. The running and cutting athlete requires proximal stability via back extensors and abdominal muscles stabilizing the pelvis. Lastly, the rehabilitation program should be progressive, and isometric stability should be accomplished before attempting isotonic (concentric and eccentric) strengthening (Chapters 5 and 6).

Specific Adaptations to Imposed Demand

Stress to healing tissue must be activity specific and must be applied in a timely manner. This is the point at which the art of functional progression enters the picture. The SAID principle governs the type of stress that must be applied to the healing injury.[3] To maximize the efficacy of the functional progression program, activities must mirror the demands that will be placed on the patient once the patient returns to work or competition. Intimate knowledge of the activity and, more importantly, the specific duties required of the patient in a given environment are necessary prerequisites for a successful program.

Obviously a football player has different physical demands than a baseball player, an ice skater has different demands than a hockey player, and a soccer player has different demands than a wrestler. When prescribing and administering a functional progression program for any of these patients, a good working knowledge of the specific activity is an absolute prerequisite. The same can be said for prescribing and advancing the functional progression program for any athlete involved in any sporting activity. It is the duty of the PT to understand the specifics of a sport well enough to confidently prescribe the functional progression program. It is also important for the PTA to understand the specifics of the sport well enough to supervise the functional progression program that is delegated to them. If the PTA does not possess this knowledge, it is incumbent for the clinician to identify and secure the resources that will provide this information. Often the athlete or coach is a valuable resource when the functional progression program is formulated.

Taking this notion one step further, the PT and the PTA must also possess a thorough understanding of the athlete's specific roles in a given sport. For example, in football the demands on an offensive lineman are different from those on a defensive back; thus, the functional progression program for each of these football players must address the individual demands. The lineman must be able to assume a down position and is involved with run blocking, pass blocking, and double-team blocking on the line of scrimmage. On the other hand, the defensive back generally engages in action away from the line of scrimmage and is involved with back pedaling, cutting, jumping, and sprinting. It is clear why the clinician must seek a depth of knowledge regarding the sport-specific responsibilities of the patient.

According to the SAID principle, for the functional progression program to be complete, stress on the healing tissue must reflect the demands of a given activity. The physical demands on the patient must be analyzed globally and then broken down by level of difficulty and progressed according to the patient's tolerance. Physical demands consist of the gross fundamental movements required for a given task as well as specific tissue function. Examples of fundamental movements include stationary positions, such as standing, squatting, and kneeling. Stationary efforts may entail open-chain or closed-chain activities and may take place with both feet on the ground (bilateral support activities) or with only one weight-bearing lower extremity (unilateral support activities). Functional requirements also include dynamic body segment movements, such as jumping (bilateral nonsupport) and hopping (unilateral nonsupport), and may involve straight-plane or multiplane activities.

Examples of tissue function are the role of the ligament as a primary or secondary stabilizer; the role of the muscle in providing dynamic restraint to the injured joint as a prime mover, synergist, or antagonist; and the role of the injured muscle as primarily generating concentric, eccentric, or isometric contractions. Activity-specific static and dynamic ROM, along with flexibility demands, must also be taken into consideration when designing the functional progression program. Finally, for activities to be functional in terms of energy requirements (anaerobic or aerobic), the duration of the drills must be sport specific.

Benefits of Functional Progression

The functional progression program provides benefits to many individuals involved in the rehabilitation program. Of course, the program provides discernible physical benefits for the patient, but it also provides less tangible psychologic benefits for the injured individual. A well-devised and efficiently implemented program is also rewarding for the rehabilitation professional and others interested in the care of the patient (coach, parent, employer, etc).

Physical Benefits for the Patient

The functional progression program promotes optimal healing of the injured tissue and maximum postinjury performance, which occur only when the program is exactly as its name implies—functional. Loading tissue in a controlled fashion promotes tissue healing. Applying loads in a graduated fashion according to the specific demands of the healing tissue promotes organization of collagen.

For example, after a first-degree proximal hamstring strain in a softball player, active-assisted hip flexion and knee extension to regain ROM and isometric, isotonic, or isokinetic hip extension and knee flexion to regain strength are certainly appropriate interventions for addressing the patient's impairment. Without focusing on deceleration activities of the hip and knee via eccentric muscle contraction in the closed-kinetic–chain, however, specific tissue function will not be addressed. Without stressing a return to running in the functional progression, the athlete risks reinjury the first time he or she is required to run in a competitive situation. Stressing the healing hamstring muscles according to functional demands in the sporting activity facilitates optimal healing. Functional demands in this case mean two joint eccentric muscle contractions for lower-extremity deceleration.

Functional progression also assists in maximizing postinjury performance. By progressing through functional skills during the rehabilitation program, the patient should be fully prepared to resume full participation. An ideal functional progression program is one in which the patient has had the opportunity to complete all activities required for the activity before actually returning to the competitive environment. For a softball player with a hamstring strain, the return to a running program should entail straight-ahead sprinting and base running and positional running. After progressing through the sport-specific running sequence, the patient should be ready to resume all competitive softball running requirements.

Psychologic Benefits for the Patient

Functional progression can also assist in minimizing the mental and emotional stress of being injured. The rehabilitation professional depends on information from the patient when designing an effective program, making the client an active participant in his or her own rehabilitation program. During the functional progression program the patient is given physical tasks to accomplish. By becoming an active, involved participant and realizing genuine progress at each step, the client regains some of the control that was lost as a result of being injured. Functional progression also enhances the patient's self-confidence. As progress is achieved through the functional progression program, the patient is provided with a sense of accomplishment. As these accomplishments build on one another, the patient becomes more confident in specific physical abilities, which in turn provide a foundation for more difficult activities in the functional progression program.

During the rehabilitation process patients who demonstrate positive psychologic factors such as positive self-talk, goal setting, and mental imagery attained desired rehabilitation goals more quickly than patients who do not demonstrate those factors.[4] Adherence to a rehabilitation program has been linked not only with the effectiveness of the program but also with social support, goal and task mastery orientation, self-motivation, high pain tolerance, and the ability to adapt to scheduling and environmental conditions.[5] Goal setting and goal accomplishment are common themes to successful programs. A functional progression program is made up of a series of physical tasks for the patient to conquer, and each step in the program is a goal for the patient to attain. The PT and PTA should work with the client to set realistic goals and prescribe a functional progression program to satisfy these goals. As the patient meets each goal, his or her self-confidence is advanced. As final functional progression activities take place in a group setting, a sense of once again belonging is a positive psychologic benefit for the patient.

CLINICAL GUIDELINES— LOWER EXTREMITY

Before initiating weight-bearing activities in a lower-extremity functional progression program, certain prerequisites must be met, including control of swelling and pain, adequate ROM and flexibility to perform the desired activities, adequate strength to perform the desired activities, and sufficiently healed tissue that can tolerate the stress of the desired activities. Care should also be taken to ensure sufficient proximal (spine and pelvis) strength, ROM, and flexibility. Soft tissue healing time constraints depend on the severity of injury. The rehabilitation professional should have a thorough knowledge of the status of the injury and how healing is progressing. Indications that activities may be overzealous and exceeding healing time constraints include increases in swelling, pain, abnormal gait, substitution in movement, loss or plateau in ROM or strength, and documented increase in laxity of a healing ligament.

The challenge of returning a patient safely to competition in the shortest time possible is made inherently more difficult because of the very nature of therapeutic exercise. As indicated, inadequate stress to healing tissue results in poor preparation for the return to activity. On the other hand, too much stress is also counterproductive. Dye's[6] "envelope of function" is an excellent way to conceptualize the advancement of the functional progression program. Dye[6] described the envelope of function as the "range of load that can be applied across an individual joint in a given period of time without supraphysiologic overload or structural failure." Activity can be described in terms of applied loads and frequency of loading. High-loading activities can be performed for only a short amount of time before exceeding the envelope of function. Low-loading activities can be performed for a longer time; however, a finite frequency for lighter loading also exists before exceeding the envelope.

A practical example of the envelope of function is the progression from bilateral nonsupport activities (jumping) to unilateral nonsupport activities (hopping) for a patient with an anterior cruciate ligament injury. As the patient progresses from jumping to hopping, the load increases; thus, to avoid exceeding the envelope, the total duration of exercise should be decreased appropriately. Overuse injuries can be prevented by scheduling periods of reduced activity during a buildup in activities. As noted, the signs of excessive loading are an increase in swelling or pain, a loss in ROM or strength, and an increase in laxity of the healing ligament. One problem is that the healthcare professional does not know that the therapeutic activities are too aggressive until after the signs of excessive loading are seen. So how does the rehabilitation professional progress the program? When does the program need to be slowed down? Perhaps the best answers to these critical questions lie in the staging of overuse injury.

Healthy tissue is in dynamic balance: Bone is constantly being deposited and reabsorbed, collagen is synthesized and undergoes catabolism, and injured soft tissue undergoes degeneration and regeneration. When these processes are in equilibrium, all is well. When bone resorption exceeds deposition or when soft tissue degeneration exceeds regeneration, normal equilibrium is disrupted. One of the symptoms of musculoskeletal disequilibrium is pain. Several authors have classified overuse injuries into stages based on pain before, during, and after activity.[7,8] In these staging systems, pain gradually increases to the point at which performance is negatively affected. As a general guideline, activities that do not cause pain during exertion and activities that cause pain for less than 2 hours after exertion are allowed. Pain during activity that negatively affects performance, pain that persists for more than 2 hours after activity, pain that affects activities of daily living, and pain at night indicate that activity restriction is required (Table 15-2).

For example, consider a grade 1 hamstring strain in a softball player. Three-quarter–speed sprinting from a stationary start, noted to cause minimal discomfort after the workout, subsided less than 30 minutes after termination of activity. Full-speed sprinting from a stationary start caused no pain during the activity but did cause localized pain in the proximal posterior thigh for 6 hours after the workout. Based on the athlete's response to full-speed sprinting, the PT and PTA determined that the activities were too aggressive and that the speeds needed to be decreased.

The PTA should now have a good understanding of the basics of the functional progression process. Each program must be individualized based on the injury and the demands placed on the patient. The following sequences and case studies will provide a better understanding of the depth that must be considered when prescribing a functional progression program. The case studies also introduce the concept of specific tissue loading. These studies are intended to provide a template for clinician reference and are not intended to be prescriptive or all inclusive. The ideal functional program is one developed by the PTA working with the PT in conjunction with the individual athlete in a specific setting.

TECHNIQUES—LOWER EXTREMITY

This section presents some of the more common functional progression activities used to train patients. As indicated, the key to an efficient and successful functional progression program is the careful progression of easier tasks followed by more difficult tasks. Therefore, this section emphasizes suggestions for the progression of a number of activities referred to as "sequences." Note that the patient does not necessarily perform each sequence independently of other sequences. Several types of sequences may overlap. For example, in one exercise session the athlete may be sprinting full speed forward in a straight plane but performing cutting activities at only half speed. Furthermore, not every sequence presented is used for all athletes. The extent to which each sequence is emphasized depends on the sport and the specific position the client plays within the sport.

Aerobic Sequence

Initially establishing a sufficient aerobic base (Chapter 12) in the functional progression program is valuable for allowing the client to demonstrate the ability to tolerate the additional stress of running. A solid aerobic base is suggested before the program is progressed to short-duration sprinting, and jumping activities.

Jogging 20 steps and walking 20 steps for a total of 20 minutes at a very slow pace is the initial stage for returning the client to aerobic activity. The client can then be progressed to jogging 4 to 5 minutes and walking 2 to 3 minutes for a total treatment time of 20 to 40 minutes at a slow pace or at the client's tolerance. Caution should be used if running around any curves or corners. Suggested frequency of the initial program is three times per week.

The jogging program can be progressed as shown in Table 15-3, which outlines a jogging program for an individual who wants to develop an aerobic base. If the client is a distance runner, he or she can be further progressed to a program similar to that presented in Tables 15-4 and 15-5. The programs in these tables are examples only—each program must be individualized according to the client's response to treatment.

TABLE 15-2 Classification System for the Effect of Pain on Athletic Performance

Level	Description of Pain	Sports Activity
1	No pain	Normal
2	Pain only with extreme exertion	Normal
3	Pain with extreme exertion 1–2 hours after activity	Normal or slightly decreased
4	Pain during and after any vigorous activity	Somewhat decreased
5	Pain during activity that forces termination	Markedly decreased
6	Pain during daily activities	Unable to perform

Reprinted with permission from Fyfe I, Stanish WD. The use of eccentric training and stretching in the treatment and prevention of tendon injuries. *Clin Sports Med.* 1992;11:601–624.

TABLE 15-3 Jogging Program

Day 1	Day 2	Day 3	Day 4	Day 5	Day 6	Day 7
0.5-mile jog on track; jog straights and walk curves	0.5-mile jog on track; jog straights and walk curves	0.5-mile jog on track; jog straights and walk curves	0.5-mile jog on track; jog straights and walk curves	0.5-mile jog on track; jog straights and walk curves	Off	0.5-mile jog on track; jog straights and walk curves
Day 8	**Day 9**	**Day 10**	**Day 11**	**Day 12**	**Day 13**	**Day 14**
1.5-mile jog on track	1.5-mile jog on track	2-mile jog on track	2-mile jog on track	Off	2-mile jog on track	3-mile jog on track
Day 15	**Day 16**	**Day 17**	**Day 18**	**Day 19**	**Day 20**	**Day 21**
3-mile jog on track	3-mile jog on track	2-mile jog on track	4-mile jog on track	4-mile jog on track	Off	Regular team conditioning

TABLE 15-4 Running Progression for Distance Runner (Every Other Day)

Day 1	Day 2	Day 3	Day 4	Day 5	Day 6	Day 7
2 miles	Off	2.5 miles	Off	3.0 miles	Off	3.5 miles
Day 8	**Day 9**	**Day 10**	**Day 11**	**Day 12**	**Day 13**	**Day 14**
Off	4.0 miles	Off	4.5 miles	Off	5.0 miles	Off

TABLE 15-5 Running Progression (Daily)

Day 1	Day 2	Day 3	Day 4	Day 5	Day 6	Day 7
5 miles	2 miles	5 miles	2.5 miles	5 miles	3 miles	Off
Day 8	**Day 9**	**Day 10**	**Day 11**	**Day 12**	**Day 13**	**Day 14**
5 miles	3.5 miles	5 miles	4 miles	5 miles	4.5 miles	Off
Day 15	**Day 16**	**Day 17**	**Day 18**	**Day 19**	**Day 20**	**Day 21**
5 miles	5 miles	5 miles	Off	5 miles	6 miles	5 miles
Day 22	**Day 23**	**Day 24**	**Day 25**	**Day 26**	**Day 27**	**Day 28**
6 miles	5 miles	6 miles	5 miles	5 miles	6 miles	7 miles

TABLE 15-6 Sprint Sequence Using Straight-plane
           Activities

Sprint at half speed.
Sprint at three-quarter speed; backward sprint at half speed.
Sprint at full speed; backward sprint at three-quarter speed;
    lateral sprint at half speed.
Backward sprint at full speed; lateral sprint at three-quarter
    speed.
Lateral sprint at full speed.

Sprint Sequence: Straight-plane Activity

Once jogging and running are painless and gait deviations
are absent, the sprint sequence should be initiated. The
client may continue the aerobic program when the sprint
sequence is added to the functional progression program.
Straight-ahead sprinting is progressed from half-speed to
three-quarter speed and finally to full speed. Once the client
is able to tolerate straight-ahead sprints at three-quarter
speed, half-speed backward sprints are added. The client is
eventually progressed to full-speed backward sprints
(Table 15-6).

When the client is able to tolerate three-quarter–speed
backward sprinting, half-speed lateral sprints (also called
carioca, braiding, or crossovers) are added. When the
client can perform the three sprints (forward, backward,

and lateral) at full speed, then other activities can be added
such as high stepping or, for a basketball player, dribbling
a ball while sprinting. These drills are limited only by the
ingenuity of the PT and PTA.

Jump–hop Sequence

Functional progression activities for the lower extremity
progress from simple to complex, from bilateral activities
(jumps) to unilateral activities (hops), from activities with
the feet on the ground (support) to activities in which the
feet leave the ground (nonsupport), from slow speeds to
faster speeds, and from straight-plane activities to multiplane activities. Specific activities and a suggested order of
progression are found in Table 15-7.

Cutting Sequence: Multiple-plane Activity

Of primary importance to the functional progression of most
athletes is the cutting sequence.[9] The cutting sequence begins
with figure-eight running and progresses to actual cutting activities in which the athlete plants the foot and accelerates in
a different direction. Gentle figure-eight running can be initiated using a distance of approximately 40 yards and running
at half-speed. For example, initially the full length of a basketball court could be used, and the athlete could change directions by running long, easy curves (Fig. 15-1). The speed
of running at this distance is then increased to three-quarter

TABLE 15-7 Jump–Hop Sequence

Loading	Activity	Intensity/Frequency
Bilateral support	Leg press Mini-squat	Three sets for 30 seconds; increase by 30 seconds until 2 minutes is reached
Unilateral support	One-leg press One-leg mini-squat	Three sets for 30 seconds; increase by 15 seconds until 1 minute is reached
Straight plane, bilateral, nonsupport	Front-to-back jumps Side-to-side jumps Vertical jumps Horizontal jumps	Multiple sets at sport-specific duration of at least 30 seconds
Straight plane, unilateral, nonsupport	Front-to-back hops Side-to-side hops Lateral stepping Lunges Vertical hops Horizontal hops	Multiple sets at sport-specific duration of at least 30 seconds
Multiple plane, bilateral, nonsupport	Diagonal jumps V jumps Five-dot drill	Multiple sets at sport-specific duration of at least 30 seconds
Multiple plane, unilateral, nonsupport	Diagonal hops V hops Five-dot drill	Multiple sets at sport-specific duration of at least 30 seconds

| Figure 15-1 | Running figure-eights in a progressively smaller maneuvering area. |

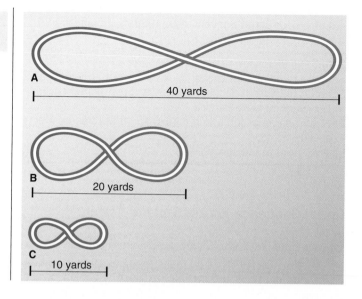

and finally to full speed. Once full-speed figure-eights can be performed at this distance, the distance is decreased to approximately 20 yards so the figure-eights are smaller and the maneuvering area is tighter; the athlete begins at half-speed. For example, the figure-eight would now be performed on only half of a basketball court (Fig. 15-1). The athlete is again progressed to three-quarter and then to full speed. The sequence is repeated at approximately 10 yards. For example, the figure-eight would now be performed between the baseline and the free throw line (Fig. 15-1). Of course, this progression could be performed in other settings besides a basketball court.

Running figure-eights can then be replaced by cutting drills in which the athlete is first asked to jog to a given spot, plant the involved extremity, and cut toward the unin-

volved side. If required, the athlete may need to perform cuts at 45, 60, and finally 90 degrees (Fig. 15-2). The speeds at which the athlete approaches the spot at which the extremity is planted is progressively increased.

After full-speed 90-degree cutting is achieved without difficulty, speeds are again decreased and the athlete begins the same cutting sequence on verbal or visual command, which more closely simulates the environment to which the individual is attempting to return. Running to a predetermined point before cutting allows the athlete to plan the movement in advance; this preparation is not available in actual practice or game conditions. Table 15-8 presents an example of a figure-eight and cutting sequence. This sample functional progression program must be individualized to the client, based on the client's response to the activity.

| Figure 15-2 | Progression for cutting activities in which the cuts become sharper and thus more difficult. 1, 45-degree cut; 2, 60-degree cut; 3, 90-degree cut. |

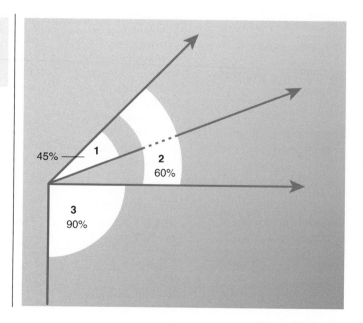

TABLE 15-8 Figure-Eight and Cutting Sequence[a]

Day 1	Day 2	Day 3	Day 4	Day 5	Day 6	Day 7
40-yard figure-eights at a jog	40-yard figure-eights at half-speed sprint	40-yard figure-eights at half-speed sprint.	40-yard figure-eights at full-speed sprint	20-yard figure-eights at half-speed sprint	20-yard figure-eights at full-speed sprint	10-yard figure-eights at half-speed sprint
Day 8	**Day 9**	**Day 10**	**Day 11**	**Day 12**	**Day 13**	**Day 14**
10-yard figure-eights at full speed sprint	Off	45-degree straight cuts at set location at half-speed sprint	45-degree straight cuts at set location at full-speed sprint	45-degree straight cuts on command at full-speed sprint	Off	60-degree straight cuts at set location at half-speed sprint
Day 15	**Day 16**	**Day 17**	**Day 18**	**Day 19**	**Day 20**	**Day 21**
60-degree straight cuts at set location at full-speed sprint	60-degree straight cut on command at full-speed sprint	Off	90-degree straight cuts at a set location at half-speed sprint	90-degree straight cuts at a set location at full-speed sprint	90-degree straight cuts on command at full-speed sprint	Off

[a]Perform two sets of ten repetitions.

CLINICAL GUIDELINES— UPPER EXTREMITY

This section will introduce a criterion-based program for progressing the patient with upper-extremity dysfunction. All patients are best served by a program that incorporates the principles of both a functional progression and a criterion-based program.

Criterion-based Intervention

The key to a criterion-based program is the interdependent, four-phased rehabilitative approach linked to a variety of exercises that guide the patient through a sequential progression of functional activities.[2] For each phase of the rehabilitation program, the PT establishes objective and functional criteria that are used to guide the patient's advancement and ensure the appropriate rate of progression. This type of program requires the patient to fulfill minimal objective criteria before attempting more advanced levels of exercise and function. This basic rehabilitative approach can be adapted for a wide variety of surgical and nonsurgical conditions.

By ensuring strict adherence to the fulfillment of the predetermined objective criteria before advancing the patient to the next phase, the PT is able to individualize the pace of the program based on the patient's age, injury, affected tis-

sue type, activity level, sport or position, and surgical procedure. It is imperative to remember that the specific exercises, positions, and progression used depend on the extent of the injury, type of surgical procedure performed, healing constraints, and tissues stressed during rehabilitation. This section provides an overview of a multiphased, criterion-based rehabilitation program for the patient with upper-extremity dysfunction. This type of program can be easily delegated to a PTA and adapted to a variety of situations as long as strict adherence to the fulfillment of the criteria before advancing the patient is maintained.

The Phases

Phase I: Immediate Motion

The three primary goals for the initial rehabilitative phase are to re-establish nonpainful ROM, to retard muscular atrophy, and to decrease pain and inflammation. It is imperative to re-establish "normal" motion. Immediately after any upper-extremity injury or surgery, motion is allowed in a safe, protected, and relatively nonpainful arc. This motion helps to minimize or eliminate the potentially deleterious effects of immobilization, which include articular cartilage degeneration and muscular atrophy.[10–12] In addition, early motion assists in aligning healing collagen fibers along appropriate stress patterns, thereby avoiding adverse collagen tissue formation.[11] Active-assistive ROM exercises are used to accomplish immediate early motion activities (Chapter 3).

Immediate motion exercises are beneficial in decreasing the client's perception of pain. When controlled movement is allowed, type 1 and 2 joint mechanoreceptors are stimulated, which presynaptically inhibit pain fiber transmission at the spinal cord level. Therefore, by allowing immediate motion, patients feel better and achieve control of the extremity sooner.

Functional decrease in the strength of musculature secondary to pain and swelling is common after injury or surgery. Frequently the pain that patients experience with ROM exercises occurs secondary to poor strength. Pain-free, submaximal isometric muscular contractions performed at multiple angles are used initially[7] (Chapter 6). Each isometric contraction should be held for 6 to 8 seconds and progressed from one or two sets of ten to 15 repetitions to four or five sets of ten to 15 repetitions, as tolerated. These exercises should be performed two to three times daily in conjunction with the active-assisted ROM exercises previously described.

After incorporation of submaximal isometrics, the exercise program should be progressed to short-arc isotonic activities. In addition, closed-chain, weight-bearing exercises are added during phase I to facilitate cocontractions of the muscles of the upper extremity (Chapter 8).

Before progressing to phase II, specific objective criteria must be exhibited by the patient on physical examination. The criteria are full, nonpainful passive ROM; minimal, palpable tenderness and pain; and good strength (4/5 on a manual muscle test).

Phase II: Intermediate

The goals of the second rehabilitative phase are to improve muscular strength, endurance, and neuromuscular control. During this phase strengthening exercises are advanced to isotonic and isokinetic activities (Chapter 6). The exercises incorporated during the first portion of the phase are low-weight, submaximal isotonic contractions. Usually the program is advanced in 1- to 2-pound intervals working up to five sets of ten repetitions for each exercise using 5 to 10 pounds of resistance.[13,14]

Submaximal isokinetic exercises can be initiated as the patient progresses during this rehabilitative phase (Chapter 6). Isokinetic exercise allows for high-speed, high-energy activities, beginning in a relatively safe and stable position.

Single-plane, submaximal isotonic and isokinetic strengthening exercises should be combined with multi-plane diagonal pattern activities using synergic movements, such as proprioceptive neuromuscular facilitation (PNF) exercises (Chapter 7). The exercise progression thus moves from basic concepts and exercises to more complex and difficult levels of physical activity. The PT and PTA should incorporate PNF patterns in a range of positions (e.g., side-lying, seated, standing, and supine) to vary the neuromuscular input and maximally challenge the ability of the dynamic stabilizers to control the upper-extremity muscles.

To progress from phase II to phase III, the patient must exhibit full, nonpainful active ROM, no pain or palpable tenderness on clinical examination, and at least 70% of the strength of the contralateral uninjured extremity. The client must exhibit these specific criteria before attempting any of the phase III exercise drills. The drills, activities, and exercises used in the advanced rehabilitative phase require greater strength, power, and endurance and prepare the patient for return to strenuous, unrestricted activities.

Phase III: Advanced Strengthening

Phase III exercises are considered dynamic strengthening exercises and drills. The goals of this phase are to increase strength, power, and muscular endurance; improve neuromuscular control; and prepare the patient for a gradual, controlled return to functional activities. These exercises include high-speed, high-energy strengthening drills; eccentric muscular contractions; diagonal movements in functional positions; isotonic dumbbell movements; resistive exercise tubing movements with concentric and eccentric contractions; isokinetic exercises; and plyometric activities.

Plyometric drills provide the patient with a functional progression to unrestricted, sport-specific movements such as throwing, swinging, and catching. These dynamic, high-energy exercises prepare the upper-extremity musculature for the microtraumatic stresses experienced during most sports activities (Chapter 9).

The patient must meet the following four specific criteria to progress to the final phase of rehabilitation: full, nonpainful active and passive ROM; no pain or palpable tenderness on clinical examination; satisfactory muscular strength, power, and endurance based on functional demands; and satisfactory clinical examination.

Phase IV: Return to Activity

Phase IV is a transitional phase directed toward returning the patient to unrestricted, symptom-free athletic activity. During this phase the patient is encouraged to continue specific exercises to address any remaining strength deficits and to improve upper-extremity muscular strength as it relates to the functional demands of the sport. In addition, the patient begins a progressive and gradual return to athletics, using a controlled program that specifically meets the patient's individual needs.

The purpose of an interval sports program is to progressively and systematically increase the demands placed on the upper extremity while the athlete performs a sport-specific activity.[15,16] A progressive program can be adapted for any functional athletic rehabilitation program. Tables 15-9 to 15–12 provide examples of interval programs for throwers, golfers, and tennis players. The interval programs presented in the tables are intended to be used as guidelines; the PT should make modifications based on the individual response of the patient.

TABLE 15-9 Phase I Interval Throwing Program

45-foot Throwing Distance
   Step 1: 50 throws with 15-minute rest[a]
   Step 2: 75 throws with 20-minute rest[b]

60-foot Throwing Distance
   Step 3: 50 throws with 15-minute rest[a]
   Step 4: 75 throws with 20-minute rest[b]

90-foot Throwing Distance
   Step 5: 50 throws with 15-minute rest[a]
   Step 6: 75 throws with 20-minute rest[b]

120-foot Throwing Distance
   Step 7: 50 throws with 15-minute rest[a]
   Step 8: 75 throws with 20-minute rest[b]

150-foot Throwing Distance
   Step 9: 50 throws with 15-minute rest[a]
   Step 10: 75 throws with 20-minute rest[b]

180-foot Throwing Distance
   Step 11: 50 throws with 15-minute rest[a]
   Step 12: 75 throws with 20-minute rest[b]
Following step 12, begin throwing off mound or return to respective position.

[a]Fifty throws consists of (a) warmup throwing, (b) 25 throws at distance, (c) 15-minute rest, (d) warmup throwing, and (e) 25 throws at distance.
[b]Seventy-five throws consists of (a) warmup throwing, (b) 25 throws at distance, (c) 10-minute rest, (d) warmup throwing, (e) 25 throws at distance, (f) 10-minute rest, (g) warmup throwing, and (h) 25 throws at distance.

TABLE 15-10 Phase II Interval Throwing Program[a]

Stage 1 (fastball only)
   Step 1: 15 throws off mound at half speed
   Step 2: 30 throws off mound at half speed
   Step 3: 45 throws off mound at half speed
   Step 4: 60 throws off mound at half speed
   Step 5: 30 throws off mound at three-quarter speed
   Step 6: 30 throws off mound at three-quarter speed; 45 throws off mound at half speed
   Step 7: 45 throws off mound at three-quarter speed; 15 throws off mound at half speed
   Step 8: 60 throws off mound at three-quarter speed

Stage 2 (fastball only)
   Step 9: 45 throws off mound at three-quarter speed; 15 throws in batting practice
   Step 10: 45 throws off mound at three-quarter speed; 30 throws in batting practice
   Step 11: 45 throws off mound at three-quarter speed; 45 throws in batting practice

Stage 3 (variety of pitches)
   Step 12: 30 fastballs off mound at three-quarter speed; 15 breaking balls off mound at half speed; 45 to 60 fastballs in batting practice
   Step 13: 30 fastballs off mound at three-quarter speed; 30 breaking balls at three-quarter speed; 30 throws in batting practice
   Step 14: 30 fastballs off mound at three-quarter speed; 60 to 90 breaking balls in batting practice at one-quarter speed
   Step 15: Simulated game, progressing by 15 throws per workout

[a]All throwing off the mound should be done in the presence of the pitching coach, who should stress proper throwing mechanics. The use of a speed gun may help pitcher control intensity.

TABLE 15-11 Interval Golf Program

Week	Monday	Wednesday	Friday	Week	Monday	Wednesday	Friday
1	Stretch 10 putts 10 chips 5-minute rest 15 chips Use ice	Stretch 15 putts 15 chips 5-minute rest 25 chips Use ice	Stretch 20 putts 20 chips 5-minute rest 20 putts 20 chips 5-minute rest 10 chips 10 short irons Use ice		10-minute rest 5 long irons 15 short irons 15 medium irons 10-minute rest 20 chips Use ice	10 long irons 10-minute rest 10 short irons 10 medium irons 5 long irons 5 woods Use ice	10 long irons 10-minute rest 10 short irons 10 medium irons 10 long irons 10 woods Use ice
2	Stretch 20 chips 10 short irons 5-minute rest 10 short irons Use ice	Stretch 20 chips 15 short irons 10-minute rest 15 chips Use ice	Stretch 15 short irons 10 medium irons 10-minute rest 15 chips Use ice	4	Stretch 15 short irons 10 medium irons 10 long irons 10 drives 15-minute rest Repeat Use ice	Stretch Play 9 holes Use ice	Stretch Play 9 holes Use ice
3	Stretch 15 short irons 15 medium irons	Stretch 15 short irons 10 medium irons	Stretch 15 short irons 10 medium irons	5	Stretch Play 9 holes Use ice	Stretch Play 9 holes Use ice	Stretch Play 18 holes Use ice

Putts, putter; chips, pitching wedge; short irons, W, 9, 8; medium irons, 7, 6, 5; long irons, 4, 3, 2; woods, 3, 5; drives, driver.

TABLE 15-12 Interval Tennis Program

Week	Monday	Wednesday	Friday	Week	Monday	Wednesday	Friday
1	12 FH 8 BH 10-minute rest 13 FH 7 BH Use ice	15 FH 8 BH 10-minute rest 15 FH 7 BH Use ice	15 FH 10 BH 10-minute rest 15 FH 10 BH Use ice		10-minute rest 30 FH 25 BH Use ice	10-minute rest 30 FH 25 BH 15 OH Use ice	30 FH 15 OH 10-minute rest 30 FH 30 BH 15 OH Use ice
2	25 FH 15 BH 10-minute rest 25 FH 15 BH Use Ice	30 FH 20 BH 10-minute rest 30 FH 20 BH Use Ice	30 FH 25 BH 10-minute rest 30 FH 15 FH 10 OH Use ice	4	30 FH 30 BH 10 OH 10-minute rest Play 3 games	30 FH 30 BH 10 OH 10-minute rest Play set	30 FH 30 BH 10 OH 10-minute rest Play 1.5 sets
3	30 FH 25 BH 10 OH	30 FH 25 BH 15 OH	30 FH 30 BH 10-minute rest		10 FH 10 BH 5 OH Use ice	10 FH 10 BH 5 OH Use ice	10 FH 10 BH 10 OH Use ice

FH, forehand ground stroke; BH, backhand ground stroke; OH, overhead shot.

CASE STUDY 1

PATIENT INFORMATION

Initial examination of a 23-year-old collegiate volleyball player indicated complaints of right shoulder pain and popping when serving and hitting. The athlete stated that she played through the pain and had not cut down on practice or competition. The patient indicated that the volleyball season was over and her goals were to play and practice the next season pain free.

Medical history indicated a previous surgery 1 year ago (arthroscopic capsular shift of anterior and inferior gleno-humeral ligaments secondary to impingement) to the same shoulder. The athlete was unable to remember any rehabilitation following surgery. Additionally the patient reported shoulder injection secondary to pain "about 2 months ago," which relieved her symptoms for 1 week.

Examination of the right shoulder by the PT indicated a painful arc during active shoulder abduction and severe pain during passive overpressure of shoulder flexion and internal rotation (positive impingement signs). Resisted movement of the shoulder caused pain during abduction and external rotation and weakness of these same muscles (3/5). Palpation indicated pain at the anterior portion of the greater tuberosity and "slight discomfort" at the bicipital groove. Tests for shoulder instability were negative. ROM of the right shoulder was equal to that of the left.

Diagnosis was consistent with shoulder impingement. Examination also suggested involvement of the rotator cuff muscles, specifically the supraspinatus muscle.

LINKS TO
GUIDE TO PHYSICAL THERAPIST PRACTICE

Using the *Guide to Physical Therapist Practice*,[17] this patient falls in musculoskeletal practice pattern 4E: "impaired joint mobility, muscle performance, and range of motion associated with ligament or other connective tissue disorders." Anticipated goals for this patient as they relate to functional progression include increasing motor function; improved joint mobility; improved weight-bearing status; improved strength, power, and endurance; and protecting the injured body part and minimizing the risk of recurrent injury.

INTERVENTION

Given the irritability of the athlete's shoulder, initial goals at this stage were to decrease pain and inflammation, maintain ROM with pain-free intervention, and initiate gentle strengthening activities (analogous to phase I in the shoulder section of this chapter). The athlete was instructed to discontinue all overhead activities. Given that the volleyball season was complete, these directions were met with no resistance. The PT discussed the plan of care with the athlete and the PTA. The athlete was to be seen three times a week in the clinic, with treatment consisting of the following:

1. Ice prior to treatment.
2. Codman's exercise.
3. Active-assistive abduction and internal and external rotation in the pain-free range (Figs. 3-10 and 3-14).
4. Isometric external rotation and abduction, performed with athlete's arm at the side.
5. Isometric elbow flexion in two parts of the ROM (Fig. 6-6).
6. Ice after treatment.

The PT asked the PTA to instruct the patient on the above exercises. The PTA was also asked to instruct the athlete on a home exercise program consisting of the following:

1. Codman's exercise.
2. Wall walking: within the pain-free ROM, standing near a wall, walk the fingers up the wall, thereby causing elevation of the shoulder.
3. Ice after treatment for 10 to 15 minutes.

PROGRESSION

Two Weeks After Initial Examination

The initial plan of care was for the athlete to perform the exercises just described for 1 week and progress to more strenuous activities. The PTA following the plan of care by the PT and, maintaining pain-free intervention, reported to the PT that although the athlete had improved, she still had significant pain and inflammation. The PT instructed the PTA not to change the program. The difficulty in decreasing the inflammation was attributed to the fact that the athlete had played through pain for more than 2 months, causing a severe inflammatory process, which required 2 weeks to subside.

Examination by the PT 2 weeks after the initial exam indicated strength of the abductors were equal bilaterally, but external rotators on the right were still weak (4/5). The athlete could actively abduct through the full ROM with no pain, and no painful arc was present. The athlete still complained of pain with overpressure into full flexion and internal rotation, but the pain was not as severe as during the initial examination. Goals were advanced to increase the strength of the muscles surrounding the shoulder (progression to phase II, as described in the shoulder section of this chapter). The patient continued to be seen in the clinic three times per week. The PT asked the PTA to progress the exercise program to the following:

1. Abduction, 0 to 90 degrees, in the plane of the scapula, with the shoulder held in internal rotation using dumbbells (Fig. 6-11).
2. Internal and external rotation with the upper arm held against body (stable position) using elastic tubing (Fig. 6-15).
3. Axial compression against table and isometric push-ups (Figs. 8-1 and 8-2).
4. Biceps curls using dumbbells.
5. Ice following treatment for 15 to 20 minutes.
6. Patient was instructed to add isometric internal and external rotation exercise to the previous home exercise program.
7. The intervention previously described was performed for 2 weeks.

Four Weeks After Initial Examination

Examination by the PT after 4 weeks of intervention indicated ROM of the right shoulder equal to left and no pain on overpressure into full flexion and internal rotation (negative impingement sign). Isokinetic examination indicated a 50% deficit in the shoulder external rotators of the right as compared with the left.

Goals at this time were to increase muscular strength in preparation for a gradual return to functional activities (progress to phase III of the shoulder section of this chapter). The PT discussed the new goals with the PTA. The PT instructed the PTA to continue the same exercises as previously described and to progress as tolerated by increasing the amount of weight used for each exercise. The PT also asked the PTA to add internal and external rotation using the elastic tubing and to progress by moving the upper arm (previously held close to body) into 45-degree abduction and to add the following exercises to the 3 days per week program:

1. D2 upper-extremity PNF patterns with manual resistance (Figs. 7-7 and 7-8).
2. Resisted axial load side to side on sliding board (Fig. 14-24).
3. Initiation of a 1-mile jogging program (Table 15-3).

Six Weeks After Initial Examination

Isokinetic examination by the PT after 6 weeks of intervention indicated a 25% deficit in external rotation. At this time the plan of care was updated by the PT. The patient was now ready for a functional progression program (phase IV). The PT asked the PTA to instruct the athlete on 3 days a week activities consisting of the following:

1. Internal and external rotation using elastic tubing in 90 degrees of shoulder abduction.
2. Jogging 1 mile.
3. Balance activities (Figs. 10-16, 10-17, 10-19, and 10-20).
4. Push-up activities (Figs. 8-1 and 8-2).
5. Overhead throwing of a volleyball (standing on two feet and progressing to one foot).
6. Serving volleyball over net at half intensity but not hitting ball inside baseline.

Eight Weeks after Initial Examination

The patient reported no pain with activities of the previous week. The PTA reported the progress to the PT, and the program was progressed as follows:

1. Continuation of jogging, balance, push-ups, and elastic band activities (two times per week).
2. Serving inside baseline, progressing to three-quarter and full intensity (three times per week).
3. Outside hitting drills with coach (two times per week).

OUTCOME

Ten weeks after the initial examination the athlete participated in supervised off-season volleyball practice with no return of symptoms, and she was discharged from formal intervention. The athlete was able to participate in the full season the next year with no complaints or return of symptoms.

SUMMARY—AN EFFECTIVE PT-PTA TEAM

This case study demonstrated an effective collaborative effort between the PT and PTA that is conducive to a busy outpatient orthopaedic clinic. The PTA was able to follow the plan of care originally provided by the PT and treat the athlete three times a week under the supervision of the PT. The PTA reported any change in the athlete's status to the PT as needed. The PT then updated the plan of care and progressed the exercise program in accordance to the re-examination and the status reports from the PTA. The PT expected that the PTA fully understood the interventions that the PT was requesting and that the PTA could treat and instruct the athlete independently, reporting any adverse effects of the intervention session. This type of working relationship allowed the PT to be aware of the athlete's status, but at the same time allowed the PT to perform examinations on other patients in the clinic, demonstrating effective and efficient teamwork while still providing quality care.

CASE STUDY 2

PATIENT INFORMATION

This case involves a 20-year-old female college cross-country runner with proximal lower left leg pain for 1 week. The athlete was currently 2 weeks into the fall season and had been running 3 to 4 miles daily during the summer. Training consisted of twice-daily practices of running 4 miles in the morning before school and 6 miles after school. The pain just below her left knee started as a dull ache after practice (3 on a 0–10 scale) last week and at the time of the appointment was much worse (8 on a 0–10 scale) with any weight-bearing activity. The patient did not remember a traumatic episode to trigger the pain, denied sensory changes, and for the last two nights had noted night pain. As per the coach's instructions, the mileage of the twice-daily workouts was decreased to 2 miles in the morning and 4 miles after school. Physical examination by the PT revealed a painful gait with no assistive device. Active ROM of both knees was normal. Passive hamstring flexibility was −20 degrees from neutral bilaterally with the hips flexed to 90 degrees. Bilateral calf flexibility was +5 of dorsiflexion bilaterally. Ober test was negative. Thomas test was positive at −5 degrees from neutral bilaterally. Rearfoot to lower-leg alignment was normal, and forefoot to rearfoot relationship revealed approximately 8 degrees of forefoot varus. The athlete also demonstrated a dorsally mobile first ray and exhibited a slight amount of femoral anteversion. Ligamentous examination of the knee and a patellofemoral joint examination were unremarkable. The athlete was referred to the physician who subsequently ordered a bone scan. Results of the bone scan were positive for a proximal tibial stress fracture.

LINKS TO
GUIDE TO PHYSICAL THERAPIST PRACTICE

Using the *Guide to Physical Therapist Practice*,[17] this patient falls in musculoskeletal practice pattern 4H: "impaired joint mobility, muscle performance, and range of motion associated with fracture." The short-term and long-term goals based on the *Guide* for this patient as they relate to functional progression include reducing the risk of secondary impairment; improving motor function; improving ventilation, respiration, and circulation; decreasing loading of the involved body part; protecting the healing injury; improving weight-bearing status; and improving sense of well-being.

INTERVENTION

At the initial visit the athlete was instructed by the PT in nonweight-bearing gait using axillary crutches. The athlete was instructed to maintain cardiovascular fitness using an upper-extremity ergometer (Fig. 12-10) and was instructed to perform daily active ROM of the knee and ankle joints (Figs. 3-5 and 3-8). The PT then discussed the patient with the PTA and delegated the patient to the PTA. The interventions on which the PT wanted the PTA to focus were reducing the risk of secondary impairment, improving motor function through functional ambulation, improving ventilation and respiration through the use of cardiovascular activities on land, decreasing loading of the involved body part through the use of aquatic environment, protecting the healing injury through education, and improving weight-bearing status by progressing to partial weight bearing and then full weight bearing per patient tolerance.

PROGRESSION

Three Weeks After Initial Examination

The PTA worked with the athlete and allowed her to bear partial weight using the axillary crutches. Over the course of the next 2 weeks the athlete was to gradually resume full weight bearing with the axillary crutches. During this time cardiovascular conditioning efforts intensified to include swimming and pool running (Fig. 16-27). Instead of traditional swimming strokes, initial efforts emphasized pool running as the athlete was not an avid swimmer. The patient performed the cardiovascular workouts supervised by the PTA in the deep end of the pool wearing a vest to minimize weight bearing. Four weeks after the stress fracture diagnosis the athlete was performing 30 minutes of pool running. The PTA communicated to the PT on the progression of the patient.

Four Weeks After Initial Examination

At this point in time the athlete was allowed to bear weight to tolerance on the affected lower extremity. Between week four and week five the athlete used one crutch for ambulation and between week five and week six transitioned to full weight bearing without an assistive device. Cardiovascular conditioning was now permitted on a stationary bicycle (Fig. 12-5). The athlete rode the bicycle initially for 20 minutes every other day between week four and five. On the days the athlete was not exercising on the bicycle, conditioning efforts continued in the pool. Over the course of a week the athlete gradually increased the conditioning time on the bike to a total of 30 minutes. The PT communicated to the PTA to begin transition back to formal running. The athlete began a conditioning program on the stationary bike based upon mileage versus total time and started a running program in which the PTA educated the patient on how to properly progress the program.

Six Weeks After Initial Examination

At 6 weeks the patient was allowed to resume running distances up to one quarter of the distance she completed prior to the injury. The initial return to a running program was performed every other day and took place on the track to utilize a level running surface. The PT fabricated a soft, full-length insert which was used in the shoe to aid in shock absorption. The initial distance covered 2 miles with the athlete alternating a quarter-mile walk followed by running a quarter mile. The distance was increased a half mile every other workout (Table 15-4).

OUTCOME

The athlete performed heel cord (Figs. 4-17 and 4-18) and hamstring (Figs. 4-7 and 4-8) stretching prior to and following her workouts as instructed by the PTA. The patient progressed without incident to the point at which she was able to run 5 miles every other day. When these every other day workouts were tolerated, the patient was allowed to resume daily running (Table 15-5) and intervention was discontinued by the PT.

SUMMARY—AN EFFECTIVE PT–PTA TEAM

This case study demonstrated effective communication of the PT and the PTA that is appropriate for good patient care. The PT should discuss the plan of care initially and expect that the PTA will continue to communicate ongoing progress with the treatment. The PT will make the determination if the PTA has the knowledge and experience to work with this type of patient and the interventions that are expected. The PT will also determine, as necessary, if ongoing reassessment is needed for updating the plan of care. In this case study the PT did not need to reassess the patient at each visit and expected that the PTA would follow the plan of care and communicate as needed. The PT must intervene as appropriate to make corrections and changes to the plan of care and interventions. In this case study the PT intervened when appropriate to make changes that were the PT's responsibility.

CASE STUDY 3

PATIENT INFORMATION

A 12-year-old U.S. Gymnastics Association elite-level gymnast presented with left upper-extremity pain and dysfunction related to an injury sustained 3 days prior to her appointment. While working on a bar routine, the athlete missed a catch (after a release move) with the right upper extremity and was left hanging/swinging by the left upper extremity on the higher bar. She lost her grasp and fell to the mat onto her buttocks. The athlete was able to continue practicing that day, but the next morning she woke up with significant medial scapular pain and general upper-extremity pain. Her mother initiated an orthopaedic exam, which occurred a day later.

The athlete was referred by the orthopaedist for intervention the next day (3 days after injury) and was wearing a sling, having had radiographs that cleared her for a fracture. The orthopaedist diagnosis was "shoulder strain." Examination by the PT on the initial visit indicated the following chief complaints:

1. Sharp aching pain (5/10) in the posterior medial scapula and glenohumeral joint.
2. Muscle pull feeling (3/10) with pain into the left side of the neck and entire left upper extremity.
3. Stiffness of entire left upper extremity with attempts at activities of daily living (dressing, grooming).

The patient was very tender to palpation to the rhomboids, levator scapulae, all parts of the trapezius, and posterior rotator cuff muscles. She was mildly tender to palpation in teres major and pectoralis major and minor muscles. Examination indicated multiple trigger points in the upper trapezius and medial scapular region.

Examination of active ROM of the left shoulder indicated flexion −95 degrees, abduction −85 degrees, external rotation −70 degrees, and internal rotation −60 degrees. All ROM was limited by pain in the scapular region. Cervical ROM was within normal limits in all motions except that right sidebending was decreased and the patient complained of pain in the left upper trapezius muscle during the motion. Manual muscle test indicated the following:

External rotation: 3/5, pain.

Internal rotation: 4/5, no pain.

Middle trapezius: 3/5, pain.

Lower trapezius: 2/5, pain.

Serratus anterior: 3/5, pain.

The elbow, wrist, hand, and cervical musculature were full strength (5/5) and pain free. In addition, all special tests for laxity and impingement were negative.

This patient demonstrated strain of the left scapular and posterior rotator cuff musculature due to a traction-type injury. The patient did not demonstrate increased laxity in the injured (left) shoulder as compared with the uninjured (right).

LINKS TO
GUIDE TO PHYSICAL THERAPIST PRACTICE

Using the *Guide to Physical Therapist Practice*,[17] this patient was classified into musculoskeletal practice pattern 4E, "impaired joint mobility, muscle performance, and range of motion associated with ligament or other connective tissue disorders." Short- and long-term goals for this patient as they relate to functional progression and return to sport are that care is coordinated among patient, family, coach, and any other medical professionals; chronic/prolonged disability is prevented; performance levels in activities of daily living, recreation, school, and sport are improved; risk of reoccurrence of the same or related condition is reduced; risk of secondary impairments is reduced (neck dysfunction); and the patient will return to high-level competitive gymnastics within 3 to 4 months.

INTERVENTION

The PT established a plan of care according to the previously mentioned goals to minimize the inflammatory response caused by the injury and initiate gentle ROM activities (phase I activities as described in the shoulder section of this chapter). Intervention included the following:

- Instruction in active-assistive ROM with support for the left upper extremity offered by the right upper extremity.
- Low-level weight bearing through bilateral upper extremities with medial lateral shifting and anterior/posterior shifting in standing at plinth.
- Isometric exercises for shoulder abduction in the plane of the scapula (Fig. 6-7).
- Active ROM for scapular protraction/retraction, abduction/adduction (Fig. 3-13), elevation, and depression.
- Removal of sling for activities of daily living at waist to chest level, avoiding abnormal scapular mechanics for overhead work.
- Manual therapy for trigger point treatment.
- Scapular PNF patterns using mild manual resistance (Figs. 7-1 to 7-4).
- Use of an exercise bicycle for maintenance of cardiovascular conditioning (Fig. 12-5).
- Ice applied to the posterior scapula for pain management.
- The PT asked the PTA to initiate the interventions listed with focus on minimizing the inflammatory response.

PROGRESSION

Two Weeks after Initial Examination

The PTA continued with the PT-directed intervention and asked the PT to reassess the patient, who had regained normal ROM but still presented with general weakness to the muscles of the shoulder. The PT changed the goals to increase strength (progress to phase II of the criterion-based program described in the shoulder section of this chapter). The intervention changed to include:

- Isotonic external rotation (Fig. 6-14).
- Supine "punches" for serratus anterior (Fig. 8-5).
- Isolated internal/external rotation using elastic tubing, arm close to side (Fig. 6-15).
- PNF diagonals with manual resistance (Figs. 7-5 to 7-8).
- Continued closed–kinetic-chain push-ups: standing with upper extremities against wall, 90 degrees on wall (Fig. 8-1).
- Begin dance routines.
- Continue exercise bicycle.

The PT communicated the interventions to the PTA and explained the expectations of the plan of care.

Four Weeks after Initial Examination

The PTA continued to work with the patient, who demonstrated normal active ROM with excellent scapular control. The PTA performed a manual muscle test of rotators and scapular stabilizers which were all 4+/5 to 5/5. No trigger points or tenderness to palpation were detected. Goals established by the PT at this stage were to continue to increase strength (progression to phase II of the shoulder section in this chapter) while progressively increasing her gymnastic activities. Interventions performed by the PTA included the following:

- Progressive increased isotonic exercise in more elevated positions (90 degrees) for external rotation and internal rotation (Fig. 6-15b).
- PNF diagonals progressing to standing with elastic tubing (Fig. 7-20).
- Closed-kinetic–chain training in the push up position (Fig. 8-2).
- Initiate quadruped program; stress neutral position of the spine (Figs. 14-15 and 14-16).
- Flexibility training to the quadriceps muscles and scapular stabilizers.

Six Weeks after Initial Examination

The PTA reported to the PT that the patient showed no signs of adverse effects of the training program for the previous 2 weeks. In fact, the patient indicated a desire to do more. The goals, as established by the PT previously, at this point were to monitor the functional progression program to full participation (phase IV of the shoulder section of this chapter). The patient was progressed to the following activities:

- Progression to quadruped program, as indicated in Chapter 14 (Figs. 14-20 and 14-22).
- Initiation of plyometric upper-extremity program using push-ups (Figs. 9-8 and 9-9).
- Progression to low-level upper-extremity closed-chain tumbling activities (cartwheels, etc).
- Swinging from the upper extremity (chin-ups, swinging from the upper bar); progress to light release and catch skills of low velocity and distance.
- Begin return to sport progression for other activities including running, jumping, and specific lower-extremity landing tasks (Figs. 9-12 to 9-18, Table 15-7).

OUTCOME

At 8 weeks after injury the PT and PTA accompanied the patient to the gym to monitor a minimal supervised workout. Supervised, gradual return to full activity followed over the next 4 weeks. Close communication by the PT with parents and coach helped with successful return to sport in this case. Caution was used and more time may have been taken in the return of this young athlete compared with the intervention of an adult. But it was important to be sure that this young athlete had excellent return of strength and endurance of musculature prior to returning to sport. At 12 weeks the athlete was released from physical therapy by the PT and allowed full gymnastic activities.

SUMMARY—AN EFFECTIVE PT-PTA TEAM

This case study demonstrated components of an effective working relationship of the PT and PTA. The communication was effective and created efficient treatment of the patient. The one area that was problematic with regards to communication was the addition of an intervention (flexibility training to the quadriceps muscles and scapular stabilizers) by the PTA at 4 weeks of initial examination without consulting with the PT. The PT must be kept informed of any change to the plan of care. The PTA should have recommended this intervention to the PT, and then the PT could have made the decision to add this or not. The patient in this case study would probably not benefit from flexibility training due to her gymnastics background and due to the nature of her injury. Strengthening and stabilization of these two muscle groups would be more important at this stage of healing.

CASE STUDY 4

PATIENT INFORMATION

The patient was a 64-year-old mildly obese college professor who presented with complaints of motor dysfunction, pain, and weakness associated with right knee arthroscopic surgery 8 weeks prior to the appointment. The patient related a history of right ankle sprain occurring approximately 2 months ago when he stepped in a hole in his yard. The patient described right calf soreness lasting for several days which the patient self-treated by walking on his treadmill for 20 to 30 minutes per day. About a week following the ankle sprain the patient reported slipping while walking on the treadmill, resulting in a twist and forward fall onto his right knee. The patient indicated feeling a sharp pain just medial to the joint line which remained constant for 2 weeks with minimal swelling. The orthopaedic surgeon's report described a right arthroscopic surgery with removal of loose body and abrasion chondroplasty of right medial condyle. The associated primary pathology was indicated to be osteochondral fracture of the right medial femoral condyle. The patient had been medically cleared to be full weight bearing and to begin rehabilitative therapy. During the 8 weeks postsurgery the patient had been performing a daily self-designed home exercise regime consisting of 20 to 25 minutes on a stationary bicycle, 10 minutes in a whirlpool bath, 20 to 25 repetitions of knee flexion to extension in sitting with free weights of varied poundage (heaviest 10 pounds), and 10 minutes on a treadmill at slow speed with no incline.

Observationally the patient appeared short of breath and flushed from the 500-yard walk into the building. The patient walked without an assistive device but with a pronounced left weight shift and right limp. Examination of the patient's knee performed by the PT indicated minimal joint swelling and calor. The arthroscopic entry portals were healed with little scarring. Palpation tenderness was reported along the medial right joint line and superior to the patella. Active ROM of the knee was 140 degrees of flexion and −20 degrees extension. Passive ROM was painful toward the end range of flexion with soft end-feel. The patient could be passively moved to −5 degrees of full extension with no indication of pain. Left knee showed no limitations related to active or passive ROM.

Resisted right knee flexion was fairly strong (4/5 using a prone manual muscle test); resisted knee extension was weak (3/5 using a sitting manual muscle test) with mild suprapatellar pain. Left knee was considered strong with 5/5 on all resisted manual muscle tests.

Balance testing revealed a probable proprioceptive deficit in single-limb stance on either extremity and diminished postural responses to disturbances. The patient opted to use a compensatory hip strategy to recover balance when nudged in standing (Fig. 10-24).

Gait analysis indicated a decreased step length on the right, limited knee flexion to extension excursion during swing, shortened stance phase on right with slight knee flexion at midstance, and decreased anterior to posterior oscillations of the pelvis. The resulting appearance was of a shuffling step on right with limited floor clearance and a hip hiking circumduction motion to advance extremity.

LINKS TO
GUIDE TO PHYSICAL THERAPIST PRACTICE

Pattern 4J of the *Guide to Physical Therapist Practice*[17] describes the present diagnosis of this patient. The pattern describes the specific patient/client diagnostic group as "impaired joint mobility, motor function, muscle performance, and range of motion associated with bony or soft tissue surgical procedures." Abrasion arthroplasty and bony debridement is included in this diagnostic category. Based on the examination by the PT and using the terminology of the *Guide*, the patient was diagnosed more specifically with joint instability associated with impaired muscle performance and motor function related to right knee arthroplasty and removal of loose bodies. The plan of care for this patient emphasized the following:

- Coordination of care and instruction with patient to develop a home program that would be acceptable and safe (given his past history of self-treatment).
- Therapeutic exercise to improve aerobic capacity, motor control, and strength.
- Gait training to improve safety and efficiency of performance.

INTERVENTION

Initially the goal of intervention was to decrease pain and associated inflammation, increase pain-free range of right knee in flexion, and increase flexion to extension excursion during swing phase of gait. The patient was instructed to discontinue all of the self-designed home exercises (a decision was made that all of the exercises were stressing the suprapatellar soft tissue, resulting in inflammation and pain). In collaboration with the patient, the PT developed a home program and asked the PTA to instruct the patient on the following program:

- Ice prior to and after treatment and at regular intervals during the day for 15 minutes each application.
- Stretching exercises with emphasis on knee flexion (prone using towel to apply *gentle* pressure toward flexion) (Fig. 4-9).
- Isotonic exercises using 2-pound weight in supine position for short arc quads (Fig. 6-29) and heel slides in pain-free range (Fig. 3-6).
- Straight-leg raises in supine position (Fig. 6-26).
- Bridging with forward and backward weight shift (Fig. 14-9).
- Begin walking 0.5 mile at slow pace using indoor track and remain aware of weight shift, foot placement, and knee flexion and extension.

PROGRESSION

One Week After Initial Examination

Examination by the PT 1 week after the initial examination indicated that the patient reported minimal pain with walking and with knee flexion. However, the patient continued to demonstrate a limp on the right which became more pronounced with increased pace of walking. The patient was measured for a leg length discrepancy and was found to have approximately a 1-inch difference between the right and left legs with the right being longer. Given this information, a recommendation was made by the PT that he consult with his physician to be fitted with an appropriate custom heel lift to correct the discrepancy.

The PT instructed the PTA to ask the patient to continue with the home program for 2 more weeks with emphasis on restoration of flexion range and strengthening. The PT instructed the PTA to increase the weight to 3 pounds in nonweight-bearing gravity-controlled positions (Fig. 6-30). The patient was instructed by the PT to return in 2 weeks.

Three Weeks After Initial Examination

The patient returned with a 0.5-inch heel lift added to the left shoe to correct for leg length difference. During examination by the PT the patient reported no pain in the right knee at end range (range increased to 155 degrees with soft tissue of thigh stopping movement) and full ROM for knee extension. Resisted right knee flexion was graded 4/5 on manual muscle test. Gait analysis revealed a more typical pattern of right knee excursion, and limp was diminished. The patient walked with weight more distributed side to side. The patient continued to have limited pelvic mobility during gait. This limited movement was judged to be an age-related learned pattern and to potentially be an indicator of limited trunk mobility, which would be addressed by including diagonal patterns in the home program. The balance limitations were improved but were noted with disturbance, especially when displaced toward the right. The home program was modified by the PT with patient input. The PT discussed the plan of care with the PTA and asked the PTA to instruct the patient on the following home exercise program and ensure proper technique and safety.

- Increased poundage on free weights to 5 pounds and ten repetitions of three sets per day.
- Walking 1 mile at usual pace (he tended to walk very fast normally), increasing 0.25 mile per week up to a maximum of 3 miles three times a week on varied surfaces—grass, sidewalk, dirt.
- Treadmill walking only if weather or time did not permit outdoor or track walking (Fig. 12-8).
- Quick stops/starts and turning during walking.
- Lunges with right foot forward and then with left foot forward (Fig. 8-10).
- Mini-squats to a semi-squat position, only if pain free, five repetitions twice a day (Fig. 8-8).
- Reaching forward and sideways within limits of stability while standing on foam cushion on floor (limits of stability are defined in Chapter 10).
- Continue ice as needed.
- Use pain as guide for progression, i.e., "if it is painful, BACK OFF the exercise."

OUTCOME

Patient was discharged from intervention by the PT. Precautionary information was provided on self-treatment without input from a trained professional.

SUMMARY—AN EFFECTIVE PT–PTA TEAM

This case study demonstrated an effective and efficient working relationship between the PT and PTA. Since the primary source of rehabilitation is a home exercise program, the PT needed to examine the patient at each return visit to assess change in status and progress the patient's program. The PT discussed the findings with the PTA and requested that the PTA treat the patient independently by instructing the patient on progression of the home program. It was expected that the PTA understood what was requested for the patient and could make sure that the patient was able to perform the home exercises with proper technique and a full understanding of the expectations of completing the home exercise program. This working relationship between the PT and PTA allowed the PT to examine other patients while having confidence that the patient was being properly instructed and supervised.

SUMMARY

- No rehabilitation program is complete without a well-devised and thoroughly carried-out functional progression program. This chapter provided the scientific basis of a functional progression program. The basic premise of the program is the need to address specific function.

- Functional progression is defined as a series of sport-specific, basic movement patterns that are graduated according to the difficulty of the skill and the client's tolerance. An intimate knowledge of the sport and, more importantly, the specific duties required of the athlete in his or her chosen sport are prerequisites for a successful functional progression program.

- Each program must be individualized, based on the injury and the demands placed on the client. The ideal functional program is developed by the PT working with the PTA in conjunction with the individual and is based on the specific setting.

PEDIATRIC PERSPECTIVES

- Functional progression should be the culmination of a complete, well-designed rehabilitation process for children, just as for adults. This progression provides the necessary link from treatment of impairments to functional return to activities of daily living or sport.

- Functional progression is particularly important in the return to sport of a child athlete. The program should provide rehabilitation by using a variety of progressive tasks related to specific sport movements or skills.

- Functional progression relates conceptually to muscular training, closed-kinetic–chain, plyometric activities, and reactive neuromuscular training. See "Pediatric Perspectives" in Chapters 7 to 9 and 11.

References

1. Keggereis S, Malone T, McCarroll J. Functional progression: an aid to athletic rehabilitation. *Phys Sports Med.* 1984;12:67–71.

2. Tippett SR. Sports rehabilitation concepts. In: Sanders B, ed. *Sports physical therapy.* Norwalk, CT: Appleton & Lange; 1990:9–14.

3. Kegerreis S. The construction and implementation of functional progression as a component of athletic rehabilitation. *J Orthop Sport Phys Ther.* 1983;5:14–19.

4. Ievleva L, Orlick T. Mental links to enhanced healing. *Sport Psychol.* 1991;5:25–40.

5. Duda JL, Smart AE, Tappe MK. Predictors of adherence in the rehabilitation of athletic injuries: an application of personal investment theory. *J Sport Exerc Physiol.* 1989;11:265–275.

6. Dye SF. The knee as a biologic transmission with an envelope of function: a theory. *Clin Orthop.* 1996;323:10–18.

7. O'Connor FG, Sobel JR, Nirschl RP. Five-step treatment for overuse injuries. *Phys Sportsmed.* 1992;20:128–142.

8. Fyfe I, Stanish WD. The use of eccentric training and stretching in the treatment and prevention of tendon injuries. *Clin Sports Med.* 1992;11:601–624.

9. Besier TF, Lloyd DG, Cochrane JL, et al: External loading of the knee joint during running and cutting maneuvers. *Med Sci Sports Exerc.* 2001;33:1168–1175.

10. Arrigo CA, Wilk KE. Shoulder exercises: criteria based approach to rehabilitation. In: Kelly MJ, Clark WA, eds. *Orthopaedic therapy of the shoulder.* Philadelphia: JB Lippincott Co; 1994:337–361.

11. Akeson WH, Woo SLY, Amiel D. The connective tissue response to immobility: biomechanical changes in periarticular connective tissue of the immobilized rabbit knee. *Clin Orthop.* 1973;93:356–362.

12. Dehne E, Torp RP. Treatment of joint injuries by immediate mobilization. Based upon the spinal adaptation concept. *Clin Orthop.* 1971;77:218–232.

13. Wilk KE, Arrigo CA. An integrated approach to upper extremity exercises. *Orthop Phys Ther Clin North Am.* 1992;1:337–360.

14. Wilk KE, Arrigo CA. Current concepts in the rehabilitation of the athletic shoulder. *J Orthop Sports Phys Ther.* 1993;18:365–378.

15. Wilk WE, Arrigo CA. Interval sport program for the shoulder. In Andrews JR, Wilk KE, eds. *The athlete's shoulder.* New York: Churchill Livingstone; 1994:569–628.

16. Khan AM, Guillet MA, Fanton GS. Volleyball rehabilitation and training tips. *Sports Med Arthrosc Rev.* 2001;9:137–146.

17. American Physical Therapy Association. *Guide to physical therapist practice.* 2nd ed. Alexandria, VA; 2003.

Unique Applications of Therapeutic Exercise

Aquatic Therapy

Jean M. Irion, PT, EdD, SCS, ATC

OBJECTIVES

Upon completion of this chapter, the reader will be able to:

■ Discuss the effect of the physical properties of water on the body and its movement in the water.

■ Discuss the influence of each of the fluid dynamic properties on the performance of therapeutic exercise in the water.

■ Discuss the indications and contraindications to aquatic therapy on clinical practice using appropriate precautions and exercise parameters.

■ Apply appropriate aquatic therapeutic techniques within the plan of care to address common physical impairments and functional deficits.

Historical documentation of the use of water as a healing medium can be traced as far back as 2400 BCE in the Proto-Indian culture. The original use of water as a healing medium solely by immersion in water does not coincide with the current use and perception of aquatic therapy. Not until the latter part of the 1890s did aquatic rehabilitation move from passive immersion to a treatment technique that involved active patient participation.[1] The purpose of this chapter is to provide an overview of the use of aquatic therapy for treatment of clients with musculoskeletal dysfunction of the spine or extremities. A discussion of the physical properties and fluid dynamics of water provides the scientific basis that substantiates the use of a water medium for rehabilitation. Clinical guidelines and specific therapeutic techniques, including the appropriate use of therapeutic aquatic equipment, are discussed next. The chapter concludes with a case study, demonstrating the physical properties, fluid dynamics, and therapeutic techniques presented in this chapter.

SCIENTIFIC BASIS

Physical Properties of Water

Several physical properties of water are introduced in this section. The effect of these properties should be considered first when determining whether a client is an appropriate candidate for aquatic therapy. The inclusion of aquatic therapy in a plan of care needs to be substantiated by one or more of these properties of water.

Relative Density (Specific Gravity)

The relative density, or specific gravity, of a substance is the ratio of the density of a given substance to the density of water.[2] The "substance" referred to in the definition of specific gravity is a human body or the extremity of a human body. Pure water has a specific gravity of 1. Generally the human body, with air in the lungs, has a specific gravity of 0.974, slightly less than the specific gravity of water.[3–5] If a person's body or extremity has a specific gravity of less than 1, it has a tendency to float; if a person's body has a specific gravity of more than 1, it has a tendency to sink. The average male body has a greater density than the average female body. The differences in specific gravity between the sexes can be accounted for by the differences in the percentage of lean body mass to fat content.

Lean body mass is made up of bone, muscle, connective tissue, and organs with a relative density close to 1.1.[6] Fat mass includes both essential body fat plus any excess fat and has a relative density of about 0.9.[6] Therefore, an individual who is highly fit and muscular and has a relatively high proportion of lean body mass has a density that exceeds 1 and thus has a tendency to sink. In contrast, a person who has a greater overall fat mass, particularly excess fat, has a body density of less than 1 and has a tendency to float.

The specific gravity of the client needs to be taken into consideration when placing him or her in an aquatic medium. The physical therapist assistant (PTA) must determine whether the client is a "sinker" or a "floater" when making safety decisions about where and in what position to place the client. The specific gravity must also be taken into consideration when choosing which flotation devices are needed to optimize therapeutic treatment in the water. Safety may be compromised if the PTA places a client who has minimal swimming skills and who has a tendency to sink in the deep end of a pool to perform an exercise without the assistance of an appropriate flotation device. Furthermore, such a client will expend excess energy just to stay afloat and maintain the body in the required position instead of maximizing the use of the water for therapeutic purposes.

Likewise, placing a flotation device on a client who already has a tendency to float may cause the client to work hard simply to gain control over the level of buoyancy when attempting to maintain the required position in the water. If the client is unable to maintain an extremity in the optimal position for exercise in the water, the clinician may add a buoyancy device to that extremity to allow it to be positioned properly.

Buoyancy

It is important for the PTA using a water environment for a therapeutic intervention to understand the concept of buoyancy. The Archimedes principle states that when a body is fully or partially immersed in a fluid at rest, the body experiences an upward thrust equal to the weight of the fluid displaced.[3,6] Buoyancy is defined as the upward thrust acting in the opposite direction of gravity and is related to the specific gravity of an immersed object.[2] As mentioned, a person or extremity with a specific gravity of less than 1.0 will have a tendency to float. In this instance, the upward thrust exerted by the water on the person is greater than the weight of the fluid displaced by the person. Therefore, the individual has a tendency to float.

Buoyancy must also be considered as a force that can assist, resist, or support movement of a person or an extremity in the water. Figure 16-1 illustrates the concept of buoyancy as a force on a lever arm (the extremity) at various angles of movement of the hip into abduction in the water. The following definitions clarify the concept of buoyancy as a force on an extremity moving in the water[3,6]:

Moment of force: the turning effect of the force about a point.

Moment of buoyancy: $F \times d$; F is the force of buoyancy, and d is the perpendicular distance from a vertical line

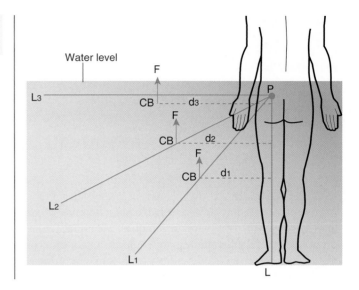

Figure 16-1 Effect of buoyancy increasing with increased hip abduction.

through *P* to the center of buoyancy (*P* is the point about which the turning-effect buoyancy is exerted).

Center of buoyancy (CB): center of gravity of the displaced liquid.

As the leg moves further into hip abduction toward the surface of the water (shown in Figure 16-1 as L_1, L_2, and L_3), the distance between *P* and *CB* (shown in the figure as d_1, d_2, and d_3) becomes greater. The longer the distance, the greater the turning effect, or moment of force, on the limb. Thus, as the limb moves closer to the surface of the water toward a horizontal position, the effect of buoyancy becomes greater.

The effect of buoyancy on the movement of an extremity is also affected by the length of the extremity and the presence of a buoyancy device at the end of the extremity. The effect of buoyancy by changing the length of the lever arm is shown in Figure 16-2 by the movement of the hip into abduction with the knee flexed to 90 degrees. In this example, shortening the length of the lever arm by shortening the limb length brings the *CB* closer to *P,* which in turn shortens the distance between *CB* and *P.* Therefore, the force of buoyancy is less.

The effect of adding a buoyancy device to the end of an extremity being moved in the water is demonstrated in Figure 16-3. If a buoyancy device is placed on the ankle while the client performs hip abduction, the *CB* moves distally, thereby increasing the distance from *P.* Thus, the effect of buoyancy on the movement of that limb is increased.

Buoyancy Assist Movements

The examples of hip abduction exercises described in Figures 16-1 to 16-3 are buoyancy assist movements; the extremity is moving from a vertical position in the water to a

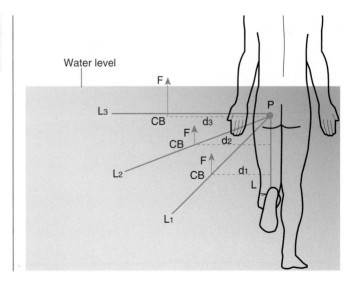

Figure 16-2 The effect of lever arm length on buoyancy, using hip abduction in a 90 degree flexed position as an example.

Figure 16-3	The effect of buoyancy is altered by the addition of a flotation device (*closed ovals*) at the end of the extremity.

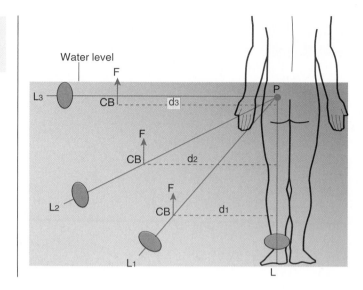

horizontal position, parallel with the water's surface (Fig. 16-4). For exercises that use buoyancy to assist movement, the clinician should use great caution when altering the length of the lever arm of an extremity or when adding a flotation device to the end of an extremity. If the patient does not have the volitional control to stop or slow the movement, any prescribed restriction in range of motion (ROM) could be exceeded. A shorter lever arm might be initially called for when using a buoyancy assist activity for a patient with restricted ROM. However, an added device that assists the effect of buoyancy on the extremity's movement might cause the patient to exceed his or her safe range, and thus caution is required.

Buoyancy assist movement can be used for isometric muscle contractions at various angles through an arc of movement of a joint or limb. For the patient to perform a buoyancy assist movement in which he or she is actively contracting, the patient must control the movement by both eccentric and concentric muscle contractions. For example, if the patient is concentrically performing shoulder

Figure 16-4	Buoyancy assist hip abduction.

PURPOSE: To improve hip abduction range of motion or initiate active-assistive strengthening of hip abductors.

POSITION: Client standing in waist-deep or deeper water with lower extremity adducted beside contralateral limb. Contralateral limb firmly planted on bottom of pool.

PROCEDURE: Client actively initiates hip abduction movement, allowing buoyancy to passively or actively assist movement of hip to fully abducted position.

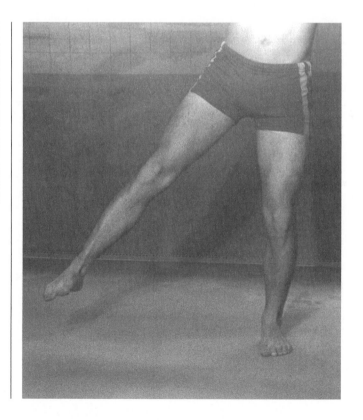

Figure 16-5 Buoyancy resist shoulder adduction.

PURPOSE: To improve strength of shoulder adductor muscles.

POSITION: Client standing in shoulder-deep water with both lower extremities firmly planted on bottom of pool. One upper extremity starts in approximately 90 degrees of shoulder abduction.

PROCEDURE: Client actively moves abducted extremity away from water's surface to shoulder adducted position, stopping when extremity contacts side of body.

abduction while standing vertically in a pool, the shoulder adductors are acting eccentrically to control the speed of the shoulder movement into abduction.

Buoyancy Resist and Support Movements

Buoyancy can provide resistance and support to movements in the water. Buoyancy resist is defined as the movement of an extremity from a starting horizontal position (parallel to the water's surface) deeper into the water (to a vertical position). This movement is directly opposite of a buoyancy assist movement. An example of a buoyancy resist movement is shoulder adduction performed from a starting position of 90-degree abduction moving toward shoulder adduction (a vertical position in the water) (Fig. 16-5). The force of buoyancy in these resist movements is greater when the limb is closer to the surface of the water, decreasing as the movement approaches a more vertical position.

Buoyancy support movements are performed when an extremity is lying on the water's surface (or just below it) and is moved parallel to the surface. For example, the patient positions the shoulder in 90 degrees of abduction and then performs horizontal abduction and adduction movements. Buoyancy support can be equated to a gravity-eliminated movement performed on land. Progression of the intensity of an exercise in the water can be achieved merely by altering a movement from buoyancy assist to buoyancy support to buoyancy resist.

Joint Loading

Buoyancy also plays a significant role in the progression of weight-bearing status in the water. Such progression performed in water is more comfortable, safer, and more easily quantifiable than any technique used for clinically determining weight-bearing status on land. Suspended vertical activities in the deep end of the pool allow exercises to be performed with no weight bearing and with minimal effects of gravity on the body. These movements, however, mimic functional movements on land, thus allowing rehabilitation to start much sooner and more safely. Harrison et al[7,8] investigated quantification of the percentage of weight bearing for immersion levels at C7, the xiphoid process, and the anterior superior iliac spine (ASIS) in a standing position and during ambulation. The subjects were able-bodied men and women with no abnormalities in gait. The weight-bearing status for men was consistently slightly higher at a given water level than for the female counterparts.

The results of the studies of Harrison et al[7,8] provide a safe range of weight-bearing status for the three water levels. Standing activities in water to C7 is 8% to 10% weight bearing for women and men, to the xiphoid process is 28% for women and 35% for men, and to the ASIS is 47% for women and 54% for men. Ambulation at a slow pace revealed the following ranges of safe weight bearing for men and women: in water to C7, up to 25% weight-bearing status; to the xiphoid process, 25% to 50%; and to the ASIS, 50% to 75%.

Clinically the use of the decreased joint-loading environment of the water allows for earlier, safer, and more comfortable rehabilitation. Clients who have pathologies that are exacerbated by gravitational forces in a vertical position of the body on land are prime candidates for early initiation of aquatic intervention. Such conditions include degenerative disc disease; facet joint pathologies; partial discectomies; spinal fusions; compression fractures of the spine from trauma or osteoporosis; degenerative joint disease of the spine or extremities such as osteoarthritis, stress fractures, and joint replacements; iliosacral and sacroiliac dysfunctions; and early open or closed reduction of fractures of the pelvis and lower extremity for which significant and lengthy weight-bearing restrictions have been imposed.

Hydrostatic Pressure (Pascal's Law)

Pascal's law states that at any given depth, the pressure from a liquid is exerted equally on all surfaces of the immersed object.[2] Hydrostatic pressure is also directly proportional to the depth of immersion of the body part below surface level. Water exerts a pressure of 22.4 mm Hg/foot of water depth.[4,9] If an individual is immersed vertically in water at a depth of 4 feet, the hydrostatic pressure at his or her feet is 88.9 mm Hg, roughly four times greater than the hydrostatic pressure at the surface of the water.

Hydrostatic pressure can be used for many purposes in rehabilitation. Pressure exerted at the feet of a patient who is standing vertically in water is slightly higher than the diastolic blood pressure, aiding in the resolution of edema in an injured part.[4,9] In addition, the hydrostatic pressure at a 4-foot depth more than doubles the pressure of the standard elastic bandage.[10] Peripheral edema in the foot and ankle, which may occur in many lower-extremity injuries, can be decreased through the use of hydrostatic pressure.

Several studies comparing cardiovascular responses to vertical aerobic exercise on land with an equivalent level of vertical exercise in water have identified hydrostatic pressure as one of the primary contributing factors for the differences noted.[11-15] The cardiovascular system appears to work more efficiently in water and therefore has a significant effect on the exercise parameters used in aerobic water exercise compared with land. This modification in parameters is discussed later in this chapter.

Because hydrostatic pressure exerts an equal force at a given level of water depth, the water provides a safe, supportive, and forgiving environment in which to start early balance and proprioceptive training. Compression on all submerged surfaces of the body by the hydrostatic pressure of the water also activates peripheral sensory nerve endings for early proprioceptive input to the trunk and extremities.

Viscosity, Cohesion, Adhesion, and Surface Tension

The combined properties of viscosity, cohesion, adhesion, and surface tension serve as a source of resistance for movement in water. All liquids share a property known as viscosity, which refers to the magnitude of internal friction among individual molecules in a liquid.[9] Viscosity affects an individual or object moving in a fluid, acting as a form of resistance when the water molecules stick to the surface of the object attempting to move through the water. Likewise, viscosity is a time-dependent property of a liquid and is described as distance over time. The faster an object moves through a liquid, the greater the viscosity and therefore the greater the resistance to movement.[9]

Cohesion is the force of attraction among molecules within the same substance, such as the attraction of one water molecule to another adjacent water molecule. Adhesion is the force of attraction among molecules of two different types of matter such as air and water at the air–water interface or water and glass molecules at the water–glass container interface. Surface tension is a force created by the cohesive and adhesive properties of the water molecules at the air–water interface. Surface tension acts as a resistance for movement in the water (e.g., when an extremity moves from the water to the air and vice versa).[7]

All four of these properties can provide a graded progression of resistive exercise. Modifications such as speed of movement, size of the surface area of the body moving in the water, and breaking of surface tension allow for a gradual progression or regression in the intensity of an exercise. Documentation of the increased tolerance to the viscosity and cohesive and adhesive properties is readily done by indicating the speed of movement, length of time the activity is performed, and extent of the body's surface area involved in the exercise. In addition, these four properties have a tendency to slow down movements normally performed on land; thus, water enables a client to practice a movement in a more controlled environment. These slower movements also allow the clinician to observe and examine movement patterns and provide feedback to the client for modification, as needed, particularly in the presence of poor movement patterns.

Refraction

Refraction causes the bending of light rays as they pass from a more dense to a less dense medium and vice versa.[4,6] In aquatic therapy, refraction occurs when light rays pass from air to water. Consideration of this property is important when the clinician is viewing the position of a body part from above the water level. The position of the trunk or extremities appears distorted and in the wrong position. Careful consideration of the true body position needs to occur before correction of the client is undertaken. An experienced aquatic therapist begins to compensate for the property of refraction and is able to correct the perception of body position before correcting the actual position of the client.

Fluid Dynamic Properties of Water

Several fluid dynamic properties must be taken into consideration before initiating an aquatic intervention: streamline versus turbulent water flow; formation of wakes, eddies, and drag force; and movement of a streamlined versus an unstreamlined object through water. The effects of these properties, in conjunction with the physical properties of water, need to be considered each time a plan of care is developed for a client.

Streamlined Versus Turbulent Water Flow

Streamlined, or laminar, flow of water is defined as a steady, continuous flow of water molecules in one direction in which the molecules are all traveling parallel to each other.[6] Once the flow of water reaches a critical velocity level, the water molecules begin to move in an irregular fashion, causing rotary movements of the molecules (known as eddies) and creating a turbulent water flow.[6] The frictional resistance to movement of an object or body provided by both a streamlined and a turbulent water flow increases with increasing velocity of flow. The resistance to movement into a turbulent flow of water is considerably greater than that of streamlined flow. In a streamline flow, resistance is directly proportional to velocity, whereas resistance is proportional to the square of the velocity in turbulent flow.[6]

When using a therapeutic pool in which turbulent flow can be created to offer resistance to an exercise or movement, progression of the velocity of the turbulent flow of water must be performed with caution. A small increase in the velocity of a turbulent flow of water significantly increases the intensity of the exercise being requested of the client.

One advantage to using a therapeutic pool in which turbulent flow can be regulated is the decreased need for various types of exercise equipment to provide increased resistance to movement. Performing exercises against or into a turbulent flow of water is an excellent means of incorporating balance and coordination activities into the plan of care.

Eddies, Wakes, and Drag Force

Movement of a body or object in water causes turbulent flow of water around and behind the object or body; these irregular patterns of water movement are known as eddy currents.[6] In addition, a pressure gradient is formed by moving a body or object through water. Pressure is increased in front of the object and decreased behind the object. The wake is an area of reduced pressure created behind a person or object moving in the water. Within the wake, eddy currents begin to form as the turbulent flow of water going around the body or object begins to flow into the lower pressure area. Flow of water into the wake also creates a drag force on the body. Drag force is the tendency for a person or object to be pulled back into the wake. As the velocity of the body or object increases, the drag force increases, creating a greater resistance to movement.[6]

Several clinical implications need to be considered when applying the concepts of eddies, wakes, and drag force to the rehabilitation process. Because the wake is an area of reduced pressure in the water, the clinician should maximize its use in gait training. To lower the resistance for the patient, allow the client to walk behind the clinician in his or her wake.[6] Gradual progression in gait training to increase the water resistance for the client during ambulation can be achieved by changing his or her position in relation to the clinician.

Many clients have a tendency to lean forward from the trunk to overcome drag force. Verbal and visual cues need to be provided to help the client overcome this and perform movement in the water in a safer neutral spine position. In addition, caution must be taken when directing a client to change direction of movement in the water. The client will be working against a turbulent flow and the water movement when starting in the opposite direction. A great deal of balance and coordination is needed to maintain an upright position against these obstacles.

Streamlined Versus Unstreamlined Movement

Turbulent flow can be created by movement of an object through water. An object can be either streamlined or unstreamlined. A streamlined object has a narrow surface area that moves through the water, demonstrated by the water paddle shown in Figure 16-6. A streamlined object disturbs the water less than an unstreamlined object. In contrast, an unstreamlined object has a broad surface area that moves through the water, demonstrated by a hydrotone bell (aquatic exercise equipment) shown in Figure 16-7. Movement of an unstreamlined object in the water causes greater water disturbance and thus greater resistance. Going from a streamlined to a more unstreamlined piece of equipment is one means of progressing the level of resistance for exercise in a water environment. This progression is also easily documented by indicating the change in the streamlined nature of the equipment being used.

A patient can alter the streamlined nature of the body by altering his or her position or the position of a body part, thus changing the resistance provided by the water. When a patient walks sideways, a narrower, streamlined surface of the body is in contact with the water. When a patient walks forward, a broader, unstreamlined surface of the body is in contact with the water. To create even more resistance, the clinician can have the patient hold a piece of unstreamlined

Figure 16-6 Movement of streamlined exercise paddle.

PURPOSE: To increase resistance to movement of an extremity through water by using a piece of equipment.

POSITION: Client standing in shoulder-deep water with both feet planted firmly on bottom of pool. Client holding onto a water paddle with one upper extremity, which is in a fully adducted, elbow extended, forearm supinated position. Paddle oriented so narrowest surface (streamlined) will be moved through water.

PROCEDURE: Client performs shoulder abduction to 90 degrees, maintaining arm position while moving streamlined water paddle through water.

equipment, such as a kickboard, in front of the body while walking forward in the water (Fig. 16-8).

Altering the position of an extremity as it moves through the water to alter the resistance provided is another means of changing the intensity of an exercise. When the shoulder is in abduction with the forearm supinated, it is more streamlined than when the shoulder is in abduction with the forearm in a neutral position. Adding a pair of aqua gloves can create a more unstreamlined surface, increasing the intensity of the exercise (Fig. 16-9). Caution must be taken when adding a piece of equipment to an exercise or changing the body position from streamlined to unstreamlined. A relatively small change in the streamline nature of

an exercise can significantly change the overall resistance level of an exercise and stress a joint or other structure beyond the patient's safe parameters.

A thorough knowledge and understanding of the fluid dynamic properties of water is vital if a physical therapist (PT) chooses to incorporate aquatic intervention into a client's plan of care. Simply applying the principles of therapeutic intervention on land, well known to the clinician, to the aquatic environment will not maximize the use of the water medium. A lack of knowledge of the properties of water may sometimes not only be an ineffective form of therapeutic intervention but also compromise the safety of the client.

Figure 16-7 Movement of unstreamlined exercise bell.

PURPOSE: To increase resistance to movement of an extremity through water by using a piece of equipment.

POSITION: Client standing in shoulder-deep water with both feet planted firmly on bottom of pool. Client holding onto bell with one upper extremity, which is in a fully adducted, elbow extended, forearm supinated position. Bell oriented so broadest surface (unstreamlined) will be moved through water.

PROCEDURE: Client performs shoulder abduction to 90 degrees, maintaining arm position while moving unstreamlined bell through water.

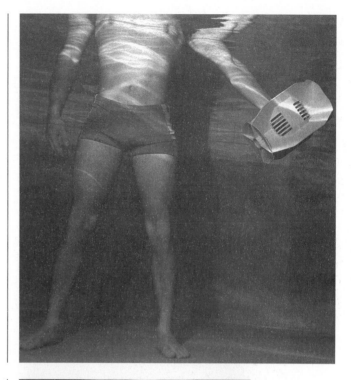

Figure 16-8 Forward walking with kickboard.

PURPOSE: To increase resistance to forward movement provided by water, increasing intensity of walking program.

POSITION: Client standing in chest- to shoulder-deep water holding kickboard parallel to front of trunk between waist and chest height.

PROCEDURE: Keeping kickboard under water, client walks forward at a pace that allows client to feel water resistance while safely maintaining upright position.

| **Figure 16-9** | Shoulder abduction with aqua glove. |

PURPOSE: To increase resistance to movement of an extremity through water by maintaining an unstreamlined body position and using a piece of unstreamlined equipment.

POSITION: Client standing in shoulder-deep water with both feet planted firmly on bottom of pool. Client wearing one or two aqua gloves with upper extremity in fully adducted, elbow extended, forearm neutral, fingers abducted position.

PROCEDURE: Client performs shoulder abduction to 90 degrees, maintaining arm and hand position while moving unstreamlined gloved hand through water.

CLINICAL GUIDELINES

Indications

The previous section emphasized the need for the clinician to fully understand and apply the physical and fluid dynamic properties of water when developing an aquatic intervention plan that best benefits the client. A knowledgeable PT can make decisions about the appropriateness of aquatic intervention for a given client. Table 16-1 lists impairments and functional limitations that indicate the use of aquatic intervention before or in conjunction with land-based therapy. Justification for reimbursement of aquatic intervention to third-party payers is enhanced when the PT is able to indicate specific impairments and functional limitations that would be more positively influenced by an aquatic medium than a land-based gravity-influenced environment. Benefits of aquatic intervention as part of a rehabilitation program are listed in Table 16-2.

History

Aquatic therapy, more than land-based therapy, requires a thorough history. The PT must always review background information on a client before initiating any therapeutic intervention. The aquatic environment presents a greater risk management environment than a comparable land-based environment. Gathering important background information assists the clinician in providing a more risk-free environment for both the client and the clinician. The background information provides specific data that can assist the clinician in developing a plan of care for a client, including safe entry and exit techniques from the pool, avoiding unsafe movement patterns, determining safe exercise parameters, and appropriately supervising the client. Table

TABLE 16-1 Indications for Aquatic Intervention: Impairments and Functional Limitations

Decreased range of motion
Pain with movement or functional activity on land
Balance, proprioception, and/or coordination deficits
Decreased strength
Cardiovascular compromise or deconditioned status
Weight-bearing restrictions on land
Peripheral edema in extremity
Gait deviations not easily corrected on land
Lack of progress with traditional land-based program
Difficulty with heat dissipation during exercise on land
Exacerbation of symptoms with land exercise
Poor movement patterns not easily correctable on land

TABLE 16-2 Benefits of Aquatic Intervention

Initiation of rehabilitation sooner than on land in many instances

Positive psychologic benefit of being able to do more in water than on land

Assist in edema control

Relaxed environment owing to warm water

Initiation of controlled active movements earlier than on land

Less pain with movement than on land

Initiation of dynamic functional movement patterns earlier than on land

Good carryover to movement patterns on land

Good environment for proprioceptive and sensory input

Forgiving environment for balance and coordination training

Options available for gradual increase of exercise intensity

Gait deviations and poor movement patterns more easily detected than on land

Easier progression of weight-bearing status than on land

Ability to completely de-weight the spine and extremity joints

Better heat dissipation and heat tolerance in below thermoneutral water temperature than on land

Enhanced cardiovascular function in below thermoneutral water temperature than on land

TABLE 16-3 History on Client

Contraindications to aquatic intervention

Safety needs and precautions of patient

Medical status and medical history

Current medications

Prior involvement in land or aquatic therapy intervention

Transferability on land

Use of assistive device on land

Weight-bearing status on land

Work, leisure, and exercise activity status before injury

Need for use of protective brace or splint during aquatic intervention

Comfort level in water

Ability to swim

Joints or structures affected

Precautions for allowable range of motion (ROM)

Pain level baseline

Psychologic status

Available active and passive ROM at affected joints

Functional limitations

Other important objective impairment information

Level of healing of surgical incision

Static and dynamic balance capabilities

Sensory status

Impairments and functional limitations determined from land-based program

Goals of aquatic intervention

TABLE 16-4 Contraindications to Aquatic Intervention

Excessive fear of water

Fever or high temperature

Untreated infectious disease

Open wound

Contagious skin disease

Surgical incision with sutures or staples in place

Partial opening of surgical incision

Serious cardiac conditions that cause cardiac compromise

Uncontrolled seizure disorder

16-3 provides a list of important information the PT should gather during history taking and before initiating an aquatic intervention.

Contraindications and Precautions

Several authors have composed lists of contraindications and precautions for aquatic therapy for various patient populations.[3,6,16,17] The contraindications and precautions most applicable to a client base with musculoskeletal and neuromuscular dysfunctions are given in Tables 16-4 and 16-5. Each facility, however, must develop and modify such contraindications and precautions based on the types of patients it serves. Knowledge and expertise of the professional and support staff affect a facility's choices in determining appropriate and safe candidates for aquatic intervention. For example, a client who has a thoracic compression fracture secondary to osteoporosis and requires the use of an oxygen tank for chronic obstructive pulmonary disease may not be accepted at all aquatic therapy facilities. One institution may not feel comfortable managing this client safely in a pool environment, whereas another facility may be able to modify an aquatic program for this client while staying within safe exercise parameters.

TABLE 16-5 Precautions to Aquatic Intervention

Seizure disorder controlled well with medications

Recently healed surgical incision

Absent or impaired peripheral sensation

Diabetes

Postural hypotension

Significant balance or vestibular disorder

Respiratory dysfunction

Colostomy

Difficulty with bowel or bladder control

Tracheostomy tube

Fear of water

Compromised vision without corrective lenses

Compromised cardiac or respiratory system (poor endurance or asthma)

Safe Exercise Parameters

Water temperature, in conjunction with depth of water, body composition, and intensity of exercise, must be considered when recommending the level of exercise for an aquatic treatment program. Water temperatures above and below thermoneutral temperature (31°C to 33°C; 88°F to 90.5°F) significantly change cardiovascular responses to exercise compared with an equal intensity and type of exercise on land. Heart rate during head out of water, light- to moderate-intensity cycling or walking/jogging in thermoneutral temperature water is not significantly different from that for the same intensity exercise performed on land. In contrast, heart rate is usually 10 beats per minute (bpm) lower for moderately heavy, strenuous, and maximal exercise in water below thermoneutral temperature.[18]

As water temperature increases above the thermoneutral level, heart rate, overall cardiovascular demands, and core body temperature all increase to potentially unsafe levels.[18,19] Evaporation of sweat is the primary means of cooling the body temperature in air, whereas conduction and convection are the primary means of heat gain or loss by the body in water. Heat exchange in water is greater than in air because heat conductance in water and the specific heat of water are approximately 25 to 1,000 times greater, respectively.[18] When water temperature is greater than skin temperature, heat gain by an immersed body is greater than heat loss. Clients should avoid exercising at moderate to high intensities in a warm-water pool to lessen or eliminate the chances of heat illness, particularly when immersed to chest level and above.

When water temperature is less than 31°C (88°F), heart rate decreases by as much as 17 to 20 bpm and stroke volume increases during moderate- to high-intensity, vertical, deep-water exercise.[11–15,18] It is speculated that immersion in cool water causes peripheral vasoconstriction so the body can maintain core body temperature. This vasoconstriction augments central blood volume, which, in turn, increases cardiac preload. The increase in cardiac preload thus increases stroke volume, which provides a strong stimulus via the baroreceptors to decrease heart rate.[11–15,18] The cardiovascular changes seen during deep-water vertical exercise are attributed to hydrostatic pressure and a more efficient cardiovascular system during exercise in cooler water. These changes are also attributed to the decreased demand on the cardiovascular system to dissipate the heat produced from exercise. Generally higher-intensity aerobic exercise is recommended at water temperatures between 26°C and 28°C (78.8°F and 82.4°F).[20]

The rating of perceived exertion (RPE) scoring system for intensity of exercise, originally developed by Borg, has been used successfully by many practitioners to accurately determine level of exercise intensity in water.[20] Wilder and Brennan[15] modified the Borg scale for water-running exercise programs. The specifics of the five-point Brennan scale are discussed later in this chapter.

Water depth affects heart rate. Heart rate is generally 8 to 11 bpm lower in chest-deep water during an aerobic shallow-water vertical exercise session compared with an equal intensity of exercise on land.[18] In addition, body composition affects a person's exercise response while immersed in water at different temperatures. Sheldahl et al[21] investigated the effect of water-immersed cycling on obese and lean women at 20°C, 24°C, and 28°C (68°F, 75.2°F, and 82.4°F). Lean women exhibited a fall in rectal core temperature during cycling at 20°C and 24°C, whereas obese women had no change. In addition, energy expenditure was greater in the lean women at the two lower water temperatures because of shivering. Shivering is a mechanism used in cool water temperatures to maintain body temperature.[21]

In summary, several factors about the client, water, and intended exercise need to be taken into consideration when determining exercise intensity levels. Water temperatures at or above the thermoneutral level are used primarily for lower-intensity exercises such as ROM; flexibility; relaxation and pain control; low-level balance, coordination, and proprioceptive training; gait training; specific low-intensity functional training; and beginning level core- and trunk-strengthening exercises. In contrast, water temperatures below thermoneutral should be used for cardiovascular endurance training, higher intensity local muscle endurance and strengthening, plyometrics training, cross-training, interval training, and some sport- or work-specific functional training. In addition, the target heart rate for land exercise should not be used to determine the target heart rate for more strenuous aerobic water exercise. The target heart rate should be modified to 10 to 20 bpm less than the desired target heart rate on land for a desired level of exercise intensity and depth of water.

Organization of Treatment Session

Generally an aquatic treatment session for a client with musculoskeletal dysfunction lasts 30 to 60 minutes. Depending on the conditioning level of the client and any comorbid conditions or precautions, the initial aquatic session may last only 10 to 15 minutes. An increase in the total time of immersion can be increased gradually over 1 or 2 weeks, as the client tolerates. Each treatment session usually consists of the following seven components, listed with the time allotted for each:

1. Warmup: 5 to 15 minutes.
2. ROM and flexibility: 5 to 15 minutes.
3. Strengthening and stabilization: 13 to 15 minutes.
4. Endurance training: 15 to 20 minutes.
5. Coordination, balance, and proprioception: 5 to 15 minutes.

6. Functional activities: 5 to 15 minutes.

7. Cooldown: 5 to 15 minutes.

The general organization of a treatment program can be modified to emphasize work in one or more aspects of an aquatic program based on the patient's impairments, functional limitations, and goals. For example, during the early phases of an aquatic therapy intervention for a patient with adhesive capsulitis of the shoulder, more emphasis may be placed on manual therapy techniques to the glenohumeral joint and the scapulothoracic articulation, in addition to ROM and flexibility exercises; less emphasis may be placed on strengthening at the shoulder. The extra time spent on ROM and flexibility alters the organization and time spent on the various components of a treatment session.

Integration with Land Activities and Return to Functional Land Rehabilitation

Emphasis in today's healthcare environment is on justification of the need for a particular intervention. This is especially true for aquatic therapy, particularly when the patient's primary functional activities are not conducted in a water environment. A definite link needs to be made between aquatic intervention and improvement in functional activities or skills on land. The plan of care chosen by the clinician—whether that intervention is performed solely in water, solely on land, or land and water in combination—needs to relate directly to the achievement of functional land goals.

The decision to include aquatic intervention in a plan of care for a client begins at the time of initial examination, during which impairments or functional limitations are determined. Then the clinician must begin to justify the need for aquatic intervention, which can be achieved by showing that a treatment program using specific physical and hydrodynamic properties of water is more effective and will achieve the patient's goals quicker than a similar land-based program. Documentation of the reasons for aquatic intervention, instead of or in conjunction with land intervention, is begun at the same time the clinician develops the plan and rationale for the specific regimen. The clinician should emphasize how the properties of water can be used to achieve land skills.

When treating patients with musculoskeletal dysfunction, the clinician generally chooses one of the following three options when deciding if it is appropriate to include aquatic therapy as part of the program: wet to dry transition, dry to wet transition, and wet only.[22]

Wet to dry transition is defined as a treatment intervention that begins in an aquatic environment and eventually transfers to a land-based intervention. This option is recommended for clients who are not able to tolerate axial and compressive forces on joint structures in a land-based program and for whom these forces are contraindicated because of a specific injury, illness, or surgical intervention.[22]

Dry to wet transition is indicated for clients for whom a land-based program exacerbates the condition.[22] Such a client is transferred to an aquatic intervention after having begun a land-based program. Gradual progression back to a land-based program is indicated once the client is ready and relatively pain free.

A *wet-only program* is recommended for clients who have a complete inability to tolerate a land-based treatment program or who prefer aquatic therapy. Patients with pathologies such as rheumatoid arthritis, osteoarthritis, fibromyalgia, spinal stenosis, significant degenerative disc disease, and chronic pain syndromes fit well into the wet-only option. Upon discharge from intervention services, a maintenance program of wet-only exercise is often the only option these clients have for continued, regular exercise.

A fourth option is a combined wet and dry program (discussed in more detail later in this chapter). Clients who need to function on land but because of their pathology cannot tolerate the rigors of a land-only intervention program prefer this option. Patients who are not progressing as quickly as anticipated in a land-only program benefit from a combined intervention, which allows the clinician to capitalize on the water's physical properties to enhance the therapy and to decrease the daily stresses on the client's affected structures. By alternating between land and water therapeutic interventions, the clinician is able to combine the best of both aquatic and land environments and to provide the client with several options for a continued home program after discharge.

In addition, clients who require variety and stimulation to adhere to an intervention program may benefit from the combined wet and dry option. Clients with long-term musculoskeletal or neuromusculoskeletal dysfunction who require years of intervention to increase function, maintain function, or prevent deterioration of function do well with this option. Understandably, these patients can become bored with a land-only program, and the clinician is challenged at every treatment session to keep these clients motivated so that functional goals in the school and home environments can be achieved in a timely manner. PTs treating clients with chronic dysfunctions report better results when using a combined land and water intervention.

The PT must re-examine the patient on a regular basis to justify the continued use of aquatic therapy beyond the initial treatment session(s). The use of aquatic intervention cannot be stagnant in nature, and its effectiveness in achieving desired functional land goals must be documented for each patient.

TECHNIQUES

Aquatic therapeutic techniques that are used to address common physical impairments and functional deficits are presented in this section. Some techniques use aquatic exercise equipment to support the trunk in a vertical or horizontal position, support an extremity in an appropriate position, add resistance to increase the intensity of an exercise, or add turbulence to increase the intensity of an exercise.

Flexibility and Range of Motion

Chapter 3 presents information on ROM. Aquatic intervention is a great supplement to those techniques. Warm water, with its buoyancy property, provides an excellent medium for enhancing and improving flexibility and ROM in the spine and extremities.[23] Immersion in warm water promotes relaxation and increases tissue temperature, enhancing the extensibility of the musculotendinous and soft tissues surrounding the joint and allowing the stretch to be more efficient.

Floating in supine is a buoyancy support position for shoulder abduction used early in an exercise program designed for improving ROM. This position is especially useful when a buoyancy assist position is too difficult for the client to control. After the client has developed the motor control needed for working within safe parameters, buoyancy assist positions for increasing ROM can be added to the program. Buoyancy devices can also be used to improve ROM (Figs. 16-10 and 16-11).

Figure 16-10   Standing shoulder abduction with buoyancy cuff.

PURPOSE: To enhance effect of buoyancy for improving range of motion at shoulder joint.

POSITION: Client standing in shoulder-deep water with both feet planted firmly on bottom of pool. Client wearing buoyancy cuff on forearm just above wrist with upper extremity in fully adducted, elbow extended, forearm supinated position.

PROCEDURE: Client initiates shoulder abduction while maintaining arm position and allowing buoyancy to perform or assist movement of upper extremity to 90-degree abducted position.

Figure 16-11 Standing knee flexion with buoyancy cuff.

PURPOSE: To enhance effect of buoyancy for improving range of motion at knee joint.

POSITION: Client standing in waist-deep water with one foot planted firmly on bottom of pool. Client wearing buoyancy cuff just above ankle on one lower extremity, which is in knee extended position.

PROCEDURE: Client initiates knee flexion, allowing buoyancy to perform or assist movement of lower extremity to allowable end point of flexion.

The use of a buoyancy assist position with or without a buoyancy device can also be used to increase the extensibility of muscles, such as the hamstrings, or for adherent nerve root stretch (Fig. 16-12).[24–27] Optimum muscle stretch on land for improving extensibility is generally thought to be 30 seconds of low-load stretching without pain for uninjured musculotendinous tissue.[28] Stretches of shorter duration repeated several times may be more tolerable during the tissue-healing phase of rehabilitation.

Gait Training

An aquatic environment is ideal for reintroducing a gait pattern to patients whose gait has been compromised by pain or other restrictions or has been minimized by injury or surgery. Early weight bearing can be initiated in the supine position in the water by use of closed-kinetic–chain weight-bearing activity (Fig. 16-13). The PTA offers unilateral weight bearing on the plantar surface of one foot. At

Figure 16-12   Adherent nerve root or hamstring stretch with buoyancy cuff.

PURPOSE: To passively mobilize and stretch adherent nerve root or stretch hamstring muscle.

POSITION: Client standing in waist- to chest-deep water with back against side of pool and one foot planted firmly on bottom of pool. Client wearing buoyancy cuff just above ankle on one lower extremity, which is in 90-degree hip flexed position.

PROCEDURE: Client allows buoyancy cuff to extend knee to limits of toleration (without causing significant discomfort).

the same time, resistance is offered to dorsiflexion of the ankle and flexion of the hip and knee on the contralateral extremity at the dorsum of the foot, mimicking the beginning of the swing phase against gravity on land.

The client can be progressed to vertical gait activities initiated with deep-water walking (a reduced weight-bearing state). If appropriate, the client can be advanced to walking in shoulder-deep water and then to shallower water to increase the weight bearing.

Water's viscosity and cohesion offer several benefits to gait training. They add resistance to, and thus help strengthen, the muscles used during gait activities. Viscosity and cohesion also have a tendency to slow cadence, which allows the clinician to carefully examine the client's gait, assess for deviations, and offer corrections via manual or verbal cuing. Furthermore, along with hydrostatic pressure, viscosity and cohesion make water much more forgiving than land for clients who have difficulty with balance. Recovery from a fall is much easier in water than on land for both the client and the clinician.

Gait training can be performed on stairs in a water environment by using an aquatic step bench (Fig. 16-14) or the pool's steps. The step bench can be placed in different depths of water, depending on the weight bearing desired by the clinician. Aquatic step benches and removable (portable) stairs are available in a variety of heights. The patient may use a kickboard or water noodle for balance and support during early gait training; as the patient gains control, the flotation device can be removed (Fig. 16-15).

Strengthening

Chapters 5 through 8 discuss enhancing muscle strength. Strengthening can also be part of an aquatic program. Progression of strength exercises can be done safely by exploring the physical and hydrodynamic properties of water. These properties, in conjunction with the physiologic properties of muscle fibers, allow the clinician to address muscle strengthening versus local muscle en-

Figure 16-13 Pregait activity in supine with tactile input.

PURPOSE: To introduce early weight bearing and sequencing of gait pattern.

POSITION: Client floating in supine supported with flotation devices about the cervical spine and pelvis. Wrists may be supported with flotation devices, if necessary. Clinician facing client's feet.

PROCEDURE: Clinician places hands on dorsum of client's feet while client flexes slightly at one knee and hip and simultaneously dorsiflexes foot of same extremity. Clinician allows client to actively flex hip and knee to about 20 degrees and dorsiflex ankle as far as tolerated. Client isometrically holds position for 5 to 10 seconds and repeats as tolerated.

Figure 16-14 Step bench with forward step-up.

PURPOSE: To initiate gait training for stair climbing.

POSITION: Client standing in waist-high or deeper water in front of step bench.

PROCEDURE: Client initiates step-up motion, leading with limb requested by clinician. Once both lower extremities are on bench, client steps off bench.

NOTE: Clinician determines the leading limb and whether client steps backward or forward.

Figure 16-15   Forward ambulation with water noodle.

PURPOSE: To initiate gait training with some assistance for balance.

POSITION: Client standing in slightly above waist- to chest-deep water, holding on to water noodle with both hands. Noodle is placed in front of client **(A)** or is wrapped under client's arms **(B)**.

PROCEDURE: Client walks forward while holding on to water noodle.

NOTE: As balance improves, client can hold on to noodle more loosely.

durance. Methods for increasing the intensity of aquatic exercises are presented in Table 16-6.

Emphasis on muscle strength or endurance can be achieved by manipulating the number of repetitions of an exercise, the work:rest ratio in a given cycle, and the total duration of a particular exercise. Both closed- and open-chain exercises for the extremities can be performed in an aquatic environment. Some examples of extremity-strengthening exercises are given in Figures 16-16 to 16-18. Trunk and multiple joint strengthening techniques are discussed in the next section.

Core and Trunk Strengthening

Chapter 14 provides background on spinal stabilization. Several clinicians have modified those concepts for use in an aquatic environment.[22,26,29–31] A spinal stabilization rehabilitation program incorporates the client's pain-free

TABLE 16-6 Methods for Increasing the Difficulty of Aquatic Strengthening Activities

Move from buoyancy assist to buoyancy support to buoyancy resist.
Increase speed of movement.
Decrease length of lever arm for active movements with buoyancy assist.
Increase length of lever arm with buoyancy resist.
Add a buoyancy device to the end of the extremity for buoyancy resist activities.
Increase size and irregularity of buoyancy device used for resistive activities.
Increase size and irregularity of resistive device.
Add turbulence to the direction of movement.
Increase the number of repetitions of an exercise.
Increase in overall time for performance of an exercise.
Decrease rest time between exercises.

Figure 16-16	Knee flexion and extension strengthening with buoyancy device.

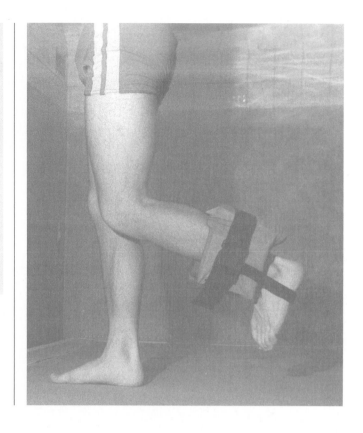

PURPOSE: To increase strength in quadriceps and hamstring muscle groups.

POSITION: Client standing in waist-deep water with one foot planted firmly on bottom of pool. Client wearing buoyancy device near ankle on one lower extremity with hip in neutral position and knee fully extended. Client holding on to side of the pool for balance and support, as needed.

PROCEDURE: Client actively flexes and extends at the knee joint while maintaining hip and spine in neutral and upright position.

NOTE: There should be no flexion or extension at hip or trunk.

Figure 16-17	Shoulder flexion and extension strengthening with aqua glove.

PURPOSE: To increase strength in shoulder flexors and extensors.

POSITION: Client standing in shoulder-deep water with arms at sides, elbows extended, forearms in full pronation, and fingers abducted. Client wearing aqua gloves.

PROCEDURE: Client simultaneously, or alternately, moves upper extremities to 90-degree shoulder flexion, back through neutral, to full shoulder extension while maintaining arm position.

Figure 16-18 Closed-chained upper-extremity push-pull.

PURPOSE: To strengthen muscle groups in closed-chain format.

POSITION: Client floating supine with shoulders fully flexed overhead and elbows maintained in almost full extension.

PROCEDURE: With hands pressed flat on side of pool or grasping railing or handles, client pushes upper extremities into pool side or railings.

NOTE: If handles or railings are available, client may alternate between pushing body away from and pulling it back into side of pool.

position of the neutral spine.[32] Neutral spine is defined as being approximately at the mid-range between the extremes of lumbopelvic spinal flexion and extension and is the position in which the patient is most comfortable.[30]

It is common for patients with spinal dysfunction to use movement patterns that take the spine out of the neutral position, especially when the extremities and spine are moved simultaneously. Patients seem to use these inappropriate patterns to compensate for pain that occurs during functional movement on land.[30] Unfortunately, these poor compensatory patterns can become habitual, perpetuating the pain and spinal dysfunction. Thus, the primary goals of spinal stabilization exercises are to facilitate and teach efficient and effective movement patterns from a sound neutral spine.[32]

The aquatic environment is an ideal medium for spinal stabilization exercises. Training the client to achieve total spinal alignment, proper posture, and neutral positioning should be the initial goal of an aquatic spinal stabilization program.[29] Once spinal alignment and proper postural awareness are obtained, the clinician uses the aquatic environment to help the client gain dynamic control over spinal movement. This control allows the client to develop better synergistic functional movement patterns and increase ROM, flexibility, and strength.

The aquatic environment enhances awareness of proper posture and body mechanics and eliminates the potentially harmful and painful compressive and shear forces that gravity places on spinal structures such as the discs and facet joints.[22,29,30] Any movement of the body in the water forces the client to stabilize at the spine and trunk to overcome the forces of the water. An aquatic-based spinal stabilization program can benefit patients with discogenic pain, nerve root impingement or irritation, postural syndrome, facet joint syndrome, chronic pain, and sacroiliac or iliosacral dysfunction. A water-based program is also recommended for patients recovering from surgical procedures such as laminectomy, discectomy, and spinal fusion.

Stabilization exercises can be performed in deep or shallow water for the cervical, thoracic, and lumbar levels of the spine. The advantage of doing these exercises in deep water, particularly for patients with lumbar spine dysfunction, is to decrease the compressive forces on bony and soft tissue structures by suspending the client in the water with a flotation device about the trunk. The disadvantage of using deep water in the initial stages of a spinal stabilization program is the lack of position sense provided by weight bearing through the lower extremities or contact of the spine and posterior trunk against a surface, such as the pool wall. For most clients, deep-water spinal stabilization techniques are more difficult because the client must rely almost completely on coordinated contractions of the muscles of the pelvis and trunk to allow pain-free movement.[30]

In contrast, for clients who are weight-bearing sensitive on land, deep water may be more comfortable and is a good choice for initial spinal stabilization activities. Strengthening the scapular stabilizers is the primary emphasis of a stabilization program for cervical and thoracic pathologies and for shoulder dysfunctions such as rotator cuff tendonitis. All exercises are performed within the client's pain-free ROM in a slowed and controlled manner.[30]

Progression is achieved in a spinal stabilization program by moving the client from small-excursion movement at one joint to large-excursion dynamic movements at multiple joints while maintaining a safe, balanced, and neutral spine position. Dynamic control of these movements is achieved through stabilization of the pelvis and lumbar spine through the cocontraction of agonist and antagonist trunk muscles (e.g., abdominals, gluteus maximus, and latissimus dorsi) in a synergistic pattern that enhances maintenance of the neutral spine position. Examples of spinal stabilization exercises for patients with lumbopelvic dysfunction are given in Figures 16-19 to 16-21. Examples of deep-water spinal stabilization exercises and their normal progression are given in Table 16-7. An example of a scapular and spinal stabilization exercise for cervical, thoracic, and shoulder dysfunctions is given in Figure 16-22.

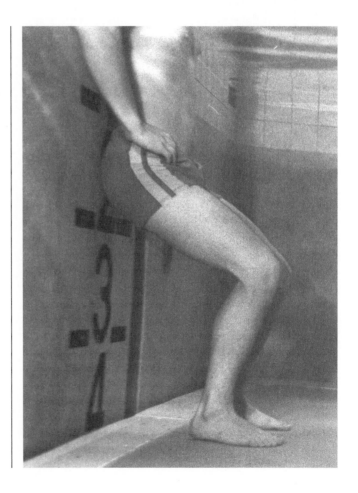

Figure 16-19 Mini-squats with back to side of pool.

PURPOSE: To experience and practice neutral spine position while superimposing functional squatting.

POSITION: Client standing in chest-deep water with back against side of pool and feet about shoulder width apart; hips and knees flexed to 20 to 30 degrees and hands on hips.

PROCEDURE: Client finds and holds neutral spine position. Client then performs isometric cocontraction of abdominal and gluteal muscles while maintaining neutral position and performing mini-squats to 50 to 70 degrees of hip and knee flexion, as tolerated.

Figure 16-20 Breaststroke with wonder board.

PURPOSE: To practice maintenance of neutral spine position in sitting position while moving upper extremities.

POSITION: Client sitting on wonder board in approximately 4 feet of water with spine in neutral position and upper extremities floating in front **(A)**.

PROCEDURE: Client maintains neutral position while performing isometric cocontractions of abdominal and gluteal muscles. Then client superimposes breaststroke movements of upper extremity **(B)**.

Figure 16-21 Abdominal strengthening in neutral lumbar spine position.

PURPOSE: To increase abdominal strength while protecting spine in neutral position.

POSITION: Client floating supine in 3 to 4 feet of water supported by flotation devices under knees and on upper extremities. Cervical spine may be supported with flotation device, if necessary. Client floating with knees flexed over barbell and hips in neutral or slightly flexed position.

POSITION: Client tucks chin and flexes slightly at hip, performing abdominal crunch while maintaining neutral spine position.

TABLE 16-7 Deep-water Spinal Stabilization Exercises[a]

Single knee to chest
Bilateral knee to chest
Side sit-ups
Hip abduction–adduction
Lower-extremity bicycling propulsion
Lower-extremity walking or reciprocal arm swing while sitting
    on barbell or kickboard
Squats while standing on barbell
Squats with quarter and half turns
Upper-extremity breaststroke forward and backward while
    standing on barbell
Forward steppage gait with lower extremity crossing midline

[a]All activities are performed while maintaining a neutral spine via co-contraction of abdominals and gluteal muscles.

Balance, Proprioception, and Coordination

Balance, proprioception, and coordination activities can be initiated in the water for the trunk and extremities. For the purposes of this chapter, balance is defined as the ability to maintain the center of gravity over the base of support, as in standing balance.[33] Proprioception is defined as the awareness of posture, movement, and changes in equilibrium and the knowledge of position, weight, and resistance of objects in relation to the body.[33] Coordination can be defined as the ability of different components of the neuromusculoskeletal system to work together to produce smooth, controlled, and accurate movements.[33] Coordination deficits occur when muscles fail to fire in sequence or when the central nervous system is unable to direct movement activities accurately. These three components are part of the entire motor control concept.

Several of the exercises used to improve balance and proprioception challenge these systems and serve as dynamic stabilization activities. Proximal stability is required of the trunk and proximal joints of the extremities to successfully and safely perform these activities, thus challenging the entire neuromusculoskeletal system.

A desired intensity of a balance, proprioceptive, and coordination activity can be achieved in several ways. One way is for the client to simply perform the skill at a faster yet safe speed. Decreasing the level of support provided by the PTA, piece of equipment, or side of pool also progresses the intensity of the exercise. Increased difficulty can also be achieved by adding turbulence, which is accomplished by increasing the speed of the water's movement, if possible.

Some exercises used in the water for balance, proprioception, and coordination are listed in Table 16-8 and shown in Figures 16-23 and 16-24. Furthermore, several more advanced plyometric activities (discussed next) can be used as well.

Plyometrics

The concept of plyometrics has its roots in Europe, where it was first known as "jump training."[34] The term was coined in 1975 by Fred Wilt, an American track and field coach; following its Latin derivation, it can be interpreted

Figure 16-22	Simultaneous alternating push-downs with buoyant dumbbells.

PURPOSE: To provide strengthening for scapular and posterior shoulder muscles for proximal stabilization in cervical and thoracic areas.

POSITION: Client standing in shoulder-deep water with shoulders and forearms in neutral position and elbows slightly flexed while holding buoyant dumbbell in each hand. Client holding spine in neutral position with cocontraction of abdominal and gluteal muscles.

PROCEDURE: Client pushes one dumbbell down toward pool floor and allows contralateral dumbbell to float toward water surface by extending shoulder and flexing elbow in controlled manner.

NOTE: Dumbbell remains submerged below water surface when client achieves full shoulder extension and elbow flexion.

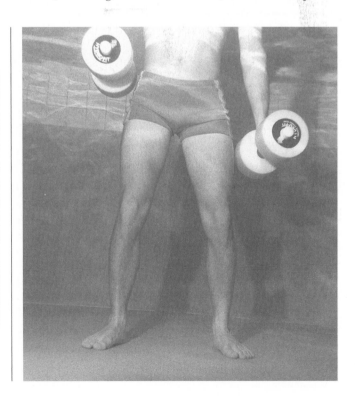

TABLE 16-8	Balance, Proprioceptive, and Coordination Activities in an Aquatic Environment

Balance

Stork-standing on injured and uninjured limbs while arms create turbulence (e.g., by breaststroking).

Stork-standing while performing a variety of levels of squats with arms held in a variety of positions (e.g., mini squats with both arms over head).

Sitting on kickboard while clinician creates turbulence.

Single- or double-leg squatting while standing on buoyant dumbbell.

Proprioception

Stork-standing on injured and uninjured limbs while moving contralateral lower extremity into different positions of hip flexion, abduction, extension, and external rotation, with and without the knee flexed.

Deep-water running for three to five strides followed by a pirouette; repeat.

Coordination

Braiding gait sideways in different depths of water with and without arm movement.

Backward and forward heel-toe walking holding on to side of pool and progressing to middle of pool.

Sidestepping while crossing arms in front and back of trunk.

Stork-standing while performing squats and asymmetric arm movement patterns.

Sitting on buoyant barbell while performing the vertical breaststroke.

Rocking horse while crossing arms in front and back of trunk.

---

to mean "measurable increases." Plyometrics are most commonly used by athletes to incorporate sports-specific jumping, hopping, bounding, and leaping skills in the rehabilitation process. Plyometric exercises enable a muscle to reach maximum strength in as short a time as possible.[34]

Plyometric exercise requires activities in which eccentric muscle contractions are rapidly followed by a movement completed by concentric contractions. It is postulated that eccentric–concentric muscle contraction not only stimulates the proprioceptors sensitive to rapid stretch but also loads the serial elastic components with a tension force from which the individual can rebound.[34]

Plyometric activities can be progressed from low to high intensity within six categories: jumping in place, standing jumps, multiples hops and jumps, bounding, box drills, and depth jumps.[34] The aquatic environment is an ideal medium for beginning plyometric training before progressing the client to training on land. Furthermore, aquatic plyometrics can be done with specificity to the requirements of sport, work, or leisure activity. Plyometric training in the water can be performed with equipment, such as aquatic step benches, elevated platforms, and balls of different sizes and weights (Figs. 16-25 and 16-26).

Cardiovascular and Endurance Training

Intervention for musculoskeletal disorders usually emphasizes regaining strength, ROM, and functional capabilities. Unfortunately, cardiovascular rehabilitation to improve the client's endurance level is seldom mentioned. Yet most clients whose physical activity level has been significantly reduced during the time of injury recovery have suffered a decline in overall cardiovascular performance. Studies have confirmed that a significant decline in cardiovascular function occurs during a period of decreased physical

---

Figure 16-23	Braiding sideways walking.

PURPOSE: To improve dynamic balance, coordination, and proprioception.

POSITION: Client standing in waist- to neck-deep water.

PROCEDURE: Client steps out sideways with leading leg and then steps with trailing leg, placing it alternately in front and behind leading leg with each step.

Figure 16-24 Rocking horse.

PURPOSE: To challenge and enhance balance, coordination, and proprioception.

POSITION: Client standing in waist- to shoulder-deep water with arms resting at side and forearms in neutral position.

PROCEDURE: Client leaps forward, shifting all weight to leading leg with hip and knee flexed while crossing one arm over the other in horizontal adduction across front midline; then client kicks trailing leg behind, with hip extended, knee flexed, and ankle plantarflexed. Next client steps back onto trailing leg (keeping hip extended, knee flexed, and ankle plantarflexed) and takes weight fully off leading leg (keeping hip and knee flexed) while crossing one arm over the other beyond the back midline. Client repeats movement.

NOTE: Trailing and leading legs and arm crossed on top can be switched or alternated.

Figure 16-25 Directional plyometric jumping.

PURPOSE: To improve power jumping skills.

POSITION: Client standing in waist- to shoulder-deep water with hips and knees slightly flexed.

PROCEDURE: Client jumps forward, backward, right, and left (north, south, east, and west).

NOTE: Clinician can determine direction pattern beforehand or randomly select and cue direction as client jumps.

Figure 16-26	Lateral box jumps.

PURPOSE: To improve lateral power jumping skills.

POSITION: Client standing in mid–trunk- to shoulder-deep water, with hips and knees slightly flexed, beside aquatic step bench.

PROCEDURE: Client jumps up and to side, placing both feet simultaneously onto step bench, and then jumps off to side, placing both feet simultaneously on pool floor.

NOTE: Client performs exercise from both sides of bench.

activity.[35,36] Thus, it is important to include some form of cardiovascular endurance training to ensure full recovery of the client with a musculoskeletal dysfunction.

Chapter 12 presents a detailed description of land-based cardiovascular programs. Cardiovascular training can also be performed in an aquatic environment. Deep- or shallow-water running, walking, and cross-country skiing are excellent choices.

Before including a cardiovascular endurance component in a treatment program, the clinician must be familiar with the client's cardiovascular and cardiopulmonary history and current medications. Some prescribed medications alter the heart rate response to a given intensity level of exercise. PTAs must also understand the cardiovascular response to immersion and exercise in the aquatic environment, as discussed earlier.

Deep-water running gained popularity as a form of cardiovascular training in the 1980s when gold medal marathoner Joan Benoit Samuelson began running in a pool during recovery from a sport-related injury. Several studies investigated the effect of cardiovascular vertical training in deep- and shallow-water running and underwater cycling. These studies showed improvement in cardiovascular function comparable to a land-based regimen of similar intensity. The studies noted that aquatic training prevented the decline in cardiovascular fitness level normally seen during an episode of decreased physical capabilities.[14,37–40] Research has also shown the importance of instruction in, and maintenance of, proper deep-water running form for optimal outcome in cardiovascular fitness training.[11,41,42]

Deep-water running is described as simulated running in the deep end of a swimming pool, avoiding contact with the bottom of the pool. Buoyancy in the water eliminates the impact with the ground experienced when running on land.[43,44] Proper form and body position are important and are described in Table 16-9. Patients may run in place by

using a tether strap or may chose to run over a given distance in the pool. It is recommended the patient wear a commercially available flotation device or vest to assist in maintaining proper form (Fig. 16-27). The motions of cross-country skiing can also be used for cardiovascular training (Table 16-10). The intensity of the cardiovascular endurance program can be increased by adding equipment (e.g., aqua gloves or fins) to increase the resistance to movement in the water by increasing the surface area of the body part.

TABLE 16-9 Deep-water Running Form

Water line at shoulder level
Head looking straight forward
Trunk slightly forward of vertical
Spine in neutral position
Upper-extremity motion identical to that used on land
Primary arm motions from shoulder
Shoulder flexion brings hands to just below water line 8 to 12 inches from chest
Extension brings hands just below hips
Hands slightly clinched with thumbs on top
Elbows primarily flexed but undergo a slight degree of extension and flexion
Lower-extremity motion requires attention to detail
Maximum hip flexion of 60 to 80 degrees
As hip flexes, knee extends
When maximum hip flexion is reached, leg should be perpendicular to the horizontal
Hip and knee extend together
Knee reaches full extension when hip is in neutral
As hip extends beyond neutral, knee begins to flex
Ankle in dorsiflexion when hip is in neutral
Ankle in plantarflexion when hip is extended beyond neutral
Dorsiflexion reassumed when hip is flexed and leg extends
Inversion and eversion accompany dorsiflexion and plantarflexion, as seen on land

Figure 16-27 Deep-water running with flotation device.

PURPOSE: To improve or maintain cardiovascular endurance.

POSITION: Client standing suspended in deep water by flotation device.

PROCEDURE: Client runs in place for designated period of time at designated pace.

NOTE: Client may wear flotation device around waist or may wear wet vest. Client must be taught proper water-running technique.

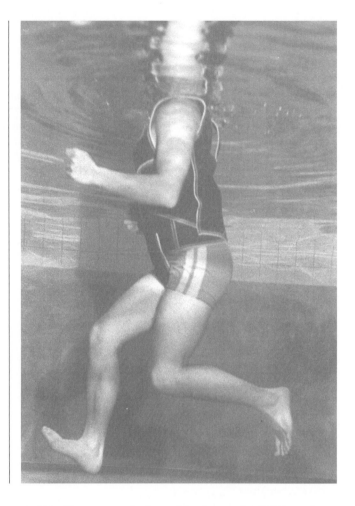

Monitoring the intensity of an aerobic endurance exercise in the water is performed in one of three ways: target heart rate, RPE, and cadence. Target heart rate should fall in the range of 60% to 90% of maximal heart rate using the following formula:

$$\text{Maximal heart rate} = 220 - \text{age (years)} - 15 \text{ bpm}$$

For the deconditioned client, it may be best to use a target heart rate in the 40% to 60% range. For more detailed information on monitoring aerobic activities, see Chapter 10.

TABLE 16-10 Cross-country Skiing Form

Use flotation belt or vest
Maintain vertical position
Reciprocal flexion and extension of upper and lower
    extremities
Very light flexion is maintained in bilateral elbows and knees
Movement occurs primarily at hips and shoulders through a
    tolerated range of motion
May add aqua gloves or paddles to upper extremities to
    increase resistance
May add fins to lower extremities to increase resistance

The Brennan scale is useful when using RPE to determine intensity of exercise in the water (Table 16-11).[43,44] The Brennan scale, an adaptation of the Borg RPE scale, is a five-point scale with increments of 0.5 that uses verbal descriptors ranging from very light to very hard. Descriptors of on-land running activities for each point on the scale are included, which makes it easy for athletes and coaches to correlate aquatic activity to an established land-based training session.[43,44]

Cadence is the third means of establishing exercise intensity for cardiovascular training in the water. Cadence is defined as the number of times the right leg moves through a complete gait cycle each minute.[43,45] Wilder et al[45] found a significant correlation (0.98) between cadence and heart rate during graded exercise testing in the pool. Cadence is most useful as a guide for exercise intensity when interval training is incorporated into a treatment program. See Table 16-11 for cadence rates appropriate for clinicians or coaches setting up interval-type training sessions for distance runners and sprinters.[43] Deep-water running interval training can closely mimic a land-based interval training session. This form of interval training has become popular not only with athletes who are recovering from injury but also with athletes who are including water running as a regular component of a cross-training program.

TABLE 16-11 Brennan RPE Scale Correlated to Cadences and Land Equivalents for Distance Runners and Sprinters

	Distance runners			Sprinters	
Brennan Score	Cadence	Land Equivalent		Cadence	Land Equivalent
1.0 very light	<60	Brisk walk		<74	>800 m
1.5	60–64			75–59	
2.0 light	60–64	Easy jog		80–84	600–800 m
2.5	65–69			85–90	
3.0 somewhat hard	70–74	Brisk run		90–94	400–600 m
3.5	75–80			95–99	
4.0 hard	80–84	5-K or 10-K race		130–134	200–400 m
4.5	85–90			135–139	
5.0 very hard	>90	Short track intervals		>113	50–200 m

RPE = rating of perceived exertion.

Cross-Training and Maintenance Programs

Many clinicians who develop rehabilitation programs for their clients incorporate a cross-training regimen when integrating water-based with land-based exercise. Some facilities are beginning to incorporate both land- and water-based exercises into work conditioning and functional restoration programs designed for injured workers. This combination maximizes the benefits of both environments, adds fun, and prevents boredom.[46]

Once a client returns to maximum improvement and is ready for discharge from services, there is no reason why the clinician cannot recommend continued individual participation in aquatic exercise in conjunction with land exercise. The clinician should recommend continuation of water exercise if the physical properties of water can be used to the benefit of the client. For clients who cannot tolerate land-based exercise (e.g., those with rheumatoid arthritis and osteoarthritis), water exercise may be the sole means of a maintenance program. For other clients, water can serve as a viable medium for cross-training. A training program of aerobic exercise such as running, walking, or cross-country skiing can be performed on both land and in water on alternating days. Even for the highly trained athlete, little to no loss in performance has been observed when water running is substituted for or performed in conjunction with land running.[11,37–39] Land and water aerobic programs can be alternated quite easily for most clients.

Strength training can be alternated between a land program (using free weights, elastic bands, circuit training, or exercise machines) and a comparable water program (using assistive and resistive buoyancy and unstreamlined equipment). Trunk stabilization exercises can continue in the water environment. Facilities around the country are beginning to offer nontherapeutic aquatic exercise classes for prevention of spine pain and for continued progress of clients who have been discharged from therapeutic services.

For many clients, aquatic exercise serves as a welcome change of pace, improving overall well-being and creating a positive attitude to exercise. Anecdotal reports indicate improved long-term adherence to exercise when a cross-training regimen that includes both land and water is incorporated. The aquatic environment may also help prevent or alleviate the exacerbation of symptoms, allowing the former patient to stay pain free and functional for leisure and work activities on a long-term basis.

Functional Training

Incorporation of functional training into an aquatic rehabilitation program is vital to transition a client to the land environment in which function will be performed on a regular basis. Functional activities performed in the water serve as initial training for carryover to safe performance on land. The type of functional training incorporated depends on the tasks and skills required by and goals of the client. Some activities used in an aquatic program are as simple as transfer skills from vertical (standing) to sitting and vice versa. Bed mobility training can be achieved by teaching transitions from supine, through side-lying to prone and back to supine on the long-body axis in a horizontal position on the surface of the water.

More complex, multitask, sport-specific, or functional work activities can also be initiated in the water. An example of functional skill training is lifting plastic crates with different numbers of holes in them to alter resistance (Fig. 16-28). Sport-specific skills include mimicking a tennis swing while holding a water paddle (Fig. 16-29).

Figure 16-28 Lifting plastic crates.

PURPOSE: To practice functional lifting technique.

POSITION: Client standing in waist-deep water in diagonal squat-lifting position (one foot slightly in front, wide base of support, and neutral spine) while holding plastic crate close to body between thighs, with elbows flexed at 20 to 30 degrees.

PROCEDURE: While maintaining neutral spine by cocontracting abdominal and gluteal muscles, client squat-lifts to 50 to 70 degrees of hip and knee flexion, keeping elbows slightly flexed.

Figure 16-29 Tennis swing with paddle.

PURPOSE: To practice a sport-specific technique.

POSITION: Client standing in mid–trunk-deep water in forehand tennis stroke position while holding on to a water paddle **(A)** or table tennis paddle **(B)**.

PROCEDURE: Client repetitively swings paddle through water, mimicking forehand tennis stroke with appropriate technique.

CASE STUDY

PATIENT INFORMATION

A 19-year-old defensive back football player presented to the clinic with a long-term history of low back pain (LBP) of insidious onset and aggravated by any sports participation. The current bout of LBP began 2 months earlier, when the patient was dead lifting as part of his weight-training program. At the time of the lifting incident the athlete stated his trunk was stuck in a forward-flexed position. A magnetic resonance imaging study, ordered by an orthopaedic surgeon within days of the onset of pain, revealed a two-level disk herniation at the L4-L5 and L5-S1 interspaces. Radiographs revealed moderately degenerative joint disease for the patient's age throughout the lumbar spine. The physician recommended "red shirting" the athlete for his freshman year and referred him to the clinic to prepare him for college football training and conditioning for the following spring's off-season training.

The patient's chief complaint was pain (7 out of 10) in the low back from the level of L1 to S1 centrally and bilaterally into the erector spinae musculature with radiation of pain into the right buttock and posterior thigh. The patient also reported pain in the lumbar spine and right buttock after sitting for a prolonged period of time during classes and while traveling in a car; he was unable to perform household chores such as vacuuming and sweeping and felt pain with lower-extremity weight training, jogging on land, and recreational sports activities such as basketball.

The initial examination by the PT revealed an altered standing posture with a forward head position and decreased lumbar lordosis on the sagittal view. Active ROM of the lumbar spine revealed decreased lumbar flexion secondary to pain in the spine and right buttock. Repeated lumbar flexion active ROM increased lumbar pain and peripheralized the radiation of pain into the right posterior thigh and calf. Myotome assessment revealed bilateral weakness and pain in the lumbar spine with resistive hip flexion, knee extension, and ankle dorsiflexion (right side more than left). Passive posterior–anterior segmental mobility testing of the lumbar spine revealed hypomobility but no pain from levels T12 through L3 with hypermobility and pain noted at levels L4 and L5. Manual muscle testing revealed weakness in the rectus abdominis and bilateral tightness in the hip flexors and hamstring musculature (right greater than left). All other examination procedures were within normal limits.

Based on the mechanism of injury, the examination findings, and the results of the diagnostic testing, the patient was diagnosed with lumbar disc disease at the L4-L5 and L5-S1 levels with associated radiculopathy into the right lower extremity.

LINKS TO
GUIDE TO PHYSICAL THERAPIST PRACTICE

Musculoskeletal pattern 4F of the *Guide*[47] relates to the diagnosis of this patient. This pattern is described as "impaired joint mobility, motor function, muscle performance, range of motion, or reflex integrity secondary to spinal disorders." Included in the diagnostic group of this pattern is intervertebral disc disorder and the anticipated goal is "ability to perform physical tasks related to self-care, home management, community and work (job/school/play) integration or reintegration and leisure activities using aquatic exercises."

INTERVENTION

The goals of intervention were as follows:

- Decrease pain by at least three levels on a visual analog scale at rest and with light activities of daily living (e.g., sweeping and vacuuming).
- Maintain a neutral spine position via better core strength of abdominal and gluteals during sitting and housecleaning activities.
- Adhere to recommended energy conservation techniques and posture and body mechanics during functional activities.
- Increase strength in the trunk and lower extremities.
- Eliminate pain during lower-extremity resistive testing.
- Obtain full pain-free repeated trunk flexion ROM.
- Return to safe and pain-free participation in off-season football training, including weight training, cardiovascular conditioning, and agility drills of running and cutting.

Football contact practice was delayed until the following fall training session. Treatment was initiated by the PTA after the PT completed the plan of care. The PT performed central posterior to anterior glides from T12 through L3, progressing from grades I through IV as tolerated to increase segmental mobility. The PT requested that the PTA assist with therapeutic exercises including spinal stabilization and education. Treatment performed by the PTA consisted of the following:

1. Prone on elbow positioning and prone press-ups, emphasizing extension at the upper lumbar levels by stabilizing the lower lumber levels with a mobilization belt (Fig. 3-31).

2. Instruction in proper posture, body mechanics, and energy conservation techniques for prolonged sitting, light housecleaning, and proper lifting.

3. No lifting during activities of daily living.

4. Use of a lumbar support cushion for sitting in class and driving and instruction on the need for frequent, short standing breaks with active trunk extension.

5. Early spinal stabilization techniques, emphasizing abdominal and gluteal sets in supine and sitting and maintenance of the neutral spine position during activities of daily living.

6. Bridging activities superimposed on a neutral spine (Fig. 14-9).

7. Gym ball activities to address spinal stabilization and core strengthening (Figs. 14-29 to 14-31).

8. Use of ice after exercise and for pain control, as needed.

PROGRESSION

Four Weeks After Initial Examination

Toward the end of the first month, the patient's pain and weakness symptoms began to subside. The PTA documented that the athlete was unable to tolerate progression to more aggressive standing, strengthening, and weight-bearing activities (e.g., jogging) because of increased symptoms. The PTA recommended to the PT that a 2-week program of aquatic therapy be initiated. The PT agreed, and the following aquatic activities were developed collaboratively by the PT and PTA:

1. Deep-water suspended vertical hanging with a flotation device under each axilla and 2.5-pound weights on each ankle.

2. Deep-water vertical suspended exercises with a flotation device under each axilla with the spine held in neutral with cocontraction of abdominals and gluteals, unilateral and bilateral knee to chest hip ROM exercises and hip abduction and adduction with knees extended.

3. Deep-water walking forward and backward.

4. Deep-water jogging or running forward and backward (Fig. 16-27).

5. Side-lying running forward and backward.

6. Shallow-water (shoulder to chest deep) exercises with the spine held in neutral position by cocontraction of abdominals and gluteals: walking forward and backward, side-stepping while wearing aqua gloves, and hamstring stretching with back against the wall (Fig. 16-12).

All of these exercises were performed under PTA supervision two times per week in the minimal pain range for the spine and lower extremities. The PTA reported to the PT after a week that there was no increase in peripheral symptoms. The PTA instructed the patient in an independent home exercise program to be performed one to two times per week.

Six Weeks After Initial Examination

After 2 weeks of aquatic intervention the PTA reported that the patient had an increase in length of time spent in sitting without pain, an increased ability to perform abdominal and gluteal cocontraction, no pain when standing in active forward flexion, and no complaints of pain into the right buttock.

Aquatic intervention was thus continued per communication with the PT for 4 weeks more. The program progressed the duration, repetitions, and speed of movement in the water, placing greater emphasis on abdominal and gluteal control in the neutral spine position and increasing the excursion of movement of the trunk and lower extremities. The patient was decreased to being seen once a week by the PTA per the plan of care, and he continued with his independent exercise program an additional one or two times per week. The following exercises were added to the aquatic program:

1. Deep-water suspended vertical exercises: side sit-ups, squats (Fig. 16-19), upper-extremity breaststroke forward and backward while standing on a barbell, and upper-extremity breaststroke or reciprocal arm swing (as during walking) forward and backward while sitting on a barbell or kickboard (Fig. 16-20).

2. Shallow-water exercises: forward and backward jogging interval training, running progression, plyometric directional drills with and without a step bench and superimposing a variety of arm positions and movements (Fig. 16-25, 16-26), and replication of running patterns and catching a football.

OUTCOMES

During the final 2 weeks of the aquatic intervention the PT prescribed a gradual return to lower-extremity and trunk weight training and a progression of jogging and running drills on land. The PTA documented at the end of the aquatic intervention that the patient had met all long-term goals and recommended discharge of the patient to the PT. The PT provided guidelines to the patient for continued progression of exercises in the water to be used for cross-training with the prescribed land exercises. The PT also gave parameters for safe progression of land weight training and running drills.

SUMMARY—AN EFFECTIVE PT–PTA TEAM

This case demonstrated ongoing written and verbal communication by the PTA. The PTA recommended several interventions and changes to the PT which demonstrated that the PTA felt confident in his or her skills. The PT in this case study took responsibility for certain aspects of the treatment such as mobilization and discharge instructions. The PTA could have completed the discharge instructions, but the PT has the responsibility for deciding what aspect of treatment is delegated. Spinal mobilization is an intervention that should be considered carefully before delegating to anyone other than the PT.

▼ ▼ ▼ GERIATRIC PERSPECTIVES ▼ ▼ ▼

- Exercising in water results in reduction of stresses on weight-bearing joints and is an ideal medium for rehabilitation of older adults with precautions and contraindications.[1-3] Before initiating a water program for older individuals, the clinician should recommend a medical checkup for blood pressure and other medical problems. In addition, a listing of current prescribed and over-the-counter medications (including vitamin and herbal supplements) should be obtained using the "brown bag" technique (the patient is told to place all frequently taken medications in a bag and to bring them in). Medications of particular concern are the antihypertensives and cardiac drugs that may limit the body's cardiovascular responses.

- With aging, the body's thermoregulating capacity is reduced and may limit the older individual's ability to adapt to central heat gain or loss. Furthermore, the patient's comfort, safety, and skill in the water should be evaluated. The clinician should determine the need for a life jacket or lift.[4]

- Most accidents in older adults involved in aquatic therapy and exercise occur when the individuals are entering and exiting the pool; the accidents are usually caused by poor balance, slow recovery time after loss of balance, dizziness, and tripping over objects left at the side of the pool. Special consideration should be given to the entry ramp in regard to hand railings, nonslip surfaces, and organization of the pool side and changing areas.

- If possible, older individuals with vision problems should wear corrective lenses during the sessions. Hearing aids, however, should not be worn in the water. Thus, instructions should be discussed with the patient before he or she removes the aid to enter the water.

- Older adults benefit from the socialization of group aquatic rehabilitative sessions; however, individualized therapy with qualified staff is more appropriate for frail older adults. Owing to the age-related increase in central processing time and response time, exercise instruction should be slow paced and clearly demonstrated.

- An emergency procedure should be carefully devised, discussed, and practiced with all staff involved in the pool area. In addition, the plan should be clearly outlined and posted near the designated telephone.

1. Heyneman CA, Premo DE. A "water-walkers" exercise program for the elderly. *Public Health Rep.* 1992;107:213–216.
2. Stevenson J, Tacia S, Thompson J, et al. A comparison of land and water exercise programs for older individuals. *Med Sci Sports Exerc.* 1988;22(Suppl 20):537–540.
3. Selby-Silverstein L, Pricket N, Dougherty M, et al. Effect of aquatic therapy on temporal spatial parameters of gait in the frail elderly. *Phys Ther.* 1999;79:S47–S51.
4. Kimble D. A case study in adaptive aquatics for the geriatric population. *Clin Manage.* 1986;6:8–11.

SUMMARY

- This chapter provided an overview of the use of aquatic therapy intervention for a client with musculoskeletal dysfunction of the spine and extremities. Several aspects of the water environment and the client must be taken into consideration before implementing aquatic techniques in a plan of care. The clinician must consider the physical properties of water each time a clinical decision is made to use an aquatic intervention for a particular patient.

- Justification for the use of the aquatic medium in a plan of care either by itself, or in conjunction with land intervention, depends on the individual needs of the client. Proper use of the physical properties of water enhances the plan of care and may speed recovery. There are many treatment options and parameters for aquatic intervention, and a careful review of the client's impairments, functional limitations, and precautions or contraindications must be undertaken before introducing specific aquatic techniques in a plan of care.

- Several types of aquatic equipment are available. Addition of any piece of aquatic equipment should have a purpose that fills a treatment need. The clinician must carefully evaluate the client's ability to safely use and tolerate a piece of equipment before adding it to the aquatic intervention program.

▲ ▲ ▲ PEDIATRIC PERSPECTIVES ▲ ▲ ▲

- Water can be an excellent and fun exercise medium for children of all ages. To increase success with children, the clinician should focus on play with therapeutic purposes.

- The principles of specific gravity and buoyancy are excellent reasons to use aquatic therapy for support during exercise interventions with children. Water can be used for assistance or resistance, depending on the exercise prescription. Specific benefits include weight relief, ease of movement, and success with activities. These benefits allow the child to explore movement more freely, strengthen muscles, and practice functional activities. Working in water may allow children to learn to perform movements and activities too difficult to accomplish on land.[1,2]

- Aquatic therapy offers children opportunities for social interaction and may help promote development of independence and a positive body image.[3] Some children (sinkers and nonswimmers) may need flotation assistance for safety and stability during aquatic exercise, depending on their height and the depth of the water. Be careful when using water wings because the buoyancy is lost if the child's shoulder musculature fatigues.[2]

- If the pool is too deep for a child to touch the bottom, a submerged table or step can be used to adjust water depth for appropriate levels for exercise. Alternatively, the child could stand on the thighs of the clinician, who stands in a partially squatted position.[2]

- Aquatic therapy can be used for both rehabilitation and general exercise for pediatric patients who have a variety of diagnoses, including cerebral palsy, spina bifida, traumatic brain injury, Waardenburg's syndrome,[1] and orthopaedic dysfunction.[3] It is an excellent choice for children with juvenile rheumatoid arthritis for treatment of both strength and flexibility impairments.[4,5] Water is also an excellent medium for general exercise in this same population because joints are supported, compressed, and protected. Aquatic exercise has been described as an appropriate and safe intervention for children with osteogenesis imperfecta.

- Be sure to monitor water temperature when children are participating in aquatic exercise. Extremes of temperature may be difficult for children to manage due to their less efficient thermoregulatory systems.

- All children participating in aquatic exercise must be carefully supervised by a qualified individual. Most aquatic therapy for children is one on one rather than in groups. Poolside charts and pictures help children remember the motions of the exercises.[2] Aquatic exercise may begin as early as 6 months of age to facilitate weight bearing and supported and assisted active exercise.[4]

1. Duval R, Roberts P. Aquatic exercise therapy: the effects on an adolescent with Waardenburg's syndrome. *Phys Ther Case Rep.* 1999;2:77–82.

2. Styer-Acevedo JL. Aquatic rehabilitation of the pediatric client. In: Ruoti R, Morris P, Cole A, eds. *Aquatic rehabilitation.* Philadelphia: JB Lippincott Co; 1997:151–172.

3. Campion M. *Hydrotherapy in pediatrics.* Gaithersburg, MD: Aspen Systems; 1985.

4. Campbell SK. *Pediatric physical therapy.* 3rd ed. Philadelphia: WB Saunders; 2005.

5. Wright FV, Smith E. Physical therapy management of the child and adolescent with juvenile rheumatoid arthritis. In: Walker JM, Helewa A, eds. *Physical therapy in arthritis.* Philadelphia: WB Saunders, 1996:211–244.

References

1. Irion JM. Historical overview of aquatic rehabilitation. In: Ruoti R, Morris P, Cole A, eds. *Aquatic rehabilitation*. Philadelphia: JB Lippincott Co; 1997:3–14.

2. Wilson JD, Buffa AJ, eds. *College physics*. 5th ed. Englewood Cliffs, NJ: Prentice Hall; 2002.

3. Haralson K. Therapeutic pool programs. *Clin Manage*. 1986;5: 10–17.

4. Becker BE. Aquatic physics. In: Ruoti R, Morris P, Cole A, eds. *Aquatic rehabilitation*. Philadelphia: JB Lippincott Co; 1997:15–23.

5. Bloomfield J, Fricker P, Fitch K. *Textbook of science and medicine in sport*. Champaign, IL: Human Kinetics; 1992.

6. Skinner AR, Thomson AM. *Duffield's exercise in water*. 3rd ed. Philadelphia: Bailliere Tindall; 1989:4–46.

7. Harrison R, Bulstrode S. Percentage weight bearing during partial immersion in the hydrotherapy pool. *Physiother Pract*. 1987;3:60–63.

8. Harrison RA, Hillman M, Bulstrode S. Loading of the lower limb when walking partially immersed: implications for clinical practice. *Physiotherapy*. 1992;78:164–166.

9. Becker BE. Biophysiologic aspects of hydrotherapy. In: Becker BE, Cole AJ, eds. *Comprehensive aquatic therapy*. Boston: Butterworth-Heinemann; 2003:17–48.

10. Genuario SE, Vegso J. The use of a swimming pool in the rehabilitation and reconditioning of athletic injuries. *Contemp Orthop*. 1990;20:81–397.

11. Butts NK, Tucker M, Smith R. Maximal responses to treadmill and deep water running in high school female cross country runners. *Res Q Exerc Sport*. 1990;62:236–239.

12. Christie JL, Sheldahl LM, Tristani FE, et al. Cardiovascular regulation during head-out water immersion exercise. *J Appl Physiol*. 1990;69:657–664.

13. Frangolias DD, Rhodes EC. Metabolic responses and mechanisms during water immersion running and exercise. *Sports Med*. 1996;1:38–53.

14. Ritchie SE, Hopkins WG. The intensity of exercise in deep water running. *Int J Sports Med*. 1991;12:27–29.

15. Wilder RP, Brennan DK. Physiological responses to deep water running in athletes. *Sports Med*. 1993;16:374–380.

16. Cole AJ, Moschetti M, Eagleston TA, et al. Spine pain: aquatic rehabilitation strategies. In: Becker BE, Cole AJ, eds. *Comprehensive aquatic therapy*. 2nd ed. Boston: Butterworth-Heinemann; 2003:73–101.

17. Cirullo JA. Considerations for pool programming and implementation. In: Cirullo JA, ed. *Orthopaedic physical therapy clinics of North America*. Philadelphia: WB Saunders; 1994: 95–110.

18. Cureton KJ. Physiologic responses to water exercise. In: Ruoti R, Morris P, Cole A, eds. *Aquatic rehabilitation*. Philadelphia: JB Lippincott Co; 1997:39–56.

19. Choukroun ML, Varene P. Adjustments in oxygen transport during head-out immersion in water at different temperatures. *J Appl Physiol*. 1990;68:1475–1480.

20. Thein JM, Brody LT. Aquatic-based rehabilitation and training for the elite athlete. *J Orthop Sports Phys Ther*. 1998;27: 32–41.

21. Sheldahl EM, Buskirk ER, Loomis JL, et al. Effects of exercise in cool water on body weight loss. *Int J Obes*. 1982;6:29–42.

22. Cole AJ, Eagleston RE, Moschetti M, et al. Spine pain: aquatic rehabilitation strategies. *J Back Musculoskel Rehabil*. 1994;4:273–286.

23. Thein L, McNamara C. Aquatic rehabilitation of patients with musculoskeletal conditions of the extremities. In: Ruoti R, Morris P, Cole A, eds. *Aquatic rehabilitation*. Philadelphia: JB Lippincott Co; 1997:59–83.

24. Babb R, Simelson-Warr A. Manual techniques of the lower extremities in aquatic physical therapy. *J Aquatic Phys Ther*. 1996;4:9–15.

25. Schrepfer RW, Babb RW. Manual techniques of the shoulder in aquatic physical therapy. *J Aquatic Phys Ther*. 1998;6: 11–15.

26. Cirullo JA. Aquatic physical therapy approaches for the spine. In: Cirullo JA, ed. *Orthopaedic physical therapy clinics of North America*. Philadelphia: WB Saunders, 1994:179–208.

27. Mickel C, Shepherd J. Towards the localization of the lumbar postero-antero mobilization technique in water in the treatment of low back pain: a clinical note. *Man Ther*. 1998: 162–163.

28. Bandy WD, Irion JM. The effect of time on static stretch on the flexibility of the hamstring muscles. *Phys Ther*. 1994;74: 845–849.

29. McNamara CA. Aquatic spinal stabilization exercises. *J Aquatic Phys Ther*. 1997;5:11–17.

30. Cercone K. Dynamic aquatic therapy for the low back. *Aquatic Phys Ther Rep*. 1995;4:6–10.

31. Konlian C. Aquatic therapy: making a wave in the treatment of low back injuries. *Orthop Nurs*. 1999;18:11–20.

32. Saal J. Nonoperative treatment of herniated lumbar intervertebral disc with radiculopathy. *Spine*. 1989;14:431–437.

33. Venes D, ed. *Taber's cyclopedic medical dictionary*. 20th ed. Philadelphia: FA Davis Co; 2005.

34. Chu D. *Jumping into plyometrics*. Champaign, IL: Leisure; 1992.

35. Coyle EF, Hemmert MK, Coggan AR. Effects of detraining on cardiovascular responses to exercise: role of blood volume. *J Appl Physiol*. 1986;60:95–99.

36. Coyle EF, Martin WH, Simacore DR, et al. Time course of loss of adaptations after stopping prolonged intense endurance training. *J Appl Physiol*. 1984;57:1857–1864.

37. Eyestone ED, Fellingham G, George J, et al. Effect of water running and cycling on maximum oxygen consumption and 2 mile run performance. *Am J Sports Med*. 1993;21:41–44.

38. Bushman BA, Flynn MG, Andres FF, et al. Effect of four week deep water run training on running performance. *Med Sci Sports Exerc*. 1997;29:694–699.

39. Wilber RL, Moffatt RJ, Scott BE, et al. Influence of water run training on the maintenance of aerobic performance. *Med Sci Sports Exerc*. 1996;28:1056–1062.

40. Quinn TJ, Sedory DR, Fisher BS. Physiological effects of deep water running following a land based training program. *Res Q Exerc Sports.* 1994;65:386–389.

41. Frangolias DD, Rhodes EC. Maximum and ventilatory threshold responses to treadmill and water immersion running. *Med Sci Sports Exerc.* 1995;27:1007–1013.

42. Michaud TJ, Brennan DK, Wilder RP. Aquarunning and gains in cardiorespiratory fitness. *Strength Cond Res.* 1995;9:78–84.

43. Bushman B. Athletes propel deep water running to prominence. *Biomechanics.* 1999;32:43–49.

44. Wilder RP, Brennan DK. Techniques of water running. In: Becker BE, Cole AJ, eds. *Comprehensive aquatic therapy.* 2nd ed. Boston: Butterworth-Heinemann; 2003:123–134.

45. Wilder RP, Brennan DK, Schotte DE. A standard measure for exercise prescription for aqua running. *Am J Sports Med.* 1993; 21:45–48.

46. Stephens-Bogard K. A dip in the pool. *Adv Directors Rehabil.* 1999;8:37–40.

47. American Physical Therapy Association. *Guide to physical therapist practice.* 2nd ed. Alexandria, VA; 2003.

CHAPTER 17

Principles of Contextual Fitness and Function for Older Adults

Reta J. Zabel, PT, PhD, GCS

OBJECTIVES

Upon completion of this chapter, the reader will be able to:

- Define the terms contextual fitness and contextual function.

- Describe the importance of training in a "real" environment such as the home, community, and work place.

- Relate the elements of fitness to the requirements of function in a given environment.

- Describe how contextual fitness impacts performance capacity.

- Apply an established plan of care to improve contextual fitness and function.

SCIENTIFIC BASIS

Physical Consideration of Function

Data from the MacArthur Studies of Successful Aging provided researchers with a means for defining important factors impacting functional changes with age.[1] The studies involved community-dwelling older individuals that were assessed on physical and cognitive capabilities, overall health status, and social, lifestyle, and psychologic characteristics from 1988/1989 to 1995/1996. Seeman and Chen[2] examined data from the MacArthur Studies to determine risk and protective factors associated with physical functioning in individuals with reported chronic diseases (hypertension, diabetes, cardiovascular disease, cancer, or fractures) and in individuals reporting no chronic disease. The researchers concluded that levels of functioning among older adults with chronic disease is dependent on disease-related health status and influenced by potentially modifiable factors such as physical exercise. Further, the researchers supported the concept that regular physical activity in adults is an appropriate means of promoting higher levels of physical functioning. Rockwood et al[3] reported data from the Canadian Study of Health and Aging defining fitness and frailty in terms of self-reported exercise and functional level. The data suggested that fitness and frailty are on opposite ends of a continuum and are predictive of survival. Through extrapolation of the results, the investigators conceptualized that if fitness was the opposite of frailty and was predictive of survival, then improving fitness through exercise influences survival (Fig. 17-1).

The relationship between functional fitness and risk factors associated with coronary heart disease in older Japanese women was examined using multiple variables.[4] Functional fitness was determined using a test battery including arm curls, walking around obstacles, side-to-side stepping, one-leg balance with eyes closed, and functional reach. Risk factors for coronary disease consisted of systolic blood pressure, total and low-density lipoprotein cholesterol, abdominal girth, oxygen uptake, heart rate, forced expiratory volume, and hematocrit. The results of the study appeared to indicate that both functional fitness and coronary function are predictive and should be clinically valued as important to the evaluation of health and functional status in the sample of older adults.

Environmental Consideration of Function

Skills involved with daily function may be divided into basic living skills (activities of daily living [ADL]) and higher-level living skills (instrumental activities of daily living [IADL]).[5,6] Performance of the majority of these skills requires that the individual demonstrate some level

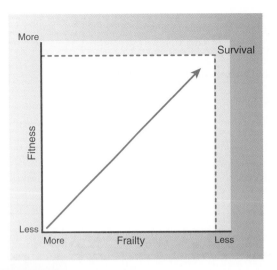

Figure 17-1 Conceptual diagram of inverse relationship between frailty and fitness. Diagram demonstrates that increases in fitness result in a decrease in frailty and therefore improvement in survival.

of mobility. Clinically, intervention strategies are developed to promote independent performance of ADL and/or IADL, and the outcome goals usually assess the level of mobility disability. However, intervention programs are likely to be short term and generally take place in a therapist-controlled setting. To function in a "real" world, the individual must be able to adapt to the demands of a continually changing environment. Several researchers have reported that the community environment is multidimensional, requiring the individual to manage a variety of special circumstances to remain safe and functional.[7–11]

In a study involving older adults with and without impaired mobility, Shumway-Cook et al[11] identified eight environmental factors that are likely to present obstacles for individuals in the community. The environmental factors were temporal (time to cross the street in the time allotted by a traffic light), physical load (carried items), terrain (stairs, curbs, slopes, and uneven surfaces), postural transition (starting/stopping, changing direction, and reaching), distance, collision avoidance (anticipate and/or compensate for disturbances and clutter in mobility path), ambient conditions (light level [bright/dim, natural/artificial] and weather conditions [rain, ice, or snow]), and attentional demands (walking and performing other cognitive or physical tasks). The researchers proposed that these factors represent the external demands that have to be met for the individual to be independent and functionally mobile in a specific environment. Further, they concluded that intervention programs should train individuals to more effec-

Shumway-Cook A, Patla AE, Stewart A, et al. Environmental demands associated with community mobility in older adults with and without mobility disabilities. *Phys Ther.* 2002;82:670–681.

TABLE 17-1	Types of Environmental Factors and Examples of Functional Tasks Impacted by the Factors
Type of Environmental Factor	*Example*
Temporal	Crossing a busy street
Terrain	Ascending and descending stairs or slopes
Loads	Carrying a bag of groceries or a child
Transitions	Starting/stopping during shopping
Distance	Walking from parking lot to door
Avoidance	Stepping around a wet floor sign in floor
Lighting	Getting up at night to use bathroom
Weather	Walking on snow-covered sidewalk
Attentional	Filling in blanks of a familiar song (e.g., *Twinkle, Twinkle Star*)

tively manage the environmental challenges inherent in the community (Table 17-1).

Contextual Fitness

The capacity to manage the physical demands of the environment without fatigue has been defined by Rikli and Jones[12] as "functional fitness." Functional fitness includes components of physical endurance, strength, balance, and flexibility sufficient to complete the activities necessary to remain independent in the community. However, the patient/client population is heterogenous in that each will have individual functional fitness needs and unique environmental demands. Consequently, intervention programs should address not only the physical components of functional fitness but also the environmental demands within the specific context of the patient/client needs. Functional fitness in terms of the performance environment may be described as "contextual fitness." Contextual fitness supports performance of meaningful tasks in an environment of importance. The meaningful tasks are typically identified by the individual or the individual's caregivers or family members as an area of training need. The context of the task is determined by elements in the performance environment. Elements in the performance environment should include community, home, and work

factors. Consideration should be given to the type of home (apartment, single floor vs multilevel structure), the setting of the home (urban vs rural), layout of the home and frequented community buildings (width of the doors, height of the countertops), and clutter (animals, toys) in planning contextual fitness training.

In summary, contextual tasks are activities that are considered meaningful and important to the patient/client and his/her family or caregivers and that take place in or close to the contextual environment. The ability to perform functional tasks like walking, preparing and consuming food, communicating with family and friends, and being productive in the home and workplace is vital to independent survival. Task-related functional movement has been suggested to be the result the interaction of three variables: the individual, the task, and the environment.[7] Therefore, successful completion of a specific task in the contextual environment is simultaneously dependent on the components of the task and factors in the contextual environment (Fig. 17-2). Intervention then should address the functional capacity, or the contextual fitness, of the patient/client to meet the demands of the interacting specific task and the environment in which the task occurs.

Contextual Function

The term function has been used widely by rehabilitation professionals since Lawton[13] included the term to define assessment. He proposed that functional assessment is "any

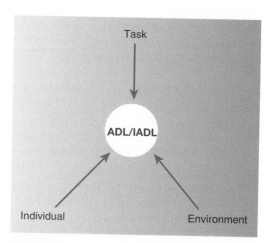

Figure 17-2   Variables impacting performance of activities of daily living and instrumental activities of daily living. Intrinsic variables associated with the individual interacting with extrinsic variables of the task and the contextual environment impact the ability of the individual to be functionally independent.

systematic attempt to measure objectively the level at which the person is functioning".[13] In more current work, Harris et al[14] discussed function from the perspective of specific tasks of ADL that were contextually, i.e., environmentally, required for the individual to be independent. The authors divided ADL into five components: walking in the home, bed to chair transfers, getting on and off the toilet, putting on and taking off shoes, and putting on and taking off socks.

Dittmar and Gresham[15] conceptualized function as a person's ability to perform ADL and IADL within his or her home, institution, or community environment. Nagi[16] first proposed that disability, or an inability to perform actions, tasks, or activities, should be defined in the context of sociocultural and physical environment. Nagi's model of "disablement" provided a classification schema with which physical therapists (PT) could organize the problems and deficits noted in patients. The Nagi model demonstrated graphically that a relationship existed among loss of physiologic function (impairments), activity deficits (functional limitations), and restrictions in function (disabilities). In 1980 the World Health Organization (WHO) developed an alternative model of disablement which used the terms of impairment, disability, and handicap.[17] However, neither model fully described the interaction of the environment on the individual's inability to function. In 2001 the WHO revised the earlier model of disablement, releasing the new version as the International Classification of Functioning, Disability, and Health (ICF) model.[18] The ICF model places more focus on the interaction of the individual, the task, and the environment related to specificity of function. In this model, impairments (decreased strength, range of motion [ROM], and endurance) are referred to as body structure and function; functional limitations (taking an object off the shelf or getting out of bed) are activity limitations; and disability (inability to perform usual roles) is described as a participation restriction. Use of such terms as activity and participation implies function within a specific context. "Contextual function" then is defined as function performed within a meaningful context or environment.

Importance of Contextual Fitness to Contextual Function

The concept of function may be defined as a person's ability to physically perform activities needed in the home, community, or institution; to understand and plan basic and higher-level tasks within the context of the specific environment; and to participate in society.[15] Fitness, as described previously, is the capacity to physically perform and participate with the least restriction.[12] A general review of the literature supports that fitness and levels of function are significantly related in that higher fitness levels have a protective effect against functional limitations in

middle-aged to older men and women.[19–25] As discussed in Chapter 10, higher levels of fitness are also related to improved psychologic function and quality of life. The physiologic capacity for older adults to manage the environmental demands also plays a role in functional limitations and disability and therefore their ability to remain independent. Lifestyle-based activities such as walking the dog, doing housework, or taking up an active hobby have been proposed as appropriate means to potentially improve contextual fitness and consequently contextual function.[15]

CLINICAL GUIDELINES

Assessment of Contextual Fitness

Contextual, or functional, fitness has been examined using a variety of impairment-based tools; however, two tools have been given the most focus in the literature.[26–30] The first tool is the Senior Fitness Test (SFT) proposed by Rikli and Jones.[12] This test consists of six different components of fitness that the developers identified as relevant to function: *chair stand* to assess lower-body strength, *arm curls* to assess upper-body strength, *2-minute step test* to assess aerobic endurance, *chair sit and reach* to assess lower-body flexibility, *back scratch* to assess upper-body flexibility, and *8-foot up and go* to assess agility and balance during movement. Normative values for each of the components have been published for men and women ages 60 to 94 years.[31] Although more research is required to confirm the connection, the SFT has been found to be predictive of disease and independence in community-dwelling adults.[32]

A second useful fitness test, the Groningen Fitness Test for the Elderly (GFE), is comprised of eight components for examination of fitness: *block transfer* to assess manual dexterity, *button push on cue* to assess reaction time, *balance board* to assess equilibrium, *grip strength* to assess maximum isometric strength of hands and arms, *right leg extension strength* to assess maximum isometric strength of the leg, *sit and reach test* to assess hamstrings and lower back flexibility, *circumduction test* as an indicator of shoulder flexibility, and *staged walking test* to assess aerobic endurance (an important indicator of cardiovascular fitness). The GFE has been found to have satisfactory reliability; however, the grip strength and block transfer tests were found to change over repeated testing.[30]

In comparing the two tests for clinical usefulness and relationship to function, the SFT appears to be more closely associated with fitness required for function in the environment, whereas the GFE selectively tests the basic motor abilities—strength, endurance, and coordination—with less consideration of context or environment. Therefore, the SFT appears more suitable than the GFE for field testing of contextual fitness. In addition, the SFT requires a minimum of specialized equipment using common, inexpensive, and easily obtained testing tools. The PT and physical therapist assistant (PTA) should find the SFT normative values published by Rikli and Jones[31] useful in determination of level of contextual fitness and need for intervention within a specific environment. The test items on both the SFT and GFE present a framework for development of a treatment plan focused on contextual fitness and functional improvement.

Training Contextual Fitness

The concept of contextual fitness necessitates that a certain level of consideration be given to requirements of functional movement and to the theoretic elements of fitness. The requirements of functional movement are stability, mobility, and adaptation.[7] The elements of fitness related to function are more physiologically-based—core strength endurance, power, agility, balance, flexibility, cardiovascular endurance, and coordination.

Requirements of Functional Movement

Stability is based on the provision of support and a diminished potential for movement. For example, the stance limb during single-limb standing is considered to have more stability than the swing limb, as a diminished potential for movement exists.[7,33] In contrast, mobility is based on motion and potential for motion.[7,33] The swing limb during gait is considered to have more mobility than the stance limb as the swing limb is in motion and has more potential for movement. Conceptually, adaptation is the ability to "grade" or alter the state of stability or mobility in response to changes in the task or environmental demands. Biomechanically, mobility requires a foundation of stability such that when one part of the body has more mobility to meet the demands, an adjacent part of the body will demonstrate more stability. Essentially, a foundation of stability with superimposed mobility in response to demands of a task within a given context is adaptation.

Elements of Fitness Related to Function

Contextual fitness requires that certain elements or components of function be present. These elements are core strength endurance, power, agility, balance, flexibility, cardiovascular endurance, and coordination.[34,35] Core strength endurance is evidenced by the ability of the postural muscles (abdominals and back extensors) to perform and maintain a tonic or holding contraction sufficient to keep the trunk upright against a force that is externally-applied (e.g., gravity). Power is demonstrated in the ability to perform rapid, strong, or phasic muscle contractions (i.e., to change the rate of work) to adapt to anticipated or unanticipated changes in the environment. The idea of agility, which may be thought of as the ability to perform side-to-side or turning-type movements in a timely manner to avoid a collision or to sidestep an obstacle in the movement path,[34] is not often considered in training of older adults for fitness but is functionally important for safety in the contextual environment. Agility may also require the ability to combine speed and coordination for movement.[12] Balance has been defined as the ability to maintain the center of gravity over the base of support involving efficient coordination among multiple sensory, biomechanical, and motor systems.[7] Flexibility is the ability to move joints through a ROM sufficient to accomplish the intended task without being impeded by soft tissue extensibility and is therefore relative to the demands of the task.[36] As previously indicated, cardiovascular endurance is the ability to effectively extract and use oxygen and efficiently remove waste products. Finally, although not of less importance, coordination is the ability to integrate the multiple components that are involved in consistent performance of functional tasks.[37]

Prior to prescribing an exercise program to improve contextual fitness, the PT should perform a standard physical therapy examination for determination of the patient's/client's overall health status; presence of pain; available ROM; any deficits associated with the neuromuscular, musculoskeletal, cardiopulmonary, or integumentary system; and examination of the elements of fitness. Once the PT develops the plan of care, the PT and PTA can work as a clinical team to implement the plan.

TECHNIQUES

Core Strength Endurance

The core muscles of focus in this chapter for improving strength and endurance are the abdominals and the back extensors. The activities occurring around the core (trunk) are back extension and flexion, side bending, rotation, and counter-rotation. In development of a treatment program to promote core strength endurance, the PT must consider the patient's needs or the amount of stress applied to the core muscles in performance of ADL.[34] By understanding the daily strength and endurance requirements of the trunk, the PT can begin the program at a level appropriate to adequately stress and therefore change the strength of the core muscles.[34] Likewise, the PTA should understand the ADL needs of the patient and the initial starting level to more effectively recognize the need for progression.

Contextual Training for Core Strength Endurance

To train the core most effectively, the specific adaptations to imposed demands (SAID) principles presented in Chapter 15 should be followed for a given functional activity. Given the myriad of functional activities required for independence, the PT and PTA should be familiar with the concept of task and subtask analysis to recognize the stability and mobility demands for a specific task.[7] In addition, prior to training within the context of function, the patient/client should perform more traditional trunk strengthening (i.e., more general strengthening preceding more specific training). Strengthening has been found to be significantly related to performance of contextual activities especially if the activities involve sufficient repetitions and loads beyond gravity.[38,39]

For ease of identifying appropriate activities to improve core strength endurance, trunk movements are divided into upper-trunk–initiated movements and lower-trunk–initiated movements.[40] Upper-trunk–initiated movements are reaching forward and upward to comb one's hair, reaching down to retrieve an object from the floor, and reaching behind to put the arm in a sleeve. Lower-body–initiated movements involve pelvic tilting forward, which results in trunk extension, and pelvic tilting backward, which results in trunk flexion. Functionally the upper body and lower body interact and are biomechanically complementary, i.e., even though the upper body initiates upward reach, the lower body follows through to extend the trunk and effectively increase the overall reach distance.[40] Examples of training core strength endurance in unsupported sitting and standing are shown in Figures 17-3 and 17-4.

Power

From a functional point of view, power is the relationship of the functional activity and time or rate of the functional performance. For example, when an individual is crossing a busy street and the cautionary signal begins to flash, the functional activity is walking and the rate of the functional performance is the walking speed; however, in this example, a rapid increase in walking speed (a rapid change in the rate of the functional performance) is required to avoid being caught in the middle of the street when the light turns green. This rapid acceleration is related to power. The SAID principle and the requirements of movement also apply here in the determination of patient-specific contextual task needs.

Contextual Training for Power

In general, activities that require rapid changes in speed as in stop/start tasks with varied task and environmental demands influence power. The activities should begin at a self-selected rate and then proceed to introduction of rapid alterations in speed. Examples of training power are walking at different speeds over grass, bark, and sand; training may be progressed by adding a load (a shoulder purse or a bag of groceries). Figure 17-5 provides an example of an activity to improve contextual power.

Agility

Agility is important functionally to sidestep and turn for collision avoidance or to manage an obstacle in the path. According to Shumway-Cook et al,[11] changing direction and anticipating or compensating for disturbances and clutter in the environment presents significant obstacles for individuals in the community. Much research has been performed on the role of obstacle management in predicting individuals who are at a greater risk of falling in the home or community.[11,41] Additionally, agility is important in performance of activities such as getting off a bus in a controlled and timely manner, going to the bathroom, or getting up to answer the telephone.[12]

Contextual Training for Agility

For a patient with a goal of independence and community participation, activities should include elements of side-to-side stepping and turning.[11] One of the tests included in the SFT is an *8-foot walk* in which the patient/client is timed as he/she rises from a chair, walks 8 feet, turns, and returns to sit in the chair.[12] If combined with obstacles or clutter in the walking path, the *8-foot walk* becomes an appropriate contextual training intervention. The path may also be varied depending on the individual needs; for example, the walk may be completed on a tiled floor and then on a carpeted floor. Community-based contextual training of agility may take place in a local supermarket at a busy time of day incorporating management of the grocery cart with walking and requiring the patient/client to sidestep to retrieve items from high and low shelves (Fig. 17-6).

Balance

Effective balance is reflected in the ability to maintain the body's center of gravity over the base of support and within the limits of stability.[7,34] Generally during functional activities the base of support is continually changing from larger to smaller as the body transitions or moves from a sitting position to standing and from standing to walking or stepping. As described in Chapter 10, balance is divided into static (or holding) and dynamic (or moving) balance. Static balance is demonstrated in the ability of the patient/client to maintain an upright position with respect to the base of support. Dynamic balance is demonstrated in the ability of the patient/client to stay upright when the base of support is changing or a displacement of the center of gravity oc-

Figure 17-3   Upper-trunk–initiated exercise.

PURPOSE: Train abdominal muscles and back extensors to improve strength and endurance for reaching up to comb hair or down to manage clothing.

POSITION: Sitting forward on sturdy chair with back unsupported and trunk in upright posture. Knees and hips are flexed to 90 degrees and feet are flat on floor. Patient is given 1-pound dumbbell (for women) or 2-pound dumbbell (for men) to hold in the right hand. Hands are placed in pronated position resting on thighs **(A)**.

PROCEDURE: Using the right arm, the patient lifts the weight up and behind the head, anteriorly tilting the pelvis and moving the lower trunk toward extension. The weight is moved down and behind the back, moving the pelvis anteriorly and extending the lower trunk **(B)**. The patient switches the weight to the left hand and repeats exercise.

NOTE: Progressively increase to 5-pound dumbbell for women and 8-pound dumbbell for men.

curs. Balance is multifactorial,[41] and the PT should identify as many of the factors as possible in development of an effective program. The PTA should be aware of the many factors impacting balance and the level of fall risk prior to intervening for contextual balance.

Contextual Training for Balance

Balance activities should incorporate both static and dynamic balance demands on varied surfaces as well as activities in different levels of lighting. Balance activities may be progressed by including an attentional demand, for example, walking and talking.[7,11,42] Safety should always be a concern in training contextual balance as the activities are directed toward challenging the patient/client by increasing the performance demands; therefore, the PT and PTA should be prepared to prevent a fall or injury. Examples of contextual training for balance are the maintenance of upright posture while standing on a block of foam or soft mat,[40] maintenance of upright posture while standing on

A   B

| Figure 17-4 | Lower-trunk–initiated exercise. |

PURPOSE: Train abdominals and back extensor muscles to improve strength and endurance for performance of functional tasks against gravity.

POSITION: Sitting forward on sturdy chair with back unsupported and trunk in upright posture. Knees and hips are flexed to 90 degrees and feet are flat on floor. Hands are placed in pronated position resting on thighs.

PROCEDURE: A 1-pound dumbbell (for women) or 2-pound dumbbell (for men) is placed on floor to front and side of patient's right foot. Patient leans forward by bending at hips to reach with left hand toward floor to retrieve barbell **(A)** and place it in lap **(B)**. Patient picks up dumbbell with right hand and places it on floor to front and side of left foot.

NOTE: Progressively increase to 5-pound dumbbell for women and 8-pound dumbbell for men.

| Figure 17-5 | Contextual power exercises with components of function and time. |

PURPOSE: Train rapid acceleration and deceleration activities in challenging environments.

POSITION: Standing at one end of tiled, well-lit hallway at least 25 feet in length. Physical therapist assistant (PTA) standing behind and to the side.

PROCEDURE: Patient is told to "walk forward at rapid pace and stop or start when instructed to do so." The patient progresses forward, and the PTA randomly instructs him/her to stop or start during the 25-foot walk. The patient repeats walk in same way but with a simulated bag of groceries.

Figure 17-6 Agility with 8-foot walk and obstacles in path

PURPOSE: Train agility for sidestepping and turning for avoidance of obstacles.

POSITION: Standing holding on to grocery cart.

PROCEDURE: Patient propels cart through and around obstacle marker cones to retrieve different size and weight objects from table, cabinet, and floor **(A–C)**.

foam and rotating to look over the shoulder, walking on a soft surface in a dimly lit hallway, management of obstacles in a simulated "real" environment,[43] and walking and performing a simple cognitive task (a math calculation or completing a sentence).[44] Examples of activities that incorporate static and dynamic balance in contextual training are depicted in Figures 17-7 and 17-8.

Flexibility

Many intrinsic and extrinsic factors affect the amount of flexibility available for performance of ADL. As presented in Chapter 3, the intrinsic factors are related to the anatomic structure of the joint and the soft tissue surrounding the joint. Extrinsic factors are more related to potential constraints or limitations placed on the joint by factors external to the joint. For example, shortening and stiffening of the muscles acting on the joint can affect the amount of range or flexibility (intrinsic factors). Likewise, factors in the environment may affect the amount of range at a joint (extrinsic factors). An example would be long periods of sitting in a soft chair (recliner) with hips flexed and knees extended. The softness of the chair results in internal rotation at the hip as the individual sinks into the surface, shortening of the quadriceps as the knees are extended, and the ankle and foot

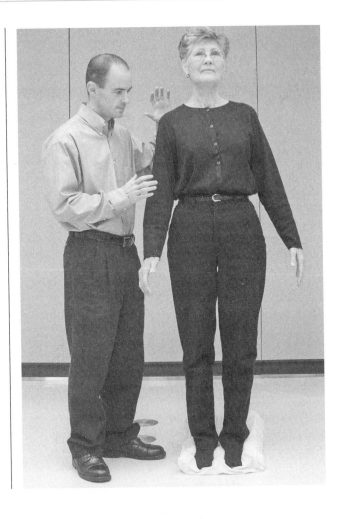

Figure 17-7   Challenging balance.

PURPOSE: Train balance reactions by challenging stability.

POSITION: Standing on 24 inch by 24 inch block of dense foam with shoes off. Physical therapist assistant (PTA) is standing, without touching patient, behind and to the side of patient.

PROCEDURE: Patient is instructed to step up onto square of foam with PTA providing support until patient appears stable. Patient is instructed to hold the stable position for 2 minutes.

moving toward supination. The eventual outcome is a combination of intrinsic and extrinsic factors limiting range and flexibility of the hip, knee, and ankle. The muscles around the hip joint may develop adaptive shortening or stretch weakness related to the prolonged positioning.[45] Therefore, to functionally improve flexibility, the flexibility of the joint (joint range) must be addressed as well as the flexibility of the surrounding contractile tissues (muscle range).[34,46] In addition, the flexibility requirements of the task and the environment or context should be fully analyzed prior to initiating a training program.

Contextual Training for Flexibility

To be most effective, the activities should address both joint and muscle range as well as consider the extrinsic factors associated with the environmental context. Placing one foot on a 6-inch step and shifting the weight forward over the limb to lengthen hip flexors and ankle plantarflexors and gain range in hip extension and ankle dorsiflexion of the forward limb is one activity to enhance flexibility (Fig. 17-9). A progression of this activity would be an increase in the height of the step.

A second activity is based on the SFT chair sit to reach test.[12] The patient/client sits on a firm surface chair with one knee positioned at approximately 45 degrees of flexion and both hands placed over the forward knee keeping the trunk aligned and pelvis at neutral (Fig. 17-10). The patient/client pushes slowly down on the knee as the foot slides further out. This activity is useful in increasing range at the joints and muscles involved in elbow, wrist, and finger extension and at the joints and muscles surrounding the hip and knee for extension.

A third activity intended to address hip adductor tightness and the hip external rotation range uses the patient/client home environment. The patient/client stands facing a counter or table that allows the hands to be in a resting position on the surface with the trunk upright and aligned over the feet. The toes should be pointing forward or slightly angled outward (based on the comfort of the patient). The patient/client keeps one foot planted and moves the other in a backward circumduction pattern as if rotating the body to place an object behind and to the side (Fig. 17-11).

Each of these activities can be progressed by changing the contextual demands: altering the sitting or standing surface from firm (tile) to soft (carpet) to unstable (foam);

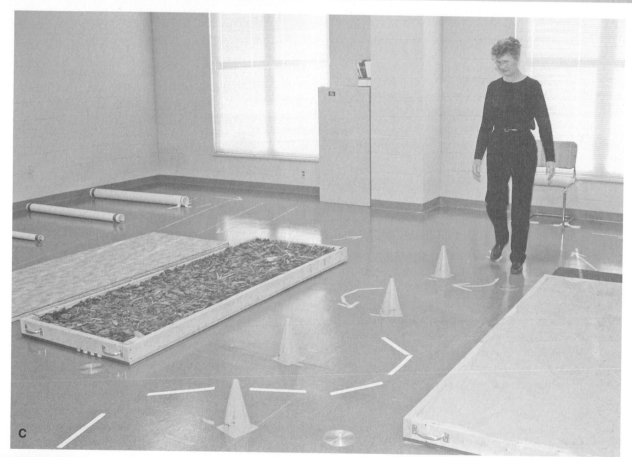

Figure 17-8 Modified obstacle course.[43]

PURPOSE: Train management of environmental obstacles using "simulated" obstacle course.

POSITION: Walking at self-selected pace through course beginning on low carpet surface. Physical therapist assistant is standing, without touching patient, behind and to the side of patient.

PROCEDURE: The clinician times patient walking through course using standard stopwatch (baseline and interval measures may be documented for comparison). The patient begins at low carpet and proceeds over different size obstacles **(A)**, high carpet, through pine bark **(B)**, sit and rise from standard chair, around cones **(C)**, through sand **(D)**, ascend and descend steps **(E)**, and up and down incline **(F)**.

Figure 17-8 Modified obstacle course.[43] *(continued)*

increasing the stretch over multiple joints (sit to reach to touch toes of outstretched limb); stepping in a circle using altering circumduction movements first in one direction and then in the other direction.

Cardiovascular Endurance

Cardiovascular endurance involves the ability of the system to perform work for a functionally sufficient amount of time. Different tasks will have different levels of cardiovascular demand, and that demand is heavily influenced by the context in which the task is performed. For example, walking across a four-lane street requires more cardiovas-

cular endurance than walking across a two-lane street. In this example, the task is similar, but the context places more demands on the cardiovascular system. If an additional contextual component like heavy traffic and a short time to cross the four-lane street is added, an even greater demand exists in the task. The most common functional activity requiring sufficient cardiovascular endurance is walking in the home and community.

Contextual Training for Cardiovascular Endurance

According to the SAID principle (Chapter 15) of training, cardiovascular endurance in walking should include the task of walking. Therefore, a progressive walking program

| Figure 17-9 | Sitting hamstring stretch. |

PURPOSE: Increase flexibility in hamstring muscles to support ease of movement in bathing and dressing.

POSITION: Sitting in sturdy chair. Patient's hips and knees of extremity not being stretched are flexed to 90 degrees and foot flat on floor. Heel of extremity being stretched is placed on stool. Hands are placed in pronated position resting on thighs.

PROCEDURE: Patient should maintain upright posture during the entire movement. Both of the hands are placed on the extended knee, and the knee is held in position while the toes are pointed toward the ceiling. Patient repeats the stretch on opposite leg.

| Figure 17-10 | Standing adductor flexibility exercise. |

PURPOSE: Stretch adductor muscles to improve rotational trunk and extremity flexibility for getting in and out of car or tub.

POSITION: Standing with one hand holding on to sturdy chair, table, or counter and the body at right angle to the surface **(A)**.

PROCEDURE: Patient's foot closest to support surface (chair) remains stable while other foot rotates out as far as patient can comfortably move. Patient's trunk rotates toward support surface **(B)**.

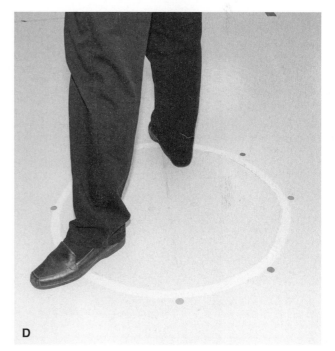

Figure 17-11   Adductor flexibility exercise with floor markers.

PURPOSE: Increase flexibility in adductor muscles to improve turning in small, constrained environments.

POSITION: Standing with upright posture and both feet directed forward in comfortable position **(A)**.

PROCEDURE: Markers (duct tape, masking tape, or sticky dots) to indicate circular pattern of foot placement. Patient moves right or left foot to place the foot on nearest marker to the right or left depending on the starting foot. Movement continues around circle until start position is attained **(B–D)**.

should be designed by the PT and implemented by the PTA. The program designed by the PT for the PTA should include alterations of the speed demands, the surface demands, the distance demands, with loads, and with management of obstacles in the environment. To improve compliance, the walking program may be incorporated into the patient's/client's lifestyle. For example, pushing and pulling a vacuum cleaner to complete housekeeping chores, taking stairs instead of the elevator, or joining a mall walking group.[12]

Coordination

Traditionally in therapeutic exercise, coordination has been defined as the ability to perform smooth, accurate, and controlled movements and having components of proper sequencing, timing, proximal stability, and balance.[37,46] However, from a broader perspective, coordination may also be thought of as the ability to bring all of the elements of function together, i.e., to integrate, manage, and synchronize strength, power, agility, balance, flexibil-

ity, and cardiovascular endurance to meet the contextual demands of a task. ADL and IADL require varied levels of elemental coordination depending on the complexity of the task and the context. In general, fine motor tasks like sewing or writing require more smooth, accurate, and controlled movements (the more traditional concept of coordination), whereas gross motor tasks like walking or running require more integration and organization of the varied elements of contextual fitness and function.

Contextual Training of Coordination

A program to train coordination should attempt to include as many of the elements of contextual fitness as possible in repeated and random succession in varied environments. The examples (Figs. 17-12 and 17-13) are simulated "real" housekeeping chores set up such that the patient/client is required to lift objects of varied weights from overhead and place them in a container on the floor; work faster and slower; perform side, diagonal, and backward steps; and turn in circle incrementally and back with trunk rotation

A   B

Figure 17-12 Retrieval and placement of varied objects.

PURPOSE: Improve coordination of extremity and trunk to remove objects from high or low shelves.

POSITION: Standing facing cabinet with varied objects on shelf at level that requires patient to reach up above shoulder level. Container is placed on floor to right or left of patient.

PROCEDURE: Patient reaches up and removes objects one at a time from shelf above shoulder level and places them in container on floor. Patient extends trunk to reach and flexes trunk to place objects in container **(A and B)**.

A   **B**

| Figure 17-13 | Physical therapy three-step exercise. |

PURPOSE: Improve coordination of lower extremities for walking and stepping over and around obstacles.

POSITION: Standing and holding sturdy chair or with hand on wall. Stepping foot is on the outside and is free to move.

PROCEDURE: Patient shifts weight to limb next to support surface and steps diagonal, backward, and to the side to touch tape markers on floor **(A and B)**. The trunk stays upright, and patient is instructed to increase speed as can be tolerated.

and lower-extremity circumduction steps (90 degrees from initial position, 180 degrees from initial position, and 360 degrees from initial position).

Precautions and Contraindications

Importance should be placed on the identification of the overall state of neuromuscular, musculoskeletal, cardiopulmonary, and integumentary health prior to initiation of activities directed toward improvement of contextual fitness. The examples presented in this chapter make the assumption that individual impairments impacting the movements and the functional performance–overall strength and ROM, joint stability, cognition, coordination, etc.–have been or are concurrently being addressed. The PTA should monitor the

patient's/client's body mechanics for appropriate alignment and to limit less efficient and potentially unsafe movements.

At no time should the activities cause pain or undue fatigue. If pain occurs, the PTA should contact the PT, who will then re-evaluate and make adjustments in the task or environmental demands to support pain-free performance; progress should then occur as the patient tolerates more activity. Most of the contextual activities described in this chapter require control of movement of the center of mass (position of the body's weight in relation to gravity) within and around a changing base of support, and therefore a higher level of fall risk is evident. The PTA must be aware of the increased risk and position himself/herself to prevent a fall. However, the patient/client should be free to move and experience some challenge to the system to progress to better performance.[8]

CASE STUDY

PATIENT INFORMATION

A 61-year-old woman presented with neuromuscular and musculoskeletal deficits associated with a hemorrhagic stroke 18 years ago. The initial interview with the patient revealed that she was involved in a motor vehicle accident (MVA) and that the stroke occurred while she was in the emergency room following the accident. The patient reported numerous musculoskeletal injuries associated with the MVA—fractures of both arms, severe whiplash, right patellar fracture, and multiple contusions and abrasions. All healed with minimal residual limitations. However, the subsequent stroke left her with right upper- and lower-extremity hemiplegia, balance, and coordination deficits. For the past year the patient had been taking part in an exercise group at her local church and had lost approximately 15 pounds. The patient indicated that she was getting married in 1 month and would like to feel more stable in walking over rough ground (her wedding was to be outdoors), develop more cardiovascular endurance to sustain activities during the long day of the wedding, increase core strength, and improve power to more readily adapt to possible changes in task demands. The patient indicated that she had become accustomed to certain patterns of movement. The patient was not currently on any prescribed medication and did not routinely take any over-the-counter medications or supplements; she was a nonsmoker and did not consume alcohol.

The physical examination performed by the PT revealed that the patient was 5 feet, 2 inches tall and weighed 115 pounds. Blood pressure was 130/80, and resting heart rate 66 beats per minute. No signs of shortness of breath were exhibited. The patient's active ROM on the left upper extremity was considered functionally normal but showed a loss of approximately 5 to 10 degrees overall; passively ROM was considered normal. The left lower extremity showed normal ranges actively and passively in both sitting and supine ranges. The patient's right upper extremity active and passive ROM was limited by dominance of flexor tone at the elbow, wrist, and fingers. The right lower extremity showed limitations of active range at the hip, knee, and foot secondary to hypotonia; passively knee extension was limited by 10 degrees. A manual muscle test[45] on the left revealed 4/5 grossly for the upper extremity, 5/5 quadriceps, 4/5 hamstrings, and ankle 5/5. Secondary to the tone changes, the Medical Research Council (MRC) scale of muscle[47] was used to rate the strength on the right with shoulder flexion and abduction, and elbow, wrist, and finger extension were all graded at 3/5. Similarly, the right lower extremity was tested using the MRC scale of muscle with all movements against gravity affected (grade 2–3). Functionally, the patient was independent and wore an orthotic on the right foot to prevent foot drop and assist with fatigue; however, when in crowded or cluttered environments, she frequently was assisted by someone supporting her on the left side after 30 minutes of walking. Walking speed was slowed with limited ability to alter her speed reactively. The patient tended to hyperextend the knee and move the right side of her pelvis back (retract) with stance on the right. The right arm was held in slight elbow flexion, internal rotation, and adduction during all activities.

This patient appeared to lack the fitness and functional ability to perform activities in different contexts and under different task demands. The upcoming wedding required that she be able to adapt her walking and management of the impairments related to the stroke. For example, the patient wanted to carry her bouquet in her left hand and walk with her son (who was much taller than she) on her right. In addition, since the wedding ceremony and reception were to be outside and on grass, more ability was required to function in the different context presented by these environmental constraints.

LINKS TO
GUIDE TO PHYSICAL THERAPIST PRACTICE

Neuromuscular pattern 5D of the *Guide to Physical Therapist Practice*[48] relates to the diagnosis of this patient. This pattern is called "impaired motor function and sensory integrity associated with nonprogressive disorders of the central nervous system—acquired in adolescent and adulthood." Included in the diagnostic group of this pattern is cerebral vascular accident, and anticipated goals include "physical capacity is increased, physical function is improved, and ability to perform movement tasks is improved."

INTERVENTION

Given the short time frame from her presentation at the clinic and the actual wedding event, a program was developed to work on the specific task of walking in varied environments, including the elements of agility, coordination, and cardiovascular endurance. The patient was seen by the PTA twice weekly for 1 hour each visit for 1 month. As per the plan of care developed by the PT, the PTA started the patient by asking her to walk over low to high carpet, through bark, and up and down four steps, sidestepping in both directions with and without obstacles and walking at varied speeds (Fig. 17-8). The PTA demonstrated alignment of posture for each activity, and the patient was asked to attempt to maintain as close to this alignment as possible during the training.

Consistent with the plan of care, the PTA also had the patient walk outside, first uphill and then downhill on a cement sidewalk. The patient was then asked to walk on grass uphill and downhill. This task was practiced initially for 5 minutes, increasing 5 minutes per session, and progressing to 20 minutes after three additional visits. Finally at the fourth visit the patient began to walk on more level grass in the shoes she intended to wear for her wedding. In this way, the task was contextually trained, increasing the patient's contextual function and fitness levels.

OUTCOME

The patient was able to walk over the grass on her wedding day holding her bouquet and her son's arm without loss of balance and in a timely, coordinated manner. She reported some carryover in the ability to maintain walking for longer periods in the community without her usual fatigue (from initial report of 30 minutes to 1 hour at discharge); however, her previous walking pattern remained unaltered as did her agility.

SUMMARY—AN EFFECTIVE PT-PTA TEAM

This case study demonstrates an effective collaborative effort between the PT and PTA. The PTA was able to follow the instructions of the PT after the PT set the plan of care. The PT expects that the PTA fully understands the interventions and the importance of putting the treatment into the context of the goals the patient is trying to achieve. The PT also expects that the PTA can instruct the patient independently and to report any adverse effects of the session.

SUMMARY

- Environmental factors like temporal demands, physical loads, terrain, postural transitions, distance demands, collision avoidance, light levels, weather conditions, and attentional demands have been found to impact performance of functional tasks.

- Contextual fitness is the capacity to manage the physical demands of a task in the specific performance environment in which the task is performed. The physical demands of a task include core strength endurance, power, agility, balance, flexibility, cardiovascular endurance, and coordination. Additional task requirements are stability, mobility, and adaptation.

- Contextual function is a task performed within a meaningful context. Conceptually, a functional patient/client is one who is able to physically perform activities needed in the home, community, or institution; to plan tasks within the specific context; and to participate in society. In other words, the patient/client can perform the functions (tasks) required to be in the home, community, or institution in a participatory manner.

- The elements of fitness related to function should be trained using as many of the aspects of the contextual environment as safely possible. For example, asking the patient/client to walk, turn, walk on varied surfaces found in the environment—tile, carpet, grass—is an appropriate intervention to train agility. If safety is a concern, the training may be initiated in a controlled, "simulated" therapy setting but should progress to include the contextual environment before discharge.

- The PT and PTA should recognize both the challenge and the necessity of contextual fitness with regard to function. The unfit patient/client is at greater risk of functional decline and possibly a catastrophic event like hip fracture. The intervention program should train the elements of fitness for older adults within the context of performance when feasible.

References

1. Seeman TE, Charpentier PA, Berkman LF, et al. Predicting changes in physical performance in a high-functioning elderly cohort: MacArthur studies of successful aging. *J Gerontol Med Sci.* 1994;49:M97–M108.

2. Seeman TE, Chen X. Risk and protective factors for physical functioning in older adults with and without chronic conditions: MacArthur studies of successful aging. *J Gerontol B Psychol Sci Soc Sci.* 2002;57:S135–S145.

3. Rockwood K, Howlett SE, MacKnight C, et al. Prevalence, attributes, and outcomes of fitness and frailty in community-dwelling older adults: Report from the Canadian study of health and aging. *J Gerontol Med Sci.* 2004;59A:1310–1317.

4. Tanaka K, Shigematsu R, Nakagaichi M, et al. The relationship between functional fitness and coronary heart disease risk factors in older Japanese adults. *J Aging Phys Act.* 2000;8:162–174.

5. Mahoney FI, Barthel DW. Functional evaluation: the Barthel index. *Md State Med J.* 1965;14:61–65.

6. Kane RL, Ouslander JG, Abrass IB. The geriatric patient: demography and epidemiology. In: *Essentials of clinical geriatrics.* 4th ed. New York: McGraw-Hill; 1999:29.

7. Shumway-Cook A, Woollacott MH. Normal postural control. In: *Motor control theory and practical applications*. 2nd ed. Philadelphia: Lippincott Williams & Wilkins; 2000.

8. Carr JH, Shephard RB. *Stroke rehabilitation: guidelines for exercise and training to optimize motor skill*. Oxford: Butterworth-Heinemann; 2003.

9. Gill TM, Williams CS, Tinetti ME. Assessing risk for the onset of functional dependence among older adults: the role of physical performance. *J Am Geriatr Soc*. 1995;43:603–609.

10. Patla AE, Shumway-Cook A. Dimensions of mobility: defining the complexity and difficulty associated with community mobility. *J Aging Phys Act*. 1998;7:7–19.

11. Shumway-Cook A, Patla AE, Stewart A, et al. Environmental demands associated with community mobility in older adults with and without mobility disabilities. *Phys Ther*. 2002;82:670–681.

12. Rikli RE, Jones CJ. Fitness testing in later years. In: *Senior fitness test manual*. Champaign, IL: Human Kinetics; 2000:2.

13. Lawton MP. The functional assessment of elderly people. *J Am Geriatr Soc*. 1971;19:465–481.

14. Harris BA, Jette AM, Campion EW, et al. Validity of self-report measures of functional disability. *Top Geriatr Rehabil*. 1986;1:31–41.

15. Dittmar SS, Gresham GE. *Functional assessment and outcome measures for the rehabilitation health professional*. Gaithersburg, MD: Aspen; 1997.

16. Nagi SZ. Some conceptual issues in disability and rehabilitation. In: Sussman MB, ed. *Sociology and rehabilitation*. Washington, DC: American Sociological Society; 1965.

17. World Health Organization. *International classification of impairment, disabilities, and handicaps*. Geneva, Switzerland: World Health Organization; 1980.

18. National Center for Health Statistics: Classifications of Diseases and Functioning & Disability: International Classification of Functioning, Disability, and Health (ICF). Available at: http://www.cdc.gov/nchs/about/otheract/icd9/icfhome.htm. Accessed October 5, 2005.

19. Gill TM, Baker DL, Gottschalk M, et al. A prehabilitation program for the prevention of functional decline: effect on higher-level physical function. *Arch Phys Med Rehabil*. 2004;85:1043–1049.

20. Topp R, Boardley D, Morgan AL, et al. Exercise and functional tasks among adults who are functionally limited. *West J Nurs Res*. 2005;27:252–270.

21. Foldvari M, Clark M, Laviolette LC, et al. Association of muscle power with functional status in community-dwelling elderly women. *J Gerontol Med Sci*. 2000;55A:M192–M1999.

22. Schnelle JF, MacRae PG, Ouslander JG, et al. Functional incidental training, mobility performance, and incontinence care with nursing home residents. *J Am Geriatr Soc*. 1995;43:1356–1362.

23. deVreede PL, Samson MM, van Meeteren NLU, et al. Functional-task exercise versus resistance strength exercise to improve daily function in older women: a randomized, controlled trial. *J Am Geriatr Soc*. 2005;53:2–10.

24. Binder EF, Schechtman KB, Ehsani AA, et al. Effects of exercise training on frailty in community-dwelling older adults: results of a randomized, controlled trial. *J Am Geriatr Soc*. 2002;50:1921–1928.

25. Brach JS, Simonsick EM, Kritchevsky S, et al. The association between physical function and lifestyle activity and exercise in the health, aging, and body composition study. *J Am Geriatr Soc*. 2004;52:502–509.

26. Simonsick EM, Montgomery PS, Newman AB, et al. Measuring fitness in healthy older adults: the health ABC long distance corridor walk. *J Am Geriatr Soc*. 2001;49:1544–1548.

27. Netz Y, Argov E. Assessment of functional fitness among independent older adults: a preliminary report. *Percept Mot Skills*. 1997;84:1059–1074.

28. Miotto JM, Chodzko-Zajko WJ, Reich JL, et al. Reliability and validity of the Fullerton Functional Fitness Test: an independent replication study. *J Aging Phys Act*. 1999;7:339–353.

29. Mobily KE, Mobily PR. Reliability of the 60+ Functional Fitness Test Battery for older adults. *J Aging Phys Act*. 1997;5:150–162.

30. Lemmink KAPM, Han K, de Greef MHG, et al. Reliability of the Groningen Fitness Test for the Elderly. *J Aging Phys Act*. 2001;9:194–212.

31. Rikli RE, Jones JC. Functional fitness normative scores for community-residing older adults, ages 60–94. *J Aging Phys Act*. 1999;7:162–181.

32. Collins K, Rooney BL, Smalley KJ, et al. Functional fitness, disease, and independence in community-dwelling older adults in western Wisconsin. *Wis Med J*. 2004;103:42–48.

33. Stockmeyer SA. An interpretation of the approach of Rood to the treatment of neuromuscular dysfunction. *Am J Phys Med*. 1967;46:900–961.

34. Bandy WD, Sanders B. *Therapeutic exercise techniques for intervention*. Baltimore: Lippincott Williams & Wilkins; 2001.

35. Malina RM, Bouchard C. *Growth, maturation, and physical activity*. Champaign, IL: Human Kinetics; 1991.

36. Spirduso WW, Francis KL, MacRae PG. *Physical dimensions of aging*. 2nd ed. Champaign, IL: Human Kinetics; 2005.

37. Schmitz TJ. Coordination assessment. In: O'Sullivan SB, Schmitz TJ. *Physical rehabilitation: assessment and treatment*. 4th ed. Philadelphia: FA Davis Co; 2001:157–176.

38. Sharpe PA, Jackson KL, White C, et al. Effects of a one-year physical activity intervention for older adults at congregate nutrition sites. *Gerontologist*. 1997;37:208–215.

39. King AC, Pruitt LA, Phillips W, et al. Comparative effects of two physical activity programs on measured and perceived physical functioning and other health-related quality of life outcomes in older adults. *J Gerontol Med Sci*. 2000;55A:M74–M83.

40. Umphred DA. *Neurological rehabilitation*. 4th ed. St. Louis: Mosby; 2001.

41. Tinetti ME. Performance oriented assessment of mobility problems in elderly patients. *J Am Geriatr Soc*. 1986;34:119–126.

42. Brauer SG, Woollacott M, Shumway-Cook A. The interacting effects of cognitive demand and recovery of postural stability in balance-impaired elderly persons. *J Gerontol Med Sci.* 2001;56A:M489–M496.

43. Means KM, O'Sullivan PS. Modifying a functional obstacle course to test balance and mobility in the community. *J Rehabil Res Dev.* 2000;37:621–632.

44. Shumway-Cook A, Woollacott M, Kerns KA, et al. The effects of two types of cognitive tasks on postural stability in older adults with and without a history of falls. *J Gerontol Med Sci.* 1997;52A:M232–M240.

45. Kendall FP, McCreary EK, Provence PG. *Muscle testing and function.* 5th ed. Baltimore: Lippincott Williams & Wilkins; 2005.

46. Hall CM, Brody LT. *Therapeutic exercise: moving toward function.* 2nd ed. Philadelphia: Lippincott Williams & Wilkins; 2005.

47. Wade DT. Motor and sensory impairments. In: *Measurement in neurological rehabilitation.* Oxford: Oxford University Press; 1992.

48. American Physical Therapy Association. *Guide to physical therapist practice.* 2nd ed. Alexandria, VA; 2003.

A

Active-assistive range of motion (AAROM): An exercise in which an external force assists specific muscles and joints to move through their available excursion. AAROM exercises are used when the patient has difficulty moving or when tissue forces need to be reduced.

Active range of motion (AROM): Amount of joint motion produced by voluntary muscle contraction.

Adenosine triphosphate (ATP): Present in all cells, it is formed when energy is released from food molecules during cell respiration.

Aerobic capacity: Ability to perform work or participate in activities over time using the body's oxygen uptake, delivery, and energy release mechanisms.

Aerobic conditioning: Performance of therapeutic exercise and activities to increase endurance.

Agility: Ease of movement; quickness.

Agonist: Muscle directly engaged in contraction as distinguished from muscles that have to relax at the same time; thus, in bending the elbow, the biceps brachii is the agonist and the triceps is the antagonist.

Airway clearance technique: Group of therapeutic activities intended to manage or prevent the consequences of impaired mucociliary transport or the inability to protect the airway (e.g., impaired cough).

Angina pectoris: Oppressive pain or pressure in the chest caused by inadequate blood flow and oxygenation to heart muscle; the single most important cause of disease and death in Western societies.

Antagonist: Muscle that opposes the action of the prime mover and produces a smooth movement by balancing the opposite forces.

Aquatic therapy: Exercises performed in water or underwater for conditioning or rehabilitation (e.g., injured athletes or patients with joint diseases).

Arteriosclerosis: Disease of the arterial vessels marked by thickening, hardening, and loss of elasticity in the arterial walls.

Arthrokinematic: Accessory or joint play movements of a joint that cannot be performed voluntarily and that are defined by the structure and shape of the joint surfaces, without regard to the forces producing motion or resulting from motion.

Asthma: Disease caused by increased responsiveness of the tracheobronchial tree to various stimuli, which results in episodic narrowing and inflammation of the airways.

Atelectasis: A collapsed or airless condition of the lung.

Atherosclerosis: Most common form of arteriosclerosis, marked by cholesterol-lipid-calcium deposits in the walls of arteries.

ATP-PC system: This system uses a molecule called phosphocreatine to produce energy very quickly and without the use of oxygen; very small stores of this substance exist in the body so this system can be used only for short-duration (about 15 seconds), high-intensity events such as sprinting.

Atrophy: Wasting; decrease in the size of an organ or tissue.

Auscultation: Act of listening to internal body sounds (e.g., heart, lungs).

Autogenic inhibition: Inhibitory signals (from Golgi tendon organs) override excitatory impulses (from muscles spindles), causing gradual relaxation.

Automatic postural reactions (APR): Highly stereotyped patterns of electromyographic activity in various muscles triggered in response to sudden disturbances of balance. It is thought that somatosensory, vestibular, and visual inputs are integrated for assessing postural equilibrium.

B

Balance: Ability to maintain the body in equilibrium with gravity both statically (i.e., while stationary) and dynamically (i.e., while moving).

Ballistic stretching: Using the momentum of a moving body or a limb in an attempt to force it beyond its normal range of motion.

Base of support: Area in which a human body can maintain its upright balance without falling/losing balance.

Body mechanics: Interrelationships of the muscles and joints as they maintain or adjust posture in response to forces placed on or generated by the body.

Buoyancy: Upward force generated by the volume of water displaced by a body fully or partially immersed in a fluid.

C

Cardiac output: Amount of blood discharged from the left or right ventricle per minute.

Cardiac rehabilitation: Customized program of exercise and education aimed at improving fitness and quality of life by attempting to regain strength, prevent conditions from worsening, and reducing the risk of future heart problems.

Center of gravity (COG): Point around which every particle of a body's mass is equally distributed. COG is located at the sacral promontory, anterior to S2 (posterior superior iliac spine), at 55% of body height in a human body.

Chronic bronchitis: Inflammation of the mucous membranes of the bronchial airways, marked by increased mucous secretion by the tracheobronchial tree and the presence of a productive cough for at least 3 months in 2 consecutive years.

Chronic obstructive pulmonary disease (COPD): Common disorder characterized by progressive expiratory flow obstruction, dyspnea on exertion, and some degree of reversible airway hyper-reactivity.

Clients: Individuals who engage the services of a physical therapist and who can benefit from the physical therapist's and physical therapist assistant's consultation, interventions, professional advice, health promotion, fitness, wellness, or prevention services.

Closed-kinetic–chain (CKC) exercises: Exercises performed when the distal end is fixed and cannot move. The distal end remains in constant contact with the surface, usually the ground or base of a machine. These exercises are typically weight-bearing exercises during which athletes or patients use their own body weight and/or external weight.

Closed-pack position: Position in which two joint surfaces fit together precisely; they are fully congruent. The joint surfaces are tightly compressed; the ligaments and capsule of the joint are maximally tight; and the joint surfaces cannot be separated by distractive forces.

Community-dwelling: Living in a personal residence; alone or with others; functioning independently or with occasional assistance.

Conditioning: Improvement of physical and mental capacity with a program of exercises or course of training.

Contextual fitness: Capacity to manage the physical demands of a task in the specific performance environment in which the task is performed.

Contextual function: Person's ability to physically perform activities in the home, community, or work; to plan basic and higher-level tasks within the context of the specific environment.

Continuous passive motion (CPM): Use of a device that allows a joint (e.g., the knee) to be exercised without the involvement of the patient/client, often in the early postoperative period.

Coordination: Working together of various muscles to produce certain movements. Coordinated movement requires sequencing of muscle activity and stability of proximal musculature.

Core strength endurance: Capacity to meet the daily strength demands of the trunk.

Criterion-based intervention: Intervention procedures performed based upon set criteria established from proven practices.

Cross-training: Use of one or more sports to train for another. For example, training in both cycling and running strengthens all of the leg muscle groups and makes them less vulnerable to injury.

Cultural competence: Set of skills necessary to understand and respond effectively to the cultural needs of each patient/client to eliminate disparities in the health status of people of diverse cultural backgrounds.

Culture: Shared attitudes, beliefs, customs, entertainment, ideas, language, laws, learning, and moral conduct.

Cystic fibrosis: Potentially fatal autosomal-recessive disease that manifests itself in multiple body systems including the lungs, pancreas, urogenital system, skeleton, and skin. It causes chronic obstructive pulmonary disease and frequent lung infections.

D

Delayed-onset muscle soreness (DOMS): Muscle tenderness, decreased strength, and decreased range of motion that develops 12 to 24 hours following strenuous exercise and peaks in intensity between 24 to 48 hours, although symptoms may persist for 72 hours or more.

Diagnosis: Process that includes the physical therapist integrating and evaluating the data that are obtained during an exam to describe the patient/client condition in terms that will guide the prognosis, plan of care, and intervention strategy.

Disability: Inability to perform or limitation in the performance of actions, tasks, and activities usually expected in specific social roles that are customary for the individual or expected for the person's status or role in a specific sociocultural context and physical environment.

E

Ejection fraction: Percentage of the blood emptied from the ventricle during systole.

Emphysema: Chronic pulmonary disease marked by an abnormal increase in the size of air spaces distal to the terminal bronchiole, with destruction of the alveolar walls.

Ergometer: Apparatus for measuring the amount of work done by a human or animal subject.

Evaluation: Dynamic process in which the physical therapist makes clinical judgments based on data gathered during an examination.

Examination: Comprehensive screening and specific testing process leading to diagnostic classification or, as appropriate, to a referral to another practitioner. The examination has three components: patient/client history, systems review, and tests and measures.

Exercise prescription: Exercise schedule usually intended to increase the physical fitness of a previously sedentary individual who has recently had a serious illness such as myocardial infarction or who is physically fit and wants to know the amount, frequency, and kind of exercise necessary to maintain fitness.

Expiratory reserve volume: Maximum volume of gas that can be expired after a normal tidal expiration.

F

Fitness: Dynamic physical state—comprising cardiovascular/pulmonary endurance; muscle strength, power, endurance, and flexibility; relaxation and body composition—that allows optimal and efficient performance of daily and leisure activities.

Flexibility: Pliability of a portion of the body that is determined by joint integrity, soft tissue extensibility, and muscle length.

Functional fitness: Capacity to manage physical demands of the environment without fatigue.

Functional limitation: Restriction of the ability to perform at the level of the whole person, physical action, task, or activity in an efficient, typically expected, or competent manner.

Functional progression: Planned sequence of activities designed to progressively stress the injured patient in a controlled environment to return him or her to as high a level of activity as possible.

Functional residual capacity: Volume of gas in the lungs at the end of normal expiration.

G

Glycolytic system: Metabolic breakdown of glucose and other sugars that releases energy in the form of ATP. This system eventually produces a substance called pyruvic acid and contributes a small amount of energy. The entire process can take place without the presence of oxygen.

Goals: Intended results of patient/client management. Goals indicate changes in impairment, functional limitations, and disabilities, and changes in health, wellness, and fitness needs that are expected as a result of implementing the plan of care.

Golgi tendon organ (GTO): Spindle-shaped structure at the junction of a muscle and a tendon. This structure is thought to function as a feedback system that senses muscle tension through tendon stretch and inhibits muscle contraction of the antagonist muscle. The purpose of this mechanism, known as autogenic inhibition, is to prevent overuse and damage to the muscle and corresponding joint.

Graded exercise test (GXT): Test that evaluates an electrocardiogram under conditions that exceed resting requirements in defined, progressive increments designed to increase myocardial workload. The GXT also objectifies the functional capacity of patients with known disease and evaluates progress after surgery or other therapeutic interventions.

H

Hydrostatic pressure: Pressure exerted by a fluid in all directions and equally on all surface areas of an immersed body at rest at a given depth.

Hypertrophy: Increase in the size of an organ or structure, or of the body, due to growth rather than tumor formation.

I

Impairment: Loss or abnormality of anatomic, physiologic, mental, or psychologic structure or function.

Inspiratory capacity: Maximum volume of gas that can be inspired after a normal expiration.

Inspiratory reserve volume: Maximum volume of gas that can be inspired from the peak of a tidal volume.

Intervention: Purposeful interaction of the physical therapist with the patient/client and, when appropriate, the physical therapist assistant using various physical therapy procedures and techniques to produce changes in the condition.

Isokinetic exercise: Exercise, usually using a specially designed machine, that controls the velocity of muscle shortening or lengthening so that the force generated by the muscle is maximal through the full range of motion.

Isometric contraction: Muscular contraction in which the muscle increases tension but does not change its length; also called a static muscle contraction.

Isotonic contraction: Muscular contraction in which the muscle maintains constant tension by changing its length during the action.

K

Kinesthesia: Awareness of movement.

M

Manual therapy: Skilled hand movements intended to improve tissue extensibility; increase range of motion; induce relaxation; mobilize or manipulate soft tissue and joints; modulate pain; and reduce soft tissue swelling, inflammation, or restriction.

Motor control: Ability of the central nervous system to control or direct the neuromotor system in purposeful movement and postural adjustment by selective allocation of muscle tension across appropriate joint segments.

Motor unit: Motor neuron and all the muscle cells it innervates.

Muscle endurance: Ability to sustain forces repeatedly or to generate forces over a period of time.

Muscle length: Maximum extensibility of a muscle-tendon unit.

Muscle spindle: Specialized sensory fiber within the muscle that is sensitive to changes in the length of the muscle.

Myocardial infarction: Loss of living heart muscle as a result of coronary artery occlusion.

O

Open-kinetic–chain exercises: Exercises typically performed when the distal end is free to move. These exercises are typically nonweight bearing, with the movement occurring at a joint. If there is any weight applied, it is applied to the distal portion of the limb.

Osteokinematics: Gross angular motions of the shafts of bones in sagittal, frontal, and transverse planes.

Overload: Planned, systematic, and progressive increase in training with the goal of improving performance.

Oxidative system: System that picks up when the glycolytic system leaves off. When the body can supply a sufficient amount of oxygen to its working muscles, most of the pyruvic acid produced during glycolysis enters a series of reactions called the Krebs cycle. This cycle produces 90% of the energy needed to sustain medium- to long-term exercise.

P

$Paco_2$: Partial pressure of carbon dioxide in arterial blood.

Pain: Disturbed sensation that causes suffering or distress.

Palpation: Examination using the hands (e.g., palpation of muscle spasm, palpation of the thoracic cage).

Pao_2: Partial pressure of oxygen in arterial blood.

Pascal's law: Pressure in a liquid increases with depth and is directly related to the density of the fluid.

Passive range of motion: Exercise in which an external force moves a joint through its excursion without any effort by the patient. It is used when the patient is unable to move or when active motion is prohibited.

Patient/client-related instruction: Process of informing, educating, or training patients/clients, families, significant others, and caregivers with the intent to promote and optimize physical therapy services.

Patients: Individuals who are the recipients of physical therapy examination, evaluation, diagnosis, prognosis, and intervention and who have a disease, disorder, condition, impairment, functional limitation, or disability.

Percussion (treatment): Procedure used with pulmonary postural drainage to loosen secretions from the bronchial walls. The therapist uses slightly cupped hands to percuss the chest wall.

Performance environment: Community, home, work, and recreational areas in which the patient/client interacts on a regular basis.

Periodization: Process of varying a training program at regular time intervals to bring about optimal gains in physical performance.

Phosphocreatine: Compound found in muscle that is important as an energy source, yielding phosphate and creatine and releasing energy that is used to synthesize ATP.

Physical activity readiness questionnaire (PARQ): Series of questions that is designed to assist individuals aged 15 to 69 in determining whether they should see their doctor before increasing physical activity or exercise.

Physical agents: Broad group of procedures using various forms of energy that are applied to tissues in a systematic manner intended to increase connective tissue extensibility; increase the healing rate of open wounds and soft tissue; modulate pain; reduce or eliminate soft tissue swelling, inflammation, or restriction associated with musculoskeletal injury or circulatory dysfunction; remodel scar tissue; or treat skin conditions. These agents may include thermal, cryotherapy, hydrotherapy, light, sound, and thermotherapy agents.

Physical therapist (PT): Person who is a graduate of an accredited physical therapist education program and is licensed to practice physical therapy. Synonymous with physiotherapist.

Physical therapist assistant (PTA): Technically educated healthcare provider who assists the physical therapist in the provision of selected physical therapy interventions. The physical therapist assistant is the only individual who provides selected physical therapy interventions under the direction and supervision of a physical therapist.

Plan of care: Statements that specify the anticipated goals and expected outcomes, predicted level of optimal improvement, specific interventions to be used, and proposed duration and frequency of the interventions that are required to reach the goals and outcomes.

Plyometrics: Stretching and shortening exercise technique that combines strength with speed to achieve maximum power in functional movements. This regimen combines eccentric training of muscles with concentric contraction.

Posture: Alignment and positioning of the body in relation to gravity, center of mass, and base of support.

Power: Work produced per unit of time or the product of strength and speed.

Prognosis: Determination of the predicted optimal level of improvement in function and the amount of time needed to reach that level.

Progressive resistance exercise (PRE): Consists of increasing the number of repetitions at a constant load until exceeding an established repetition range.

Proprioception: Reception of stimuli from within the body (e.g., from muscles and tendons); includes position sense (awareness of joint position) and kinesthesia (awareness of movement).

Proprioceptive neuromuscular facilitation (PNF): Approach to therapeutic exercise directed at increasing joint range of motion and regaining function by using spiraling diagonal patterns of movement.

Pulmonary postural drainage: Placing the body in a position that uses gravity to drain fluid from segments of the lungs.

Pulse oximeter: Electronic device that selectively measures oxygen saturation of "pulsed" (arterial) blood.

R

Range of motion (ROM): Arc through which movement occurs at a joint or a series of joints.

Rate of perceived exertion (RPE): Category ratio scale, in which a patient reports his or her level of effort during exercise. The corresponding written descriptions range from "very light" to "very, very hard."

Reactive neuromuscular training (RNT): Specialized training program designed to re-establish neuromuscular control after injury. This training program manipulates the environment to facilitate an appropriate response in the patient, making use of balance and proprioception.

Reciprocal inhibition: When an agonist muscle contracts, the antagonists are inhibited from contracting to cause the desired motion.

Refraction: Bending of a light ray as it passes from one medium to another medium of different density.

Relative density/specific gravity: Ratio of the mass of a given volume of a substance to the mass of the same volume of water.

Residual volume: Volume of gas remaining in the lungs after forced expiration.

Rhythmic initiation: Proprioceptive neuromuscular facilitation technique using a progression of initial passive, active-assistive, and active range of motion through the agonist pattern.

Rhythmic stabilization: Proprioceptive neuromuscular facilitation technique using an integrated function of neuromuscular systems requiring muscles to contract and fixate the body against fluctuating outside forces, providing postural support with fine adjustments in muscle tension.

S

SAID principle (specific adaptations to imposed demand): Principle which explains that a certain exercise or type of training produces adaptations specific to the activity performed and only in the muscles (and energy systems) that are stressed by the activity.

Slow reversal: Proprioceptive neuromuscular facilitation technique using an isotonic contraction of the agonist followed immediately by an isotonic contraction of the antagonist.

Specific gravity: Weight of a substance compared with the weight of an equal volume of water. For solid and liquid materials, water is used as a standard and is considered to have a specific gravity of 1.000.

Specificity of training: Adaptations in metabolic and physiologic functions that depend upon the type of overload imposed. Specific exercise elicits specific adaptations creating specific training effects.

Static stretching: Sustained, low-intensity lengthening of soft tissue (e.g., muscle, tendon, or joint capsule) performed to increase range of motion. The stretch force may be applied continuously for as short as 15 to 30 seconds or as long as several hours.

Strength: Muscle force exerted by a muscle or a group of muscles to overcome a resistance under a specific set of circumstances.

Strengthening: Process of making stronger; any form of active exercise in which a dynamic or static muscular contraction is resisted by an outside force. The external force may be applied manually or mechanically.

Stroke volume: Amount of blood ejected by the left ventricle at each heartbeat.

T

Therapeutic exercise: Systemic performance or execution of planned physical movements, postures, or activities intended to enable the patient/client to remediate or prevent impairments, enhance function, reduce risk, optimize overall health, and enhance fitness and well-being.

Tidal volume: Volume of gas inspired or expired during each respiratory cycle.

Treatment: Sum of all interventions provided by the physical therapist and physical therapist assistant to a patient/client during an episode of care.

Total lung capacity: Amount of gas in the respiratory system after maximal inspiration.

V

Vibration: Therapeutic shaking of the body used with pulmonary postural drainage to loosen secretions from the bronchial walls.

Vital capacity: Maximum volume of gas that can be expelled from the lungs after a maximal inspiration.

$\dot{V}O_{2max}$: Maximum ventilatory oxygen extraction; a measure of the exercise capacity of a patient.